CULTS and New Religious Movements

Committee on Religion and Psychiatry

Marc Galanter, M.D. (*Chairperson*)
Herzl Spiro, M.D. (*Vice Chairperson*)
Walter Christie, M.D.
Edgar Draper, M.D.
Paul Hamburg, M.D.
David Hoffman, M.D. (*APA-Burroughs-Wellcome Fellow*)
Klaus Hoppe, M.D. (*Consultant*)
Cathy Laue, M.D.
Paul Mohl, M.D.
Richard J. Thurrell, M.D. (*Assembly Liaison*)
Brant Wenegrat, M.D. (*Consultant*)
Paula Dobbs-Wiggins, M.D.

CULTS and New Religious Movements

A Report of the
American Psychiatric Association

Edited by
Marc Galanter, M.D.
Committee on Psychiatry and Religion

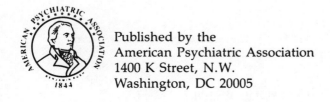
Published by the
American Psychiatric Association
1400 K Street, N.W.
Washington, DC 20005

NOTE: The authors have worked to ensure that all information in this book concerning drug dosages, schedules, and
routes of administration is accurate as of the time of publication
and consistent with standards set by the U.S. Food and Drug
Administration and the general medical community. As medical research and practice advance, however, therapeutic standards may change. For this reason and because human and
mechanical errors sometimes occur, we recommend that
readers follow the advice of a physician who is directly involved in their care or the care of a member of their family.

The findings, opinions, and conclusions of the report do
not necessarily represent the views of the officers, trustees, or
all members of the Association. Each report, however, does
represent the thoughtful judgment and findings of the committee of experts who composed it. These reports are considered a substantive contribution to the ongoing analysis and
evaluation of problems, issues, and practices in a given area of
concern.

Copyright © 1989 American Psychiatric Association
ALL RIGHTS RESERVED
Manufactured in the United States of America
First Edition

92 91 90 89 4 3 2 1

The paper used in this publication meets the minimum requirements of American National Standard for Information Sciences—
Permanence of Paper for Printed Library Materials, ANSI Z39.
48-1984.   ∞

Library of Congress Cataloging-in-Publication Data

American Psychiatric Association. Committee on Psychiatry and
    Religion.
      Cults and new religious movements: a report of the
    Committee on Psychiatry and Religion of the American
    Psychiatric Association/edited by Marc Galanter.—1st ed.
        p. cm.
      Includes bibliographies and index.
      ISBN 0-89042-212-5
      1. Cults—Psychological aspects. 2. Cults—United States.
    3. Psychology, Religious. 4. United States—Religion—1960-
    I. Galanter, Marc. II. Title.
    BP603.A46 1989   88-7817
    306'.6—dc19   CIP

CONTENTS

CONTRIBUTORS

Ted Bohn, M.S.W., J.D.
The Firm of Levy, Gutman, Goldberg & Kaplan

David G. Bromley, Ph.D.
Professor of Sociology,
Virginia Commonwealth University

Richard Delgado
Professor of Law
University of California Law School
Los Angeles

Alexander Deutsch, M.D.
Clinical Associate Professor of Psychiatry
New York University School of Medicine

Marc Galanter, M.D.
Professor of Psychiatry
New York University School of Medicine

Jeremiah S. Gutman, LL.B.
Former President, New York Civil Liberties Union
The Firm of Levy, Gutman, Goldberg & Kaplan

David A. Halperin, M.D.
Assistant Professor of Psychiatry
Mount Sinai School of Medicine

Paul Hamburg, M.D.
Department of Psychiatry
Harvard Medical School

David Hoffman, M.D.
APA–Burroughs-Wellcome Fellow
Department of Psychiatry
Harvard Medical School

Brock K. Kilbourne, Ph.D.
NATO Fellow
Psychology Institute
University of Heidelberg

Saul V. Levine, M.D.
Professor of Psychiatry
University of Toronto

Paul C. Mohl, M.D.
Associate Professor of Psychiatry
University of Texas
San Antonio

Robert C. Ness, Ph.D.
Associate Professor
Department of Psychiatry and Health Behavior
Medical College of Georgia

E. Mansell Pattison, M.D.
Professor and Chairman
Department of Psychiatry and Health Behavior
Medical College of Georgia

James T. Richardson, Ph.D., J.D.
Professor of Sociology
University of Nevada

Anson Shupe, Ph.D.
Associate Professor of Sociology
University of Texas, Arlington

J. Thomas Ungerleider, M.D.
Professor of Psychiatry
University of California, Los Angeles

David K. Wellisch, Ph.D.
Associate Professor of Psychiatry
University of California
Los Angeles

Brant Wenegrat, M.D.
Assistant Professor of Psychiatry
Stanford University School of Medicine

Louis Jolyon West, M.D.
Professor and Chairman
Department of Psychiatry
University of California
Los Angeles

Henry Work, M.D.
Clinical Professor of Psychiatry
Georgetown and George Washington Universities

PREFACE

This volume is the culmination of a three-year project designed
to prepare a comprehensive report on the contemporary phenomenon of cults and new religious movements. The project
was undertaken by the Committee on Psychiatry and Religion
and the American Psychiatric Association at the request of the
Board of Trustees of the Association, and the Board itself acted in
response to concerns raised in the Association's elected Assembly. The emergence of cultlike movements over the previous
decades posed troubling questions regarding individual psychology and group behavior. It also raised questions regarding
the proper role of the psychiatrist in addressing zealous religious
and social movements. Groups such as the "Moonies," Hare
Krishnas, and even quasi-therapeutic ones like Synanon often
left the mental health profession uncertain about how to apply
its expertise.

From the outset, our Committee appreciated that we were
dealing with a highly controversial phenomenon about which
thoughtful and well-intentioned observers often came to opposing views. We were aware that conclusions drawn on this issue
were often determined by the nature of the groups themselves;
that principles of individual freedom and society's responsibility
to protect its members were often cast against each other; that
the basic psychology of group behavior encountered in cults was
not yet understood.

Because of this, we planned this report with three goals in mind: 1) to bring together the contributions of scientists and scholars who could shed light on the complexity of the phenomenon, 2) to strive for a balanced view on the controversies that had arisen, and 3) to make recommendations only on issues where standards of clinical practice and legality were clear. We did not feel it appropriate to force a consensus position where there were legitimate differences of opinion. It is therefore our position that informed readers should draw their own conclusions on many of the issues presented. This meant that divergent views were often represented, sometimes without integration. In the Committee we labored at length over this issue as we were aware that there were conflicting perspectives on the field, sometimes not easily reconciled. We decided to include such perspectives, and to distill observations and recommendations of the Committee in areas where consensus could be reached. These are included in the beginning of the report and represent those matters that we felt could be reasonably presented to the mental health professional by the Association.

To assure the reader sufficient material, we invited leading contributors in the field. The volume begins with an Overview on the Issues by our Committee focusing on concerns related to psychotherapy with members and their families, and on civil liberties of members. It includes recommendations where we felt that a consensus view was clear. The ensuing chapters then offer a perspective on the following issues: the psychology of cultlike groups; the impact of memberships; group function and social control; entry and departure from these groups; and legal and social implications. On most all of these issues the reader is offered a thorough body of knowledge as well as a contrast in views. We anticipate that most of these chapters will be of direct value to the clinician, while others will serve more to adumbrate some of the theoretical issues raised by cult and new religious movements. The clinician generally does not have easy access to the latter material on an issue as unusual as this and may want to reference this without resorting to an extensive library search. We felt it important to include this latter material in the text.

It should also be noted that there is a very important place in the understanding of cults and new religious movements for a perspective from organized religion and religious scholars. Ideally such views should be presented in depth and with a full balance of their diversity. In framing our own report, however, we appreciated our own limitations in drawing such a perspective, and the diversity of valid views. We therefore hesitated to choose among religious leaders and scholars for representative opinions, and elected to limit ourselves to scholars in the psychosocial sphere. We look to other sources for religious views.

The issue of cults and new religious movements raises many compelling legal and political problems. Although important, many of these are beyond the scope of this volume, which focuses primarily on the psychiatric issues that impinge on clinical phenomenology and practice. Where appropriate, however, these legal and political problems are raised by chapter authors, and appropriate references have been cited for further reading.

Another important area that was not dealt with at length was that of the psychology of religion more broadly. Certain authors included material on psychodynamics of religion and cults, but the extensive and scholarly material that might be introduced on the issue of religious psychology was felt to be beyond the scope of this report. The reader, however, is encouraged to read further on this in pursuing the issue of cults.

In addition to the members of the Committee and the chapter authors, each of whom contributed with thoughtfulness and concern to the preparation of this report, I would like to express appreciation to Dr. Clark Aist, of the Association of Mental Health Clergy, a group that has long collaborated with this Committee; Dr. Richard Thurrell, the Assembly liaison of the Committee; Ms. Linda Roll, Executive Staff of the Committee; and also those who contributed to the review of this manuscript, most prominent among them Drs. Allen Beigel and John McIntyre of the Joint Reference Committee of the American Psychiatric Association and Drs. Mortimer Ostow and Stanley Cath, members of the Association.

Altogether, we hope that this volume will not only inform the reader on contemporary cults and new religious movements, but also serve as a basis for understanding new zealous groups that will no doubt emerge in the coming years.

Marc Galanter, M.D.
Chairman, Committee on Psychiatry and Religion
American Psychiatric Association

OVERVIEW ON THE ISSUES

Chapter 1

PSYCHOTHERAPY OF CULT MEMBERS

Paul Hamburg, M.D.
David Hoffman, M.D.

Context of Psychiatric Intervention

Faced with the complex religious, social, and psychological dimensions of cults, a psychiatrist asked to treat a cult member
might well feel perplexed. How is it possible to distinguish the
etiologic roles of religious quest, developmental impasse, underlying psychopathology, family disruption, group coercion, and
the seductive power of a charismatic leader? How can the psychiatric history be extended to encompass religious and social phenomena that arouse such intense controversy and passion? Despite these undeniable difficulties psychiatrists are nevertheless
in a unique position to provide substantial help to cult members
and their families. We are trained to comprehend complex clinical situations with several layers of meaning, and we know how
to relieve suffering in situations where a cure is not immediately
at hand. The psychotherapy of cult members can be based upon
the traditional psychiatric assessment, if we are willing to extend
our concern into some less familiar realms.

Few situations require more suspension of disbelief than the
evaluation of an individual who is involved with a religious cult.
Depending upon our own beliefs, we may tend to tolerate unusual religious phenomena and risk ignoring the coerciveness of
a particular cult: our desire to see the normative value of cults

3

may blind us to their dangerousness. Alternatively, we may see only psychopathology in any spiritual quest: our disdain for religion may prevent us from understanding the spiritual motives for cult affiliation. A repugnance toward totalitarian groups might lead us to discount the search for community that drives some young people to enter cults; a habitual attention to the individual psyche may let us ignore the import of group phenomena. We may be drawn into a family drama, seeing a young person struggle for freedom from a stifling family, or a family defend its integrity against an alien group. In collecting information prior to an intervention, the psychiatrist must postpone judgment despite an atmosphere of crisis (1).

The available data may be sorely limited. The cult member may not agree to a direct interview, or may appear psychologically removed and resistant. An important aspect of the evaluation is to acknowledge these limitations, and restrict the certainty of conclusions accordingly. Ideally, the psychiatric evaluation of a cult member should include a thorough psychiatric and developmental history, supplemented by specific information about the motivations for cult affiliation and the nature of the particular cult.

Through an attitude of compassionate, open inquiry, the psychiatrist is in an ideal position to help a cult member and his or her family understand the complex dilemmas of cult affiliation.

Psychiatric Evaluation of the Cult Member

Important information to gather about the cult member includes: age, sex, past religious involvement, length of time with the group, extent of involvement, the member's stated reasons for joining and staying with the group, the member's precult personality, mental health, and state of mind, precult experience with school, work, friends, drugs, and sex, and precult relationships to family and other social groups. It should also include the degree and kind of change in personality, activities and relationships since joining the cult, the member's present status in the cult, willingness to cooperate with treatment, degree of subjugation to the group, and degree of autonomy. Important information to gather about the group itself includes: the nature of leadership (group versus charismatic leader), established versus fringe, old versus new, Eastern versus Western derivation, degree of tolerance and intolerance, openness versus suspicion and secrecy. Also relevant are the degree of authoritarianism, bizarreness of rituals, presence of violence or threats of violence, asceticism versus hedonism, degree of dishonesty in fund-raising, degree of absolutism, ethnocentricity, rigidity, promises of salvation, and degree of social control over the individual. Individuals who join cults vary enormously one from another, and range from the severely disturbed to the apparently normal. Cults themselves vary from those that are barely distinguishable from normative religious groups to those that are severely coercive, totalistic, and demand absolute obedience to a leader (2).

The goals of an evaluation are to place in perspective the multiple determinants of an individual's joining and remaining in a cult. These include the following.

1. *The biomedical context.* Does this person have major affective disease or psychosis? Included is an assessment of current competency and need for medical interventions such as antidepressants, anxiolytics, neuroleptics, and hospitalization (voluntary or involuntary).
2. *The psychological context.* Included is an assessment of personal relationships, significant losses, developmental impasses, and current self-capacities.
3. *The family context.* Included is a formulation of family dynamics prior to cult membership and the impact of this event upon family life, with an emphasis on the family's current needs for support and intervention.

In addition to these three familiar contexts in the psychiatric evaluation, several extensions of concern are required. Given our unfamiliarity with religious and group phenomena in day-to-day practice, we may be tempted to doubt their authenticity, and try to explain away the spiritual quest or the search for community that has inspired cult affiliation. Understanding cult phenomena requires a willingness to value an individual's search for religious meaning and for community. At the same time, the psychiatrist must respect the extraordinary power that these realms, particularly in conjunction, can exert upon individuals, and recognize that this power can be either beneficial or destructive. In this regard, the following three questions demand attention in evaluating a cult member.

1. What is the nature of personal change since joining the cult? How has the person's ability to work and love been affected by joining the cult? How has his or her sense of well-being changed? What aspects of cult membership have facilitated or stifled personal growth and autonomy?
2. What was the quality of previous religious experience, and what might motivate a current spiritual quest? How has cult membership fulfilled or betrayed this search?
3. What is the balance of personal and group forces that currently hold this person in the cult? How did the desire for group affiliation motivate the decision to join a cult? How does this particular cult restrict the individual's freedom to make choices? In what ways has the cult inflicted psychological damage upon this individual?

The psychiatric evaluation of a cult member must include careful attention to religious and group phenomena in addition to the usual assessment of biological, psychological, and family contexts.

Psychiatric Intervention During Active Cult Membership

Occasionally, a psychiatrist may have the opportunity to intervene before a person has made a commitment to join a religious cult. If the psychiatrist is asked to intervene, and if the results of an evaluation suggest that there is a significant risk of psychological harm, then the situation demands an extremely active approach, including an attempt to make empathic contact with the individual in the hope of delaying a decision to join and exploring other alternatives for a personal, spiritual, or communal quest (2).

More often the psychiatrist first hears about cult membership after affiliation has occurred, from a family in crisis. This situation engenders acute frustration. Collecting an adequate data base may be difficult. The cult member may refuse to be interviewed, or come to an interview full of open hostility, with an unapproachable benevolence, or with a view to convince the psychiatrist to join the cult as well. The cult may subject the psychiatrist to harassment. It may be hard to find a thread of empathic connection with the unwilling, unfree patient.

Within the limits of possibility, the goal should always be to inform and to relieve suffering. Parents may consult a psychiatrist hoping to rescue a child from a cult; even if this proves impossible, there is no justification for therapeutic nihilism. The psychiatrist has an ideal opportunity to help the family cope with its loss, and the ensuing guilt, anger, and disruption, thereby facilitating further intervention with cult member and the family as it becomes possible (2). By placing this disruptive event in its various contexts, the psychiatrist can help the family avoid undue self-blame or harshness with their child, encouraging them to maintain channels of nonjudgmental communication with the cult member. The psychiatrist can help to focus concerns on the general welfare of the individual rather than on the specific dilemmas of cult membership. Even if the cult member does not decide to leave the cult immediately, maintaining contact with a supportive family leaves the door open for reconsideration should the cult member develop doubts about his or her affiliation. In this way, the process of psychiatric inquiry itself provides a measure of relief. Additional interventions might include placing the family in touch with self-help groups and sources of information about cults such as the Cult Awareness Network. Psychiatrists can help to temper the anticult fanaticism that often afflicts a distressed family, which itself can become a barrier to communication with the cult member.

Intervention during active cult membership strives to maintain open, supportive nonjudgmental communication between the psychiatrist, the family, and the cult member.

Deprogramming, Guardianship, and Legal Intervention

The family of a cult member may be driven by their frustration and concern to contemplate direct action to terminate cult involvement. Such interventions include coercive persuasion (de-

programming), court-sanctioned guardianship, conservatorships to grant the family control over the cult member's use of
financial assets, and child custody proceedings (in the unusual
case where one parent is actively involved in a cult). Psychiatrists are often asked to participate in these interventions. This
poses some unfamiliar clinical issues.

The term "deprogramming" has been so widely used that its
meaning has become imprecise. In this discussion the word
refers specifically to coercive efforts to force a cult member to
give up his or her beliefs and renounce allegiance to the cult
(Chapter 13). Psychiatrists should be aware that deprogramming is still being employed, although with decreasing frequency. Deprogramming should not be considered as a potential clinical intervention, as its fundamentally coercive nature
raises serious legal and ethical questions.

Other appropriate roles do exist for the psychiatric physician
in situations involving involuntary treatment. The family of a
cult member often seeks the psychiatrist's advice and intervention as an expert witness in a guardianship or conservatorship
proceeding. The definition of these terms varies by jurisdiction,
but for the purposes of this discussion, a *guardianship* is an
arrangement wherein a court, having found a person incompetent to care for himself or herself, appoints an agent, who may be
from the court itself, from the person's family, or a third party, to
make decisions on behalf of the incompetent person on matters
in which he or she has been deemed incompetent. Guardianship
may involve a general determination of legal incompetency, or
be specifically limited to one area, such as the use of medication.
A *conservatorship* is a more restricted arrangement where the
incompetency is limited to assets, property or financial affairs,
and the conservator may act on behalf of the cult member in
matters of money and property alone.

It is important to remember that the psychiatrist's primary
tasks are the evaluation, diagnosis, and treatment of mental
disorders, and the fostering of increased knowledge, understanding, and communication among those who seek his or her
assistance. Nevertheless, the impact of a family's struggles to
extricate their child from a cult has sometimes prompted psychiatrists to step beyond these usual clinical tasks. Two principal
questions confront the psychiatrist who is considering the ap-
propriateness of involuntary intervention.

1. Does the cult member suffer from a psychiatric disorder?
2. Is the cult member's judgment impaired, either as a direct result of a psychiatric illness or due to the coercive persuasion experienced during indoctrination into the cult, to the extent that he or she is unable to make rational, sound decisions in his or her own interest?

Standard diagnostic methods will generally provide an answer to the first question. The second question requires a more subtle finding, but is the more crucial one, since involuntary intervention or vicarious decision-making can only occur after a finding of incompetence has been made. In endeavoring to evaluate the cult member's judgment and decision-making ability, the clinician should pay particular attention to impairments of abstract thinking, an area that often yields the most discriminating information in these cases (Chapter 15).

Clinical decisions concerning the use of any type of involuntary control of a person or property must be based on a consideration of the relevant legal issues. Unfortunately, there has been little consensus among experts in the legal and psychiatric community concerning the limits of appropriate intervention, perpetuating an aura of intense controversy surrounding these proceedings. Psychiatrists who have testified against a cult member's mental competency, and by extension against the cult itself, have been the targets of civil suits and even threats of physical harm. To help negotiate the confusion, complexity, and apprehension these cases create, the clinician would be well advised to obtain specialized consultation from a psychiatrist and an attorney with expertise concerning cults.

Psychiatric intervention that involves involuntary evaluation or treatment must follow careful ethical and legal guidelines and should generally include a consultation with attorneys and psychiatrists who have special expertise in the field.

If the family of a cult member decides to seek legal intervention, a careful psychiatric history may clarify long-standing family dynamics in a way that fosters increased understanding, tolerance, and communication. Sometimes this will obviate the need for a court proceeding. Should the family remain convinced that legal action is necessary, and the psychiatrist concur, there are three guidelines that should govern psychiatric intervention.

1. Expert psychiatric testimony relevant to a permanent guardianship should not be rendered without an in-person evaluation of the person in question, who should be informed and aware of the nature and purpose of the evaluation.
2. If a temporary guardianship or conservatorship is sought in the cult member's absence for the purpose of mandating a proposed thorough in-person psychiatric evaluation, such a mandated evaluation should only take place in a medical setting (Chapter 13).
3. Psychiatrists should not participate in any involuntary action directed toward changing a person's religious or political orientation when it is conducted under coercive circumstances (Chapter 7).

Involuntary psychiatric intervention should be based on an in-person evaluation, performed in a medical setting, and should not include coercive attempts to alter a person's religious or political orientation.

Psychiatric Treatment of the Former Cult Member

For the cult member who has left a cult, whether voluntarily through a process of doubt and disaffiliation or involuntarily through court-ordered treatment and deprogramming, the re-entry into ordinary life is a difficult experience. Psychotherapeutic intervention at this time can make an enormous difference (1). In many respects the situation resembles that of former hostages, prisoners, exiles, soldiers, or those emerging from divorce or the death of a spouse. In each of these instances the terms of life have drastically altered, and issues of loss, reintegration, and transition need to be addressed in order to turn a potentially fragmenting experience into an opportunity for psychological growth.

Beyond the general framework of facilitating grief work and reintegration, several specific issues affect the psychotherapy of former cult members. The psychiatrist must be willing to consider "both the positive and negative aspects of experience" in the cult, and to "transcend the traditional bias against religion as psychopathological and religious experience as purely regressive." At the same time, we must guard against "naivete about the uses of coercion, deception, and manipulation [which] may make it difficult for the clinician to understand the eroding effects of an authoritarian system on individual values or the ways some groups promote and shape individual psychopathology" (1). The appropriate psychotherapeutic stance encompasses sensitivity to spiritual issues and to the extraordinary power of groups. It allows for the positive and negative effects of both religious and communal phenomena.

Psychiatric treatment that is conducted involuntarily under a court-ordered mandate, whether in hospital or in the clinic, should focus on the mental disorder that justified the declaration of incompetency. It should not include attempts to indoctrinate, coerce, or convert the former cult member to a new religious or political viewpoint. Such coercive efforts duplicate the loss of autonomy experienced during the cult experience. They also violate the patient's personal freedom.

Work with families during this period can help to mitigate the overprotection, anxiety, blame, and vigilance that are the legacy of the traumatic experience of cult membership (Chapter 7). The psychiatrist can continue the supportive, educational work begun during the earlier phase of cult membership, to further trust within the family, promote individuation and development, and to recognize pathologic elements of family structure that may require more intensive treatment. In addition to individual and family therapy, therapeutic groups composed of former cult members can provide mutual validation and support, becoming an example of a noncoercive group experience that contrasts to the authoritarian structure of the cult (3).

Specific psychotherapeutic impasses may occur (4). Former cult members sometimes lapse into fanatical anticultism, which may preclude more integrative resolutions. Alternatively, they may wish to simply forget the entire experience, increasing the likelihood of delayed depressive reactions akin to pathologic grief. Transference phenomena may be accentuated in former cult members who have lived in the shadow of charismatic leaders. Termination may recall the anxiety of departure from the cult and re-entry into a world whose openness may seem unsustaining. As in other directed, brief psychotherapies, complex personality issues, and chronic problems may emerge to justify a longer, deeper exploration. Optimally, psychotherapy enables the former cult member to recapture the authentic quest for understanding and spiritual growth that led to cult membership, while coming to terms with the painful as well as the beneficial aspects of the cult experience (1).

Psychotherapy with individuals who have left cults strives to achieve the integration of a difficult experience with an appreciation of its positive and negative aspects.

References

1. Gordon JS: The cult phenomenon and the psychotherapeutic response. J Am Acad Psychoanal 11:4, 603–615, 1983
2. Levine SV: Role of psychotherapy in the phenomenon of cults. Can J Psychiatry 24:593–602, 1979
3. Galanter M: Charismatic religious sects and psychiatry: an overview. Am J Psychiatry 139:1539–1548, 1982
4. Maleson F: Dilemmas in the evaluation and management of religious cultists. Am J Psychiatry 138:925–929, 1981

Chapter 2

CIVIL LIBERTIES, CULTS, AND NEW RELIGIOUS MOVEMENTS: THE PSYCHIATRIST'S ROLE

Paul C. Mohl, M.D.

If any conclusion can be drawn with certainty from a review of the chapters in this report, it is that sophisticated, knowledgeable professionals can come to widely disparate opinions about cults and new religious movements (NRMs), with each opinion seemingly solidly based on an extensive review of data. We see this disparity of opinion in the two chapters addressing legal issues. In Chapter 14, Bohn and Gutman argue that any group that self-labels itself as a religion must be so regarded by the government. They further argue that the constitutional guarantees on freedom of religion are absolute and the only question is why the state and federal governments have tolerated certain legal attacks on cults and NRMs. Delgado, on the other hand, argues in Chapter 15 that freedom of religion does not entail the right to do physical and psychological harm to oneself nor to others. Nor does it entail acceptance of fraudulent misrepresentation during proselytization designed to reduce a citizen's truly free exercise of choices. He proposes a variety of legal remedies such as "truth in proselytizing" laws, suits against cult leaders for mental distress, peonage, unlawful imprisonment, and so on. He also suggests that it may be possible to carefully craft laws based on a sophisticated social-psychological appreciation of social influence and informed consent, limiting induction techniques that seem designed specifically to limit a person's autonomous choices.

The implication of these widely divergent opinions about cults from so many perspectives is that we are dealing with an area more complicated than it would at first appear, one in which what data we possess have not resulted in a clear line of knowledge and understanding. Such a situation is ripe for countertransference to dictate psychiatrists' behavior. This countertransference may take the form of overly hostile or overly sympathetic stances toward cults and NRMs. However, psychiatrists are used to dealing with such situations: changes in sexual mores, "recreational" substance use, unusual ideologies, or adolescent social rebellion. It may be a truism to say that a psychiatrist must be aware of and carefully monitor his or her own emotional biases about cults, but it must be the starting point for any guidelines about dealing with cults in any fashion. We are dealing with an area in which what we feel and what we believe may be at variance with what is truly known.

This is particularly important when contemplating involvement with the legal system and its dealings with cults and NRMs. This is a situation rife with the danger of psychiatrists doing damage to psychiatry's image by appearing not to be the sober, informed professionals they must be. Indeed, as Bohn and Gutman note, several mental health professionals and physicians have testified in court on the mental status of an individual who was never even interviewed. Each situation must be dealt with by psychiatrists, in their professional roles, on an individual basis. **Under the current situation of limited knowledge and widely differing opinions, each individual patient must be evaluated carefully and testimony offered based solely on that individual's current clinical status, a knowledge of the particular cult's induction practices and daily habits, and an expert understanding of the social psychological literature on social control.** Any sweeping generalizations about cults, cult members, and cult practices run the risk of reflecting the psychiatrist's personal bias, not his or her truly expert professional opinion.

When encountering the legal system, a whole new set of parameters are added to the ones noted above. The legal system must first ensure certain civil rights, responsibilities, and procedures before considering (and sometimes in lieu of considering) the dimensions of primary concern to psychiatrists. This is as it should be, but it is not always a comfortable position for the clinical psychiatrists with their (often passionate) commitment to mental health values. Justice and civil liberties are not necessarily intrinsically empathic, supportive, trusting, interpersonally open, and so forth. This is, no doubt, why so many psychiatrists avoid forensic work.

The particular issues raised by cults and NRMs are ones which the legal system must guard especially carefully: the freedoms of religion, speech, and association. Clearly, Bohn and Gutman implicitly give the benefit of the doubt to cults and NRMs as religions and regard the constitutional guarantees as absolute. Delgado seeks to respect those guarantees while proposing some legal remedies for *some* of the features of *some* cults and NRMs that may distinguish them from religions. The legal issues for nonreligiously defined cultlike groups are somewhat less stringent but are still involved with issues other than those of strict concern to psychiatrists. The point here is that psychiatrists must be prepared to yield control and final decision-making to judges, juries, and legislatures, not permitting personal passion to prevent mental harm to interfere with our expert, consultative, essentially advisory role. **The psychiatrist can offer expert testimony on the mental status of a given individual and the physical and psychological effects of particular practices, but courts and legislatures have the power and responsibility to define the boundaries of legal and societal tolerance for such effects.** With these general guidelines in mind, we may turn to the specific roles and issues a psychiatrist may be asked to become involved in: conservatorships, damage suits alleging mental abuse, forced treatment, and laws attempting to limit abusive practices.

Conservatorships

Conservatorships have been sought by distraught families seeking to gain custody of an adult child whom they believe to have been rendered mentally incompetent by involvement in a cult or NRM. Psychiatric testimony becomes absolutely crucial in such a judicial proceeding. Psychiatrists will be asked to render expert opinions on the mental status of the cult member. This is not really different from the psychiatrist's role in most states' commitment procedures. However, the task may be considerably more complex than identifying the incapacity of a delusional schizophrenic or suicidally depressed patient. As Halperin suggests in Chapter 7, the psychiatrist may be caught in a familial individuation struggle, in which the NRM member is self-destructively seeking autonomy by immersing himself or herself in a controlling group, while the family is failing to grieve and trying to crudely but legally reassert its control. Nonetheless, many states use criteria for conservatorship that bear similarity to their criteria for commitment. As both Bohn and Gutman and Delgado note, deprivation of liberty in our country demands extraordinary cause.

It is important in these and other instances for the psychiatrist to base his or her testimony on a careful, thorough evaluation of the patient, with cult membership not regarded as prima facie evidence of diminished capacity. A thorough knowledge of the particular state's laws on conservatorship and scrupulous adherence to their guidelines is central. It is probably a good idea for the psychiatrist to ask, "Would I support hospital commitment of this patient if I were unaware of the cult membership?" If the state's laws define appropriate conditions for conservatorship less stringently than do most commitment laws, a solid knowledge of the particular cult's practices may help the psychiatrist determine the degree of genuine disability. It will be useful to keep in mind that the very use of these laws in this situation is of questionable constitutionality and the court may well be more concerned about this issue than with the psychiatric testimony.

Damage Suits Alleging Mental Abuse

Psychiatrists may also be called upon to offer somewhat similar testimony in court proceedings in which an ex-cult member sues an NRM or cult leader for alleged mental damage. The responsibilities of the psychiatrist are similar to those involved in conservatorship proceedings: careful clinical evaluation of the patient's status at the time of exit from the cult, careful ancillary history of the patient's status prior to cult induction, and sufficient knowledge of the particular cult's practices and their relationship to modes of social control. Just as each state's criteria for conservatorship may differ from those of commitment, so may the legal definition of what constitutes mental abuse. Independent legal advice may assist the psychiatrist in rendering an expert opinion as to the extent to which his or her clinical findings conform to that state's definitions of mental abuse.

Forced Treatment

Some instances may arise in which family members of a NRM member ask a psychiatrist for assistance in bringing the cult member in for treatment. Again, this is not terribly different from other situations in which a psychiatrist is asked to "get" a resistant patient into treatment by concerned friends or family. The psychiatrist's role is to advise the family about his or her availability and their options for using suasion or legal compulsion. An awareness of the state's laws on conservatorship or outpatient commitment, together with Bohn and Gutman's caveats about their use with respect to cults, is important.

The more difficult dilemma comes afterward, when a court may have ordered a conservatorship and remanded the cult member to treatment. On the one hand, this is similar to other forced treatment situations (prisons, outpatient commitments, military psychiatry, certain school referrals), but on the other, the family and court may be seeking to use the psychiatric treatment as a form of deprogramming. Many psychiatrists are uncomfortable with any forced treatment situation and would shy away from this one as well. Others will be willing to consider it. Forced treatment is most comfortable for the therapist when the court's, society's, or the institution's agenda is very close to the psychiatrist's (e.g., "cure this schizophrenic's delusions"). But the more variance there is the more conflictual will be the therapy (e.g., "keep this normally rebellious late adolescent from disrupting our military unit"). **In considering whether to accept such a case, familiarity with the ordering authority's agenda, perhaps including consultation with judges, family members, and so on, and comparison of this to one's own clinical findings on the presence, nature, and causes of any mental disorder is crucial.** Margaret Singer's work on the passivity and dependency found in some ex-cult members may be an important consideration, as well (1). The psychiatrist, having evaluated these issues, is in a position to make an intelligent clinical decision on participating in treatment.

Most psychiatrists would probably have some ethical con-

cerns about being used strictly as a kind of deprogrammer, in the absence of any mental disorder.

Forced treatment of any sort demands tremendous effort in dealing with therapeutic alliance issues, which become the first issues once treatment is begun; they may well be the central issues throughout treatment, especially if Halperin's hypothesis about cult membership and separation-individuation issues in the family is accurate. It will take all of a psychiatrist's subtlety and skill to maneuver himself or herself away from the "agent of controlling family" position into "agent of my own best interest" without seeming to collude with the "controlling cult leader." Singer's use of groups of ex-cult members may be useful in this regard (1).

Legislating Boundaries on Cults and NRMs

This chapter and, to a great extent, this entire volume has taken a cautious approach to the psychiatrist's interactions with cults, NRMs, and their members. We have emphasized the legal and ethical position that it is preferable to accept some, albeit tragic and painful, disruption, rather than violating certain values of autonomy, free choice, and free belief. Yet, it is amply clear that some psychiatrists believe firmly, even passionately, that at least some cults do not deserve the benefits of this cautious, conservative approach. These psychiatrists argue, often persuasively, that autonomy and free choice become jokes when cult membership evolves out of subtle, planful, and systematic undermining of these very principles. What is the appropriate legal avenue for advocates of this position, which has substantial data to support it?

Probably, the most suitable professional role for the psychiatrist is as an expert witness before courts, legislative committees, and executive regulative agencies as they interpret laws, write laws, or create regulations as suggested by Delgado (Chapter 15). The psychiatrist's role would be to provide expert information documenting the clinical damage to individuals, and expert opinion on the boundaries between "brainwashing" and legitimate proselytizing. Such testimony can be based on the extensive social psychiatry and social psychology *data* on social influence and social control, especially the work of Lifton

(2), Andersen and Zimbardo (3), and Milgram (4). Drawing this line intellectually is not easy, and drawing it legally is further complicated by constitutional issues. However, there is a sense within some of the chapters here that many of the cults and NRMs have responded to social and legal pressure, evolving toward institutions more readily recognized as noncoercive religions.

Particularly in reading the historical chapters of this book, I found myself wondering how I would have regarded the Mormons in the 1830s. Without an empty West for new, cultish, religious groups to escape to, our society faces a dilemma on how to protect the freedoms of deviant groups while limiting unnecessary physical and psychological harm by them. The dilemma facing psychiatrists is how to balance what we really know professionally with what we may strongly feel personally, and to find an appropriate professional role amid society's larger, often legal, struggle with this very same issue.

These issues are highlighted by situations where a psychiatrist may be asked to testify even though he or she has not interviewed the party involved. This is indeed done at times (although not without some controversy) on wills and estates, diagnosis, and psychopharmacology. Since such testimony may be solicited in relation to cults and new religious movements, too, it is essential that the clinician exercise appropriate reserve. The clinician should provide useful, expert information but at the same time avoid excessive inference from the material presented if he or she has not been able to personally interview the cult member.

References

1. Singer MT: Coming out of the cults. Psychology Today, January 1979, pp 72–82
2. Lifton RJ: Thought Reform and the Psychology of Totalism. New York, WW Norton, 1961
3. Andersen SM, Zimbardo PG: On resisting social influence. Cultic Studies Journal 1:196–219, 1984
4. Milgam S: Obedience to Authority. New York, Harper & Row, 1974

PERSPECTIVE ON CULTS AND NEW RELIGIOUS MOVEMENTS

INTRODUCTION

Chapter 3

CULTS AND NEW RELIGIOUS MOVEMENTS

Marc Galanter, M.D.

Cults and new religious movements have come to public attention in the last two decades, but they may be subsumed under a broader phenomenon which can be termed charismatic groups (1). The *charismatic group* generally contains more than a dozen members, typically many more. Participants adhere to a consensual belief system, sustain a high level of social cohesiveness, are strongly influenced by group behavioral norms, and impute charismatic (or divine) power to the group or its leadership. This phenomenon includes most of contemporary cults and new religious movements, but also other nonreligious zealous groups which range from certain self-help groups to radical political organizations. Such groups may operate for the good or detriment of their members, depending on the nature of the particular group and the observer's perspective as well.

The concept of a cult, more specifically religious, connotes religious deviancy and, often, transcendental experience. Most cults would fall within our definition of the charismatic group. The cult has been characterized as a "religious movement which makes a fundamental break with the religious traditions of the culture and which is . . . composed of individuals who had or seek mystical experiences" (2). Troeltsch (3), in his classical discourse on the Christian Church, distinguished the established Church from Church sects. He then characterized a third entity, "spiritual and mystical religion," akin to the cult phenomenon,

which conveys "the direct inward and present religious experience." This latter subtype of religious experience has also been
described from a sociologic perspective, as a "mystic collectiv-
ity . . . understood to refer to all people who hold the tenets of
mystical religion and consequently have a sense of common
solidarity and obligation, even though they do not interact" (4).
Such a community provides consensual validation for its own
system of beliefs.

A study of the social origins of cults leads to the observation
that their growth is often promoted by a crisis within the culture.
Other zealous groups may emerge because of focal failings in
the culture. But when the plausibility of a society is diminished
because of crisis, or fails to meet the needs of a group, its
ideological underpinnings cease to be credible (5). Individuals
may then become deprived of a meaningful orientation to their
lives.

Members' Experiences

Most reports have characterized subjects of contemporary cults
and new religious movements as coming predominantly from
middle- and upper-middle-class social backgrounds (6–9). In
our studies of members of two sects, the Divine Light Mission,
an Eastern sect, and the Unification Church ("Moonies"), a neo-
Christian group, the majority of members had attended college,
as had one or both of their parents (10–13).

Many of the sect members have been reported to be troubled,
on the basis of member's self reports (12, 14, 15). Psychological
distress among potential members is also found to be an important antecedent to joining. Based upon interviews with members, ex-members, and relatives, a number of clinicians have
described members as emotionally disturbed. They have been
seen as predominantly "depressed, inadequate, or borderline
antisocial youths" (16), or as "lonely, rejected and sad" (8).
Inductees are also reported to have limited social ties before
joining the sect (14). Some are thus described as using these
sects to reduce a sense of personal incompleteness, often at a
time of normative crisis.

The recruitment techniques employed by these groups has
been the focus of much concern. Lofland and Stark (17) pro-

posed a model for this based on their observations of a small millenarian Christian group. They emphasize acutely felt tension on the part of a convert, experienced within the context of a religious problem-solving perspective. This lends itself to acquiring the role of a "religious seeker." Alternatively feelings of meaninglessness and deprivation may also be addressed (18–21). The encounter with the cult then becomes a turning point in the person's life as members shower the convert with affection (16, 17). In a controlled assessment of these issues (22), for example, we found that a cohort of persons entering a workshop sequence for induction into the Unification Church scored below the general population on psychological well-being, and those who ultimately joined scored lower than the ones who did not. In addition, the joiners were found to score lower than the nonjoiners on affiliative ties outside the group.

The role of transcendental or mystical experiences in both individual conversion and in group induction procedures can be very important. This was, of course, emphasized by both James (23) and Freud (24). The importance of transcendental experiences in conflict resolution has also been noted, even to the point of precipitating acute hallucinatory episodes in nonpsychotics (25, 26), as well as in psychotics (27, 28). In any case, these experiences are integral to conversion and to continuing membership (10, 29) for many charismatic sect members. Explanatory models for the appearance of "psychotic-like" phenomena in normal individuals within the context of religious experience have not, however, been fully developed.

An orientation toward communal living is characteristic of many charismatic sects. This is typical of both contemporary sects and of ones in previous centuries, such as the Shakers and the original Mormons. In the Unification Church, for example, 94 percent of members we studied in the late 1970s lived in Church-owned residences. Some sects, on the other hand, such as the Meher Baba movement, do not have a tight-knit communal structure. This group, studied by Anthony and Robbins (30), consisted of local autonomous groups with members developing independent living arrangements. Nonetheless, most followers of Meher Baba were found to associate primarily with other members of the group, and constituted an informal community, based on close friendships and social affiliations.

Sect members frequently think of each other as "family," and often refer to fellow members as such. This style also emerges in charismatic groups directed primarily toward therapeutic purposes. For example, Ofshe (31) studied patterns of relating in Synanon, a self-help group which was initiated in 1958 for the treatment of drug abusers. Shared residential facilities and economic resources and a "family-like atmosphere" underlie a considerable degree of intimacy within this group.

The behavioral norms of many sects appear to express a reaction to the sexual permissiveness characteristic of the 1960s and 1970s. Harder, Richardson, and Simmonds (32), for example, studied courtship, marriage, and family style in one segment of the Jesus movement. They describe the express avoidance of situations that may be sexually charged and outline specific sect regulations regarding courtship and bodily pleasures. Dating, for example, was considered inappropriate because it might lead to temptations and possible transgression. This phenomenon has clearly moved closer to the mainstream with the upsurge of contemporary fundamentalism.

Norms for residence and sexual behavior reflect the profound influence that charismatic groups may bring to bear on the lifestyle of their members. More compelling examples, of course, for the impact of cults on members' behavior have been reported in the popular press in settings where leaders have driven members to participate in deviant behaviors. The impact of psychotic behavior of a charismatic sect leader was undertaken from a psychiatric perspective by Deutsch (33). Because of the grandiose role vested in this charismatic leader, members' reality testing was suspended in the face of the avowals presented them. When necessary, rationalizations emerged so that the leader's bizarre commands might be perceived as reasonable and then accepted.

The belief systems that characterize many contemporary sects may seem confusing to the outsider. Many are based on transcendental and mystical experiences. Some are drawn from unfamiliar Eastern traditions, and others embellish on established religions to the point of reconstructing Biblical doctrine. Singer (12) divided the many cult orientations into nine types, although many typologies are possible. One common orientation is based on neo-Christian ideas, as illustrated by the True World Evangelical Christian Church associated with the Pentecostal movement (34). This group accepts the Bible as the literal word of God, and members have been observed to speak in tongues and believe in personal prophecy and faith-healing.

Eastern groups typically emphasize meditation and transcendental experiences. The most common Eastern orientation is based on Hindu concepts, as in the Divine Light Mission and the small Meher Baba group discussed above, as well as the Hare Krishna movement (35). Some groups are based on Zen or other Sino-Japanese practices. Soka Gakkai (36), for example, is a Buddhist sect which originated in Japan and now has headquarters in major American cities; their belief system emphasizes religious chanting and a positive attitude, but does not impose extensive behavioral restrictions on its followers.

Not all charismatic groups are religiously oriented. Some emphasize contemporary psychology as an ideologic perspective, to the point of a charismatic commitment. The ideologies of groups like these, however, such as Synanon (31) before its descent into deviant behavior, and est (37), may be more palatable to the mental health professional.

According to Richardson (38), the term "deprogramming" refers to " a set of techniques for removing persons from new religious groups and involving them in a rigorous and even coercive resocialization process in an attempt to get them to renounce their beliefs and accept more traditional ones." Psychiatric options for deprogramming have been discussed by Etemad (8). He suggests that the process be preceded by a physical examination and a comprehensive psychiatric evaluation, and recommends that it take place in a "pleasant psychiatric facility"; when possible, the family should be firm but gentle and should accompany and support the patient.

There is, however, no clear basis for estimating how many sect members leave under coercion and how many do so voluntarily. There are also no controlled observations of the deprogramming process. Ungerleider and Wellisch (39), however, did contrast a sample of members who left their groups subsequent to deprogramming with another sample who had been "unsuccessfully" deprogrammed and returned. They found that the majority of those who did leave the sects had been members for less than a year. Conversely, the majority of those who returned after deprogramming had been members for more than a year.

We studied persons who had left the Unification Church. After an average of 3.8 years, members had apparently achieved

a stable social adjustment. Most had left because they saw themselves at odds with the operating principles of the Church,
usually after being frustrated in their work or relationships
within the Church. Those who left voluntarily retained a notable
fidelity to the sect, in contrast to those who were deprogrammed. Significantly, 36 percent of the sample reported they
had experienced serious emotional problems shortly after leaving. This latter phenomenon probably reflected in Singer's experience (12) with therapeutically oriented groups for persons who
have left, a majority of whom experience deprogramming. She
suggests that people who join were troubled to begin with and
have difficulty with their subsequent community adjustment.
Problems of depression, loneliness, and uncertainty were frequent among ex-members.

Psychological Perspectives

Members of cults and new religious movements generally state
that joining has a positive effect on their psychological state.
Interviewers describe reports of new strength and "spiritual
resources," as well as reduced "self-hatred" (14). Increased feelings of calm, happiness, and a capability for better relationships
are also noted (16, 40). In our studies of the Divine Light Mission
and the Unification Church, members reported considerable
amelioration of emotional state over the course of joining, with
stability in this improved state apparently maintained over the
course of long-term membership (13, 22, 41–43). Interestingly,
however, despite the reported improvement, long-term members' scores on the psychological General Well-Being Schedule
were still somewhat below those of an age- and sex-matched
sample from the general population. This was compatible with
the finding of a notably low level of psychological well-being
measured in a separate sample of nonmembers who had registered for the sects' workshops prior to joining. These studies
support the hypothesis that, at least for certain sects, many of
those attracted to joining are in a state of significant emotional
distress, and do indeed experience an amelioration of their affective status upon conversion.

These findings, based on self-report data, should be compared with the impressions of certain observers who report their

own assessments of members' status (6, 12, 44). Clark (6), for example, states that, "Converts often seem drab and dreamy outside the group, stereotyped, and somewhat expressionless when discussing anything other than their new experience. They lacked mirth and richness of vocabulary." If such observations do reflect a negative impact of membership in charismatic groups, they should be considered in relation to studies of psychopathology induced within certain groups in more controlled settings. Yalom and Lieberman (45), for example, in a carefully controlled study, noted a 7.5 percent incidence of psychological casualties in time-limited encounter groups, a setting with much less prolonged, directed interpersonal input. Similarly, casualties have also been reported among members of est (46), a self-help group involving commitments generated in a large-group setting, based on teachings of a charismatic secular leader.

The diagnosis of major psychopathology among converts is difficult to undertake because interviewing of volunteer members does not necessarily reach a more dysfunctional minority and more widely distributed self-report instruments may not accurately tap more severe symptoms. Nonetheless, certain findings do shed light on this issue. For example, in our studies, emotional problems among Divine Light Mission respondents had led 38 percent to seek professional help prior to joining and 9 percent to hospitalization. For the Unification Church, corresponding figures were 30 percent and 6 percent, respectively. A number of members to whom we gave clinical interviews were found to have experienced amelioration of symptoms of major psychopathology subsequent to joining.

It appears that certain sects attract members with considerable psychopathology. For example, among the small band of 24 devotees of Meher Baba, "virtually all gave histories of chronic unhappiness and unsatisfactory parent relations" (47). Similar findings were reported with regard to the Subud sect, which appeared to attract individuals in considerable distress. Kiev and Francis (48), who studied the sect, also described members of this group with known psychiatric illness. They observed that although the group appeared to offer temporary remission to such persons, it would likely contribute to a later exacerbation of their illness because the pressure for personal change promoted anxiety in those who did not achieve clear-cut progress.

Mystical experiences associated with religious conversion

have, conversely, been described as having a salutary effect on psychopathology. Thus, there have been reports of schizophrenic adolescents emerging from transcendental religious experiences with a resolution of suicidal impulses (49), bizarre behavior (50), and psychotic decompensation (10).

Another area to be considered is that of substance abuse. Remission in patterns of abuse are frequently reported, along with rapid changes in attitudes toward drugs upon conversion (10, 11, 16, 51–53). These changes occur among young people who were acculturated into patterns of rather heavy drug use during the "counterculture" period of the 1960s and 1970s. The apparent potential of charismatic groups to enforce new behavioral norms is well illustrated by their impact on intoxicant use.

Behavioral conformity is often the *quid pro quo* which members must yield for the emotional relief they experience. In considering the marital practices of the Unification Church, for example, we examined the remarkable conformity to group norms evident in their group engagements (13, 44). Members had agreed to placement into marital engagement in a highly unusual fashion: their partners were assigned to them by the group's leader as a part of a religious ritual. Significantly, the abrogation of contemporary norms for mate selection was not associated with increased psychological distress. Church-related life experiences, however, were perceived as being of considerable psychological impact. Multiple regression analyses further revealed that the vulnerability of respondents to perceived life disruption was relieved by their affiliation to the sect.

This "relief effect" (41) is associated with social and religious ties to the sect. It apparently reinforces compliance with the group's behavioral norms by means of operant reinforcement: When members distance themselves from the group's membership or beliefs, they experience or anticipate experiencing distress. Conversely, closeness and conformity lead to reinforcement by perceived diminution in vulnerability to disruptive life events and the reduction of stress.

A similar pattern of operant reinforcement was evident for long-standing members of two sects that we studied (41, 53): the Unification Church and the Divine Light Mission. Those closer to the group were found to experience enhanced psychological well-being. It appears, therefore, that a system of operant reinforcement is built into the group's function such that members are conditioned to respond to the group's expectations. The group's social structure operates so as to generate a self-sustaining pattern of reinforcement, which comes to be internalized within the members.

The "relief effect" may also be understood from the perspective of the new discipline of sociobiology. Sociobiology (54) posits that observable behavior is rooted in biologic traits which have persisted in the species because of their adaptive value. On this basis, the question may be raised as to whether individual's valency for such large-group experiences may be based in biologically grounded adaptive social behavior.

The issue of thought control or "brainwashing" in sects has been raised in both the popular press and the scientific literature (8, 39, 55, 56). Lifton (57) originally studied this process as applied by Chinese Communists to Western prisoners of war during the Korean conflict. Richardson and Stewart (58) drew on a number of these traits in their own study of the Jesus movement. Milieu control, for example, entails establishing constraints over all facets of communication; the degree of such control varies among religious sects, usually contingent on the proximity of residential and work arrangements. A shared belief that members' work is devoted to some grand plan (whether revealed or not) is the basis for the mystical manipulation of members' activities; all planned and observed events are thereby rationalized on the basis of the group's mystified goals. The sect is presumed to maintain a sacred science, whereby unquestioned dogma can explain all facets of life; this effectively eliminates the difference between the sacred and secular spheres.

Another perspective helpful in understanding how the individual begins to experience the influence of the large-group has emerged from studies on the attribution of meaning in experimental contexts. Attribution theory (59) defines a model for an individual who achieves understanding of a situation which is not easily understood on the basis of his or her previous attitudes. For example, an individual may experience either cognitive dissonance or emotional disruption in a given social context. The person may then accept a new explanatory model for his or her experiences based largely on its availability within that context. In the setting of induction into religious sects (11, 60), a dissonant context may be produced by the intense and supportive interpersonal input provided by persons espousing an unfamiliar belief system: "How can people who are so kind maintain a threatening or incorrect perspective?" This, then, generates the psychological pressure to make sense of the experience and place it in an acceptable cognitive framework. This may ultimately be accomplished by accepting the religious perspective offered by the conversion context. There is a subsequent need to sustain the stability of this new perspective. This is achieved by attributing the meaning of later experiences to the same perspective, thereby (apparently) providing external validation for the beliefs, albeit circular in nature.

A Systems Approach

If the charismatic group is to be conceptualized as a functional whole, a number of social-psychological issues must be integrated. This model can be drawn from systems theory. From this perspective, an aggregate of interacting components is considered a system. In studying the system, the relationships among these components is emphasized, rather than the effect of each component directly on another. An open system is one that is in active exchange with its environment. We may consider the charismatic group as an open system, as it contains a number of interacting functional components, and also conducts exchanges with the environment (primarily in the form of interpersonal exchanges). In this respect, the group's environment is defined as the broader society in which it is lodged, one with a contradictory set of beliefs, and often hostile to it.

Open systems are characterized by the function of boundary control (61). By means of boundary control, the potential components of the system (people and beliefs, in this case) are defined as either part of the system or outside it. In the charismatic group, that is particularly important because of the dissonance between the group's perspectives and those of the general population.

The function of boundary control, like other ones inherent in the open systems, may help to explain puzzling behaviors observed among members of charismatic large-groups. For example, a glazed and withdrawn look has been described among sect members by some observers critical of these groups (6, 12) and not reported by others (10, 16, 40). This description may reflect a psychological response, perhaps of a dissociative nature, which members may experience when they perceive their affiliation to the group being threatened. Although this response may appear pathologic when observed in a given individual, it may be an appropriate response with regard to sustaining membership in the group. It can be understood as a component of the group's boundary control function, evinced as a demand characteristic of the group. Although such responses may be engendered through membership in the group, they may only emerge in settings which threaten the group's integrity. Thus, an observer perceived as an antagonist of the group might be more likely to report this than one who is not.

For charismatic groups, boundary control is also facilitated by the development of the group's distinctive character, whether in dress, custom, or ideology. It is also assured if the group develops a fearfulness of outsiders and their beliefs. For example, we found that members had experienced a relief of neurotic distress upon joining. Variables related to social cohesiveness were examined to ascertain which were correlated with this relief in distress; the most highly correlated among these variables was found to be suspiciousness toward outsiders (41). It predominated over positive feelings toward the sect's own members as a component of this psychological "relief effect."

All open systems must maintain homeostasis. This role is supported by the conversion process: In addition to the need of the group to maintain its members, the acquisition of new members is perceived as legitimation of its own ideology, thereby consolidating the commitment of its long-standing members.

The needs of the group help to explain the need for certain aspects of the conversion process. In the first place, its cognitive underpinnings must be developed by the charismatic group. Individuals' acceptance of unusual beliefs may be puzzling in terms of their antecedent personalities; the panoply of ideologies outlined above bears little obvious relationship to the psychological or social needs of one group's individual members as distinguished from those of another. With regard to a system's needs, however, such ideologies do serve as a cognitive basis for implementing the conversion process. Boundary control is also necessary to the survival of the large-group; here, too, a cognitive substrate must be elicited to help members differentiate the group's own members from nonmembers.

The emergence of transcendental experiences in the context of conversion is very puzzling from the perspective of individual psychological function. For the group, however, the emergence of these phenomena assures greater commitment, since meaning for these experiences is attributed to the potency of the belief system and the charismatic leader, thereby lending the group enhanced credibility. The group may be expected to establish a context that promotes such experiences.

We have found that each of these three traits, adherence to the group's cognitive framework, cohesiveness toward members, and the experience of transcendental states all served as significant predictors of members' enhanced psychological well-being upon conversion. They are the "vehicles" for implementation of the sociobiologic "relief effect" just described.

The open system must also observe and regulate its own operations, a process called *monitoring* (61). This is accomplished in the charismatic group by an individual leader or a hierarchical structure which defines work assignments and goals, interpreting them in relation to the group's ideology. As noted above, such leadership may be either technical or charismatic in style (62). In addition, monitoring is also conducted by means of the close interpersonal bonds and the physical proximity characteristic of the members of a charismatic group; these latter traits tend to assure regulation of deviancy and implementation of group norms.

As noted above, the behavior of members directed at the larger society is considered as the output of the charismatic group. It is the product of both conversion of new recruits and of the monitoring of long-standing members. This output has a defensive character, inevitable in light of a typically antagonistic relationship with the social context. The output may therefore reflect an autistic seclusiveness, as seen in certain sects, such as groups that withdraw into social and even geographic isolation. Alternatively, other groups embark on compensatory grandiose schemes, planning to address major international issues, such as achieving world peace or eliminating hunger. Most of the ideologies described above anticipate a role for the group that will shape future events in an important way.

This is important to the group because of the feedback it produces. Feedback describes a phenomenon in which a portion of the output is returned to the system so as to assist in regulating the group function or maintaining homeostasis. In this way, the charismatic group's behavior is typically used to validate its own perspectives. Thus the very undertaking of a grandiose scheme may be perceived as evidence of the divine powers of a charismatic leader. The zeal observed in new recruits is similarly understood as feedback, to validate the group's ideology.

Describing the charismatic large-group in terms of a system model has certain advantages. It helps to understand members' deviant beliefs and behaviors as responses to the demand characteristics of the group, and thereby obviates a need to ascribe them to individual psychopathology. The importance of maintaining the group's homeostasis, for example, helps to explain why attention may be invested in recruitment practices and in rituals which define the group's distinct character. Certain areas are also highlighted in which a large-group may demonstrate unexpected behaviors. For example, aggressive paranoia may emerge as a function of boundary control, when the group is threatened from without; seemingly impractical or grandiose plans may be undertaken when internal monitoring functions define a need for stabilizing feedback; and surprisingly zealous commitments can be produced in initially uncommitted recruits as part of the group's transformation function.

References

1. Galanter M: Charismatic religious sects and psychiatry: an overview. Am J Psychiatry 139:1539–1548, 1982
2. Nelson GK: The membership of a cult: The Spiritualists National Union. Review of Religious Research 13:170, 1972
3. Troeltsch E: The Social Teaching of the Christian Churches. London, George Allen and Unwin, 1931
4. Campbell C: Clarifying the cult. Br J Sociol 28:376, 1977
5. Eister AW: An outline of a structural theory of cults. Journal of Scientific Study of Religion 11:319–333, 1972
6. Clark JG, Jr: JAMA 242: 279–281, 1979
7. Cox H: Turning East: The Promise and Peril of the New Orientalism. New York, Simon & Schuster, 1977
8. Etemad B: Extrication from cultism. Curr Psychiatric Ther 18:217–223, 1979
9. Davis R, Richardson JT: The organization of functioning of the Children of God. Sociological Analysis 37:321–339, 1976

10. Galanter M, Buckley P: Evangelical religion and meditation: psychotherapeutic effects. J Nerv Ment Dis 166:695–691, 1978
11. Galanter M, Rabkin R, Rabkin J, et al: The "Moonies": a psychological study of conversion and membership in a contemporary religious sect. Am J Psychiatry 136:165–170, 1979
12. Singer M: Therapy with ex-cult members. National Association of Private Psychiatric Hospitals Journal 9:14–18, 1978
13. Galanter M: Engaged "Moonies": the impact of a charismatic group on adaptation and behavior. Arch Gen Psychiatry 40:1197–1201, 1983
14. Nicholi AM: A new dimension of the youth culture. Am J Psychiatry 131:396–401, 1974
15. Schwartz LL, Kaslow FW: Religious cults, the individual and the family relations of schizophrenics. Psychiatry 21:205–220, 1958
16. Levine SV, Salter NE: Youth and contemporary religious movements: psychological findings. Canadian Psychiatric Association Journal 21:411–420, 1976
17. Lofland J, Stark R: Becoming a world-saver: a theory of conversion to a deviant perspective. American Sociology Review 30:862–875, 1965
18. Glock CY, Stark R: Religion and Society in Tension. Chicago, Rand McNally, 1965
19. Gordon D: The Jesus people: an identity synthesis. Urban Life and Culture 3:159–178, 1974
20. Simmonds RB, Richardson JT, Harder MW: A Jesus movement group: an adjective check list assessment. Journal of Scientific Study of Religion 15:323–337, 1976
21. Adams RL, Fox RJ: Maintaining Jesus: the new trip. Society 9:50–56, 1972
22. Galanter M: Psychological induction into the large-group: findings from a modern religious sect. Am J Psychiatry 137: 1574–1579, 1980
23. James W (1902): The varieties of religious experience. New York, Modern Library, 1926
24. Freud S (1921): Group psychology and the analysis of the ego, in Standard Edition of the Complete Psychological Works of Sigmund Freud. Edited and translated by Strachey J. London, Hogarth Press, 1955
25. Sterba R: Remarks on mystic states. American Imago 25:77–85, 1968
26. Jacobsen F: The Self and the Object World. New York, International Universities Press, 1964
27. Sedman G, Hopkinson G: The psychopathology of mystical and religious conversion experiences in psychiatric patients, I. Confina Psychiatrica 9:65–77(a), 1966
28. Sedman G, Hopkinson G: The psychopathology of mystical and religious conversion experiences in psychiatric patients, II. Confina Psychiatrica 9:65–77(b), 1966
29. Buckley P, Galanter M: Mystical experience, spiritual knowledge

and a contemporary ecstatic religion. Br J Med Psychol 52:281–289, 1979

30. Anthony D, Robbins T: The Meher Baba movement: its effect on post-adolescent social alienation, in Religious Movements in Contemporary America. Edited by Zaretsky II, Leone MP. Princeton, NJ, Princeton University Press, 1974, pp 479–571

31. Ofshe R: Synanon: the people business, in The New Religious Consciousness. Edited by Glock CY, Bellah RN. Berkeley, University of California Press, 1976, 116–137

32. Harder MW, Richardson JT, Simmonds R: Lifestyle: courtship, marriage and family in a changing Jesus movement organization. International Review of Modern Sociology 6:155–172, 1976

33. Deutsch A: Tenacity of attachment to a cult leader: a psychiatric perspective. Am J Psychiatry 137:1569–1573, 1980

34. Hardyck JA, Braden M: Prophecy fails again: a report of a failure to replicate. Journal of Abnormal Social Psychology 65:136–141, 1962

35. Nagy IB, Stark G: Invisible Loyalties. New York, Harper & Row, 1973

36. Kumasaka Y: Soka Gakkai: group psychologic study of new religiopolitical organization. Am J Psychother 20:462–470, 1966

37. Simon J: Observations on 67 patients who took Erhard Seminars Training. Am J Psychiatry 135:686–691, 1978

38. Richardson JT: Conversion careers. Society 3:47–50, 1980

39. Ungerleider JT, Wellisch DK: Coercive persuasion (brainwashing), religious cults, and deprogramming. Am J Psychiatry 136:279–282, 1979

40. Wilson EO: Mental health benefits of religious salvation. Diseases of the Nervous System 33:383–386, 1972

41. Galanter M: The "relief effect": a sociobiological model for neurotic distress and large-group therapy. Am J Psychiatry 135:588–591, 1978

42. Galanter M: "Moonies" get married: a psychiatric follow-up study of a charismatic religious sect. Am J Psychiatry 143:1245–1249, 1986

43. Galanter M, Gleaton TJ, Marcus CE, et al: Parent self-help groups for youthful drug and alcohol abuse. Am J Psychiatry 141:889–891, 1984

44. Shapiro E: Destructive cults. Family Physician 15:80–83, 1977

45. Yalom ID, Lieberman MA: A study of encounter group casualties. Arch Gen Psychiatry 25:16–30, 1971

46. Kirsch MA, Glass LL: Psychiatric disturbances associated with Erhard Seminars Training: II. Additional cases and theoretical consideration. Am J Psychiatry 134:1254–1258, 1977

47. Deutsch A: Observations on a sidewalk Ashram. Arch Gen Psychiatry 32:166–175, 1975

48. Kiev A, Francis JL: Subud and mental illness: psychiatric illness in a religious sect. Am J Psychother 18:66–78, 1964

49. Horton PC: The mystical experience as a suicide preventive. Am J Psychiatry 130:294–296, 1973

50. Levin TM, Zegans LS: Adolescent identity crisis and religious conversion: Implications for psychotherapy. Br J Psychol 47:73–82, 1974
51. Simmonds RB: Conversion or addiction. American Behavioral Scientist 20:909–924, 1977
52. Robbins T: Eastern mysticism and the resocialization of drug users: the Meher Baba cult. Journal of Scientific Study of Religion 8:308–317, 1969
53. Galanter M: Sociobiology and informal social controls of drinking. J Stud Alcohol 42:64–79, 1981
54. Wilson EO: Sociobiology: the new synthesis. Cambridge, MA, Belknap Press, 1975
55. Clark JG, Jr: Problems in referral of cult members. National Association of Private Psychiatric Hospitals Journal 9:27–29, 1978
56. Richardson JT, Harder M, Simmonds RB: Thought reform and the Jesus movement. Youth and Society 4:185–200, 1972
57. Lifton RJ: Thought Reform and the Psychology of Totalism. New York, WW Norton, 1961
58. Richardson JT, Stewart M: Conversion process models and the Jesus movement. American Behavioral Scientist 20:819–838, 1977
59. Bem DJ: Self perception: an alternative interpretation of cognitive dissonance phenomena. Psychol Rev 74:183–200, 1967
60. Proudfoot W, Shaver P: Attribution theory and the psychology of religion. Journal of Scientific Study of Religion 14:317–330, 1976
61. Miller EJ, Rice AK: Systems of Organization. London, Tavistock, 1967
62. Robbins T, Anthony E, Richardson J: Theory and research on today's "new religions." Sociological Analysis 39:95–122, 1978

THE SOCIAL CONTEXT

Chapter 4

NEW RELIGIOUS MOVEMENTS IN HISTORICAL PERSPECTIVE

E. Mansell Pattison, M.D.
Robert C. Ness, Ph.D.

New religious movements, some termed sects and cults, have attracted enormous attention in the last two decades in the United States, among the public, the media, the academic community, mainline religious groups, the legal profession, and the mental health professions. The ensuing debate about the meaning, value, and social role of these religious movements has been intense and often polemical. Within psychiatry we find a tangled admixture of technical-clinical observations about individual members of these religious movements interposed with social-political rhetoric about the value of such groups for society (1–6).

We wish to distance ourselves in this chapter from both these components of psychiatric commentary. Instead we draw upon an array of studies in history, sociology, political science, and anthropology in order to develop a social and historical perspective from which to interpret the current clinical and social responses of psychiatry to the new religious movements.

A decade ago the historian Hillel Schwartz (7) set out a research agenda much like what we envision here. Reviewing previous work, Schwartz noted a sharp distinction in perception of the critical issues between the first generation of scholars of this century, and the current second generation.

What the first generation of collectors, typologists, and crusaders had originally found to be sporadic frontier phenom-

> ena, the birthright second generation has found to be the
> constant center of religious life. . . . The first generation had
> regarded end-of-the-world hopes and movements as symp-
> tomatic of social or personal illness. The second generation
> describes millenarian beliefs and actions less often as products
> of disease, more often as an arsenal of world-sustaining forces.
> (p. 1)

We believe current psychiatric debate is still substantially re-
liant upon the "first generation" of scholarship. Therefore we
wish to explicitly shift psychiatric discourse toward the second,
broader, more theoretically informed analysis of religious movements. We depart from the familiar pattern of discrete empirical
data analysis; instead we strive to comprehend what Mauss
terms "total social facts" that are simultaneously religious, legal,
moral, economic, and aesthetic.

Specifically, we shall address the following questions.

1. What is the nature of fundamental social relations?
2. How does the development of increasingly complex social
   organization disrupt human relations, and how is this re-
   dressed in religious forms?
3. How are religion and politics related to social organization,
   thus influencing the religious formulation of sect and cult?
4. How does the current pattern of religious forms in America
   reflect general patterns of social and political organization?
5. How do we differentiate between fact and value assessment
   of religious movements?

In the process of addressing these issues, we proffer an un-
abashed original attempt at synthesis and theory-building. This
chapter is unavoidably, however, a synopsis of our much larger
study where the reader is urged to turn for a more detailed
discussion of supportive and substantiative data (8).

Finally, we wish to note that we follow an approach that
Foucault (9) has called an "archaeological methodology"; that is,
we are in search of artifacts that embolden a reconstruction. We
do not hold that we present "scientific truth," but rather a
heuristic framework that may provoke further research. The
historian David Chidester (10) aptly expresses the essential
point of view of our study:

[W]e do not seek to establish explanation in terms of causes
. . . the archaeological method describes configurations. Such
an approach does not carry the awesome responsibility of
being correct: it must only be *interesting, illuminating,* and
perhaps even *disturbing.* (p. 2)

The Quest for Cosmological Communion and Its Equivalents

We begin with a basic observation: humans everywhere "band
together," forming voluntary social bonds between people of
"like-mindedness." These universal social relationships are a
reflection of fundamental biopsychosocial components of the
human organism, not simply culturally patterned modes of living. This structure of social relationships is named by anthro-
pologists as a "communion." Persons participating in "communion" experience others as reciprocal to themselves; that is,
social and psychic bonding occurs. As the early social theorist
Schmalenbach (11) describes it,

communion cherishes and perhaps even demands unreserved
devotion, complete sacrifice, and unreserved giving, not only
of material things, but also of oneself.

The social structure of "communion" is described in the current social science paradigm as the "intimate psychosocial network" consisting of approximately 25 people whose voluntary
and daily interactions are characterized by a high level of psy-
chic-emotional bonding and an equally high level of instrumen-
tal-social bonding (12). The communion appears to be not only
an ancient form, but also an enduring and universal form of
social relations.

A central organizing feature of communion has been cosmological, or religion in the broadest sense: a shared set of
beliefs, values, and behavioral orientations. This persistent confluence of communion and cosmology has been explained by the
anthropologist Clyde Kluckhohn (13) in the following terms.

There is a need for a moral order. Human life is necessarily a
moral life precisely because it is a social life, and in the case of
the human animal the minimum requirements for predic-

tability of social behavior that will insure some stability and
continuity are not taken care of automatically by biologically
inherited instincts, as is the case with the bees and the ants.
Hence there must be generally accepted standards of conduct,
and these values are more compelling if they are invested with
divine authority and continually symbolized in rites that appeal to the senses. (p. ix)

Thus, social and psychic bonding is functionally related to
both a commonality of shared beliefs and an interdependent
social existence. We shall therefore refer to a "cosmologically
constituted communion" wherein "religion" is the cosmological
glue that binds together the fabric of social relations within the
communion.

It should be apparent at this point that the structure of social
organization called a "communion" is the ideal type sought by
conventional religions, but rarely achieved in social fact. In contrast, the "communion" achieves its fullest social expression in
the intimate small religious cult. In this sense the cult represents
the purest form of a "cosmologically constituted" group in
which cosmological ideals and social relationships approach veridicality.

It is critical to stress that our concept of "religion" departs
from conventional current usage because many cosmologically
constituted communions do not adhere to conventional beliefs
even though they do ascribe to complex and explicit cosmologies. Religion in the everyday sense is therefore but one
way of framing a cosmology.

This observation leads us to consider the issue of "equivalent
cosmological groups" which may be totally dissimilar from each
other in terms of the content of cosmological beliefs or content of
interaction, yet still demonstrate the identical structure and
functional characteristics of a cosmologically constituted communion. People the world over "quest" for cosmological communions as they search for, create, join, and maintain relationships which afford social and psychic bonding, while the specific
content of interaction and belief will vary with time, place, and
circumstances.

When we examine the social history of equivalent cosmologically constituted groups we note that these equivalent
forms become more numerous as social organization becomes
more complex (14, 15). In addition, as social organizations be-

come more abstract, impersonal, and utilitarian, the communions people create represent but a small segment within the larger impersonal social universe. In other words, communions are organized around selected segments of the social universe, while other aspects of social existence may be perceived as secondary to the primary communion. In order to demonstrate this theme we can identify a variety of equivalent communions based in one dimension of the social universe as we move from one level of social complexity to another.

1. In a *village or tribal setting* we may find a male agricultural solidarity centered in fertility rituals.
2. In a more complex *feudal society* we may find a merchant guild or a religious cult.
3. In the early stages of *industrialization* we may identify fraternal brotherhoods, labor unions, or atheistic sects.
4. In *postmodern urbanized society* we may find flying saucer groups, self-help groups, and various health cults.

We have taken time to emphasize the analytic significance of equivalent cosmologically constituted communions because the concept underscores the pervasive quest for this fundamental social form throughout history. Thus, as we begin our historical and social analysis of religious cults we cannot confine ourselves to only those "communions" that have been explicitly labeled "religious" or "cults," for this orientation would severely distort the data. Rather, we must examine the entire range of cosmologically constituted communions.

The Ethos-Cosmos Strain and Religious Forms

We have found Lamert's comprehensive definition of religion to be particularly useful for describing the structure of cosmologically constituted communions: "A religion is to be found where persons take it for granted that their own ethos corresponds to the meaning of the cosmos" (16). Applying this definition to our concept of communion, we recognize three analytical dimensions: 1) the creation of an *ethos*, 2) a process of cosmization, and 3) the reification of ethos with cosmos.

The empirical set of social relations in any social group is the "ethos." The term refers then to the roles, behaviors, and patterned interactions through which a group defines its "peculiarly ordered relationship to reality." The process of "cosmization" refers to the process of imputing meaning to the general order of existence that transcends the empirical reality of social relations (ethos). This process provides coherent meaning and value to social relationships, both rationalizing and sustaining them. Berger and Luckman have referred to this process as "the social construction of reality" (17). And finally, reification is the attempt to create an "isomorphic fit" between meaning and value (cosmos) with actual behavior (ethos). Through the process of "reification" veridicality is, to some degree, established between the empirical social order (ethos) and the system of explanatory meanings (cosmos).

There is, however, always some degree of incompleteness or strain between cosmos and ethos: normative structure and ultimate values are never fully isomorphic with specific patterns of behavior. In fact, the effort to reify cosmos (transcendent meaning) with ethos (social relations) becomes increasingly difficult at each subsequent level of social organization. Attempts to reduce the strain between cosmos and ethos, thus approximating veridical reification, are the wellspring of experimentation in religious forms throughout history.

From this perspective the concepts of *church*, *denomination*, *sect*, and *cult* are really variations in form around the theme of *strain reduction*. Utilizing the framework developed by Swatos (18) we diagram these four basic religious forms and their orientations toward strain between ethos and cosmos (Figure 1).

1. In Type 1, *monopolistic religion*, there are two variants. One is the relatively isolated, small face-to-face village where cosmos and ethos tend toward concrete veridicality, thus approximating total reification. The second variant is the "universal church," a structural monopoly which is ostensibly isomorphic with a geographically defined social universe. Historically this type may be seen in the "monarchial state-church" of medieval Europe or the country of Iran under the Ayatollah Khomeini. In this variant the state maintains a cosmological hegemony and there is officially no strain between cosmos and ethos.
2. In Type 2, the *denomination*, there is recognition of a pluralistic

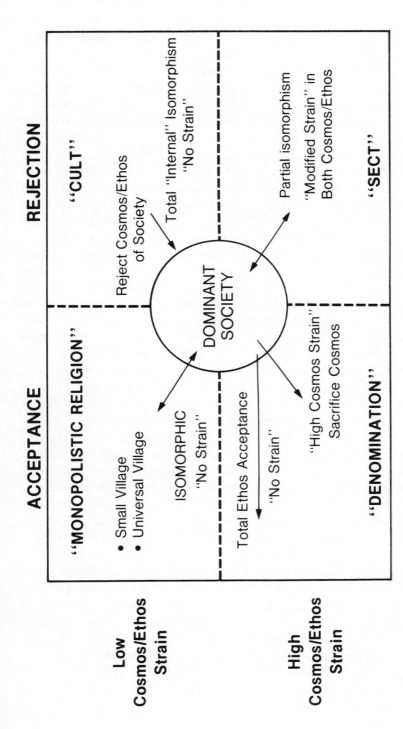

Figure 1. Religious forms vis-à-vis society.

social universe and recurring social change. Strain reduction is attempted by ongoing redefinitions of the cosmos to match the ethos. This process of accommodation is popularly termed secularization as the cosmos becomes increasingly less transcendent and more "this-worldly" or "civil religion." The cosmos emerges in this process as a rationalization of the status quo (ethos).

3. In Type 3, the *sect*, there is a rejection of the dominant society (ethos) and retention of a strong cosmology that exists in substantial strain with the concurrent ethos. The phrase "we live in the world, but are not of the world" summarizes this orientation. Sects assert that their cosmology is the true cosmology and typically attempt strain reduction by confirming cosmos-ethos veridicality in their private, sect meetings. Outside of these communal gatherings the strain between cosmos and ethos is viewed as a constant burden that cannot be eliminated but must be tolerated.

4. In Type 4, the *cult*, we find a full rejection and withdrawal from the dominant ethos, an attempt to create a new social universe completely veridical with an explicit cosmos. In Bainbridge's terms, "a cult is a culture writ in small terms" (19). Through self-established isolation, strain reduction is attempted by rejection and withdrawal from the dominant society, or the proclamation of a revolutionary ideology.

We recognize that some cults do proselytize and have members who live in the "mainstream" society. The central point is that the cult member gives cosmological allegiance to the cult, the "separate reality" of the cult social universe. In contrast, sect members conceive of both a sacred and secular world and shoulder the strain in everyday life.

In review, we believe that the quest for "cosmologically constituted communions" is a perpetual social process linked to fundamental biopsychosocial components of the human organism. In the ideal form, communions achieve a veridicality between ethos and cosmos which is integrative for both individual members and the group. However, as the structure of society becomes increasingly complex, the strain between ethos and cosmos also increases. We have described four social experiments in religious forms which represent attempts to reduce the strain and reestablish communion.

Social Organization and Religious Forms

In this section we describe the relationships between levels of social organization and concomitant religious forms as they manifest themselves through time and space. As we identify five levels or "epochs" of social organization we will briefly consider how social relations are organized during that epoch and influence the religious and political structure. Our intent here is to trace out the implications of increasing complexity and differentiation of social life through history, not to suggest that each succeeding level of social organization reflects an evolutionary progression toward the "refinement" of human society. Figure 2 illustrates a summary of our analysis.

Level 1: Village Organization

The village is a self-contained social universe where social relations are based upon a contiguity of time, space, place, and consanguinity. Role differentiation is low and social relations combine high affective and instrumental bonding. The cosmos and ethos tend to be veridical and isomorphic, but the cosmology is not formalized. This level of organization is a religio-culture in that political, social, and religious activities are coterminous. Deviance, either political or religious, is rare and individualized. "Secret societies," often misnamed cults, exist as specialized groups that concretize key aspects of the cosmological order. Although relatively infrequent (20) they are harbingers of cosmologically specialized communions that will appear much more elaborately at later levels of social organization.

Level 2: Tribal Organization

Kinship, ethnicity, and economic interdependence are the fundamental structures of tribal organization. Although daily interaction is typically face-to-face, there is the nascent separation of ascriptive and instrumental roles, as well as primary and secondary loyalties, which are functionally linked to an increasing division of labor.

At the tribal level, there is still a universal cosmology, but daily social interaction (ethos) reflects increasing pluralism. Thus,

	Village	Tribe	Monarchial State	Federalism	Post-Modern State
Basis of Social Structure	Time, place, physical contriguity, consanguinity	Kinship Ethnicity Economic barter	Religious/political hegemony	Economic Interdependence	Abstract "Social contract"
Character of Social Relations	Personal affective/instrumental	Primary and secondary groups	Social differentiation (local vs central)	Localized relationships	Anomic Instrumental
Religious Form	Inchoate belief in communion	Universal Cosmology	State Church	Sect/denomination	Denomination, Civil religion
Political Form	Consensual communion	Tribal loyalty	Monarchy	Weak democratic pluralism	Strong democratic centralization
Source of Social Stability	Isolation Sense of place Oral tradition	Kin/tribal ties	Central authority, monopoly	Economic well-being	U.S.: politics Europe: religion
Source of Social Change	Communion	Variant social loyalties	Religious/political dissent	Voluntary organizations	U.S.: religion Europe: politics
Patterns of Deviancy	Personal idiosyncrasy	Sect variants Foreign cosmology	Low sect High cult	High sect "Hidden" cults	High sect High cult
Social Response to Deviancy	Tolerance, extrusion	Tolerance Inter-tribal warfare	Oppression, Persecution	Tolerance	Official tolerance Unofficial oppression
Examples	Small rural village	Third World Africa	China, Iran, South America	India	Western nations, Japan

Figure 2. Levels of social organization and religious forms.

specialized social roles for religious leaders are required to publicly maintain the constancy of the cosmology and its reification
with the ethos.

We first observe the emergence of sects at the tribal level of
organization. These sects do not reject the universal cosmology
but do compete with ethos. Sects arise at this level of organization because of geographic dispersal, growing complexity of the
intratribal division of labor, and intertribal competition.

There are several empirical studies that document the appearance of sects at the tribal level of organization. Barratt, for example, has argued that contemporary tribal Africa has a religious
sect rate six times higher than the United States (21). If, however,
we include the proliferation of "equivalent cosmological communions,"the highest rate of communions is in fact found in
postmodern American society.

Level 3: The Monarchial State

The transition from tribal society to a centralized social hegemony is marked by the appearance of the monarchial state—the
feudal baronies of medieval Europe. The basis of social organization at this level is a pervasive political and economic hegemony
rationalized by a cosmology which is officially promulgated by
the state church.

Under these circumstances the solidarity of everyday relationships is severely compromised: social and psychic bonding is
eroded by role specialization, geographic dispersal, and an increased division between private affective relations and public
instrumental roles. Religious leaders, bishops, and cardinals are
distanced from everyday life and symbolize the growing irrele-
vance of the official cosmology. The voice of the state and the
church are identical and dissent of either type is heretical. Here
then a functional relationship between ethos and cosmos has
disappeared. No communion can be found within the official
parameters of the monarchial state, thus setting the stage for the
appearance of a new religious form: the emergence of true cults.
In contrast to the sect strategy of strain reduction which is
content to tinker with the extant cosmos and ethos, cults emerge
now in an attempt to reestablish communal groups with veridical cosmos and ethos. Medieval cults typically sought to reframe
the extant cosmology and either withdraw from the corrupt

ethos, or they attempted to destroy or overthrow the social order.

Level 4: Federalism: The Industrial State

The transition from the monarchial state to the industrial state is marked by the Reformation Movement. During this period a "federation" of smaller political and geographic units into an abstract political unity is attempted in order to strengthen the economic viability of each participating unit. This federalist form did not seek total hegemony over the daily lives of people; rather, explicit sociocultural "pluralism" was the basis of social organization for the first time. Each city or locale explicitly recognized and promoted its distinctiveness within the federation and meaningful instrumental and affective bonds were tied to specific local social settings.

The motif of pluralistic federalism fostered the emergence of both denominations and sects, each a local variant of larger denomination groupings in the federation. The denomination form, we recall, is characterized by acceptance of social diversity, eschewing the establishment of a universal cosmology. Sects, in turn, reject certain features of the ethos but accept the necessity of the external world. This religious form of communion reflects the social order of federalism where the "locale" was the center of daily life and participated only partially in the federalist alliance.

Finally, we note that without a universal cosmology, federalist forms of communion were not invariantly religious, but also emerged in relationship to the workplace, the marketplace, and recreation. In addition, a growing literacy spawned a variety of intellectual forms of spiritualism and mysticism which became the cosmological foundation for communions. Thus, within the federalist level of social organization, with religious and political pluralism, sects were created apart from a purely "religious" cosmology. Thus at the federalist level, we observe the emergence of "equivalent communions" without explicit religious cosmology (24–26).

Level 5: The Postmodern State

This level of social organization is exemplified by the Western industrialized nations. The central principle of organization is a set of universal, abstract principles of political organization disjoined from economic or affective-personal relationships. Rather than networks of personal commitments to other individuals, the utilitarian performance of tasks specified by social contracts link anonymously with the related tasks of others. Beliefs, values, ideologies, and religious cosmology are not critical for the articulation of contractual job performance or the production of goods and services. The ethos of everyday life has been totally disembodied from any overarching set of transcendant principles which inform the daily life of people. In the postmodern state performance, regardless of "race, color, or creed" is what counts.

Within these social parameters of the postmodern state, the denominations emerged as perfect reflections of the larger social process: an acceptance of the extant ethos and cosmological pluralism. However, the wane of denominational cosmologies as potent transcendental structures from 1850 to 1950, and the inability of other thought-forms such as science to provide a grounding for human behavior have set the stage for the emergence of the postmodern state, particularly America, as a primary setting for a virtual panoply of efforts to construct cosmologically constituted communes. In short, the pervasive strain between ethos and cosmos in the postmodern state has generated the rampant construction of new cosmologies and associated communions. From 1850 to 1900, for example, Clark counted the appearance of 300 new sects (27). Then, from 1900 to 1950 a second form of communion, the quasireligious "equivalent" forms appeared (28, 29). Thus, while America was "officially" becoming secularized, communions of all types were forming, setting the stage for the explicit "religious resurgence" after 1950.

Summarizing this section, we wish to underscore the idea that at each of the five levels of social organization there are different features of social organization that "strain" the veridicality of cosmos and ethos. Different types of "strain" emerge at different levels of organization, thus evoking different cosmological forms to "reduce the strain." In historical perspective, then, we conclude that "religion" is a pervasive social process that strives toward the construction and maintenance of "cosmologically constituted communions." These relationships are summarized in Figure 3.

Level of Social Organization	Degree of Cosmos-Ethos Strain	Solutions
Village	Very Little	No Solution Required
Tribal	Mild	Sect Variants of Universal Cosmology
Monarchial State	High	Withdrawal or Revolutionary Cults To Re-establish Cosmos/Ethos Veridicality
Federalism	Low	"Localized Competing Sects" General: High Tolerance in Democratic Pluralism Local: High Intolerance
Post-Modern State	High	Denomination: Sacrifice Cosmos Secular Ethos Sect: Privatized Cosmos/Ethos Cult: Establish New Cosmos/Ethos

Figure 3. Level of social organization, cosmos-ethos strain, and social solutions.

America: Home of the Sect and the Cult

In the previous section we have described a general framework for identifying the relationships between levels of social organization and religious forms. In this section we will illustrate briefly how the general principles described above also hold true in the history of the United States.

Our discussion is summarized in Figure 4, which details the patterned relationships among the five historical epochs, geographical regions, and religious forms in America from 1607 through the present.

During the period of early colonization from 1607 to 1680 the American social structure was characteristically a Puritan *village* with a universal, transcendent cosmology carefully articulated (reified) with the ethos of everyday life. In essence, America had been founded by a cult to form a series of cultic communes! Ahlstrom (30) has called these villages "Holy Commonwealths."

Religious deviance in this context was, ipso facto, also social and political deviance, and that which threatened the social order of the village was dealt with harshly. Roger Williams, for example, fled Puritan New England labeled a heretic and established his own cultic commune (the Baptists) in Rhode Island. Thus we note that the Baptist denomination of today took roots in America as a cult.

The second level of organization, *tribal*, reaches across the period from 1680 to 1776. In 1680 the British monarch developed a plan to bring political hegemony to the expanding colonies. In terms of our general schema these colonies can be viewed as tribal, based as they were on intracolony networks of kinship, ethnicity, and economic interdependence. This tribal base, "unified" by England, supported a pluralism of religious sects: Catholics in Maryland, Quakers in Pennsylvania, and Calvinists in New York.

Tribal social organization continued throughout the westward expansion of our country, providing the social base for the proliferation of sectarian groups across the Alleghenies from 1800 to 1860 and for the revivalistic sect religion (The Great Revival) between 1820 and 1840 on the frontiers of West Virginia, Ohio, Kentucky, and Tennessee. Later, between 1840 and 1860 the Midwest was settled by immigrant tribes, each establishing their

Level of Social Organization	Dates	Geographic Areas	Dominant Religious Form	Sect/Cult Pattern
Village	1607-1680	New England	Universal Church Universal Cosmology	Personal Idiosyncracy
Tribal	1680-1776	New England (Latent-Far West)	Universal Cosmology	Variant Sects on Christian Cosmology
Monarchial State	1776-1865	New England Mid-Atlantic South	Church-State	Low Sect High Cult
Federalism	1865-1950	Mid-West	Denominational Democratic Pluralism	High Sect Low Cult
Post-Modern State	1950-Present	Cosmopolitan Urban U.S.	Civil Religion	High Sect High Cult

Figure 4. Levels of social organization and religious forms in the United States: a historical perspective.

own religious sects: Scandinavian Lutherans in Minnesota and Germanic Catholics in Illinois, for example.

After 1900 immigrants carried the tribal form into the mountain and Pacific coast states. Interestingly, new sects have their highest rate of origin in *the Far West* today, while mainline denominations have the least appeal there (31).

Thus the predominant prerevolutionary and pioneer westward social structure in America was tribal, a form of social organization particularly prone to spawning sect forms of cosmologically constituted communions.

The *monarchial state* is the term most characteristic of the third level of social organization in America from 1776 to 1865. We have chosen this term because during this time each state exhibited a rather distinctive religious homogeneity, a heritage of the earlier immigration pattern. Although the separation of church and state was officially declared by the Constitution, the original colonies (states) all had a variety of religious regulatory statutes and it was not until almost 1850 that such monarchial statutes were removed. Thus, de facto monarchial states with a unitary religious and political structure were prevalent during this pre--Civil War epoch.

Our general framework predicts that cults emerge within the context of the monarchial state. Congruent with our expectations the historical record indicates that utopian and apocalyptic cults and communes first appeared as a major religious form in the United States during this epoch (1776–1865). The Shakers, the Oneida community, the Orwellians, Fournierists, Mormons, and Millerites are all examples (32, 33).

Just as the vestiges of tribal organization can be found in the ethos of the Far West, the vestiges and ethos of the monarchial state are still present in the South. Under these conditions we expect to find an "official" monopolistic church, dissident sects, and a proliferation of dissident cults which are vigorously persecuted.

As we examine the social organization of the South today we find the (unofficial) sprawling Southern Baptist array, a few dissident sects, and a variety of cults which attempt to avoid official persecution. Poor white and black cults of snake-handlers, Pentecostals, "primitive" churches, and "root-workers" remain secluded in the rural hinterland. Finally, reflecting a pattern typical of medieval times, satanic and witch cults "mirror" the dominant Christian cosmology and find their highest incidence in the South (34).

Our fourth level of social organization, *federalism*, spans the period 1865–1950 and began as the Civil War united a diversity of state economic interests. Our framework identifies the following structural features of federalism: the promulgation of social diversity, the growth of voluntary association, new forms of sectarian affiliation in quasireligious or particularistic communions, and the emergence of denominations that support democratic pluralism. Within this context we expect high sect development but low cult development.

Examining the Federalist epoch (1865–1950) we find: 1) proliferation of over 300 new sects founded prior to 1900 (27). In fact, Stark and Bainbridge have noted that 64 percent of all existing sects were founded prior to 1950 (31). 2) The growth of membership in mainline denominations from 16 percent to 57 percent of the population, concurrent with a transmutation of a transcendent cosmology into a social gospel (35, 36). 3) The appearance of quasireligious sects (Christadelphians, Christian Science), metaphysical sects, and non-Christian sects drawing on Asian, Indian, and Middle Eastern traditions (37–39). 4) The proliferation of "cosmologically equivalent" communions (voluntary association) focused on particularized interests (e.g., labor unions, fraternal orders, farmer cooperatives, and social welfare associations) (40, 41).

Finally, the fifth level of social organization, the *postmodern state*, emerges from 1950 onward. We have described above how this contemporary social structure creates a pervasive strain between ethos and cosmos. Concurrently the mainline denominations have lost membership as a transcendent Christian cosmology, and lost potency in their recasting as "civil religion."

Under these circumstances, Christian sect development flourishes in multiple attempts to reestablish a viable reification of cosmos and ethos. Cults, too, have emerged during this epoch because the cosmology of the past has been so universally ineffectual. In strong confirmation of our thesis we note that a full 75 percent of current American cults were formed after 1950 (34). The new cults and older sects represent a persistent and hardy thrust toward the rediscovery of the original form of human communion—the cosmologically constituted community.

The Current American Scene:
A Cross-sectional Analysis

Up to this point we have presented an historical analysis of social organization and religious forms. Now we turn to in-depth discussion of current religious forms in the United States.

Our approach must be analytical, rather than merely descriptive, because 1) the manifest features of cults and sects belie their latent qualities and 2) we wish to include the nominally religious, the nonreligious, and equivalent cosmological forms in our discussion.

Glock and Stark have proposed a five-factor typology of religion based on a factor-analysis reduction of descriptive variables (42). These five dimensions can be considered as major organizing motifs of ethos within any given religious form. For example, in Figure 5 we list and describe these five dimensions of ethos as they are elaborated by current American denominations.

Unlike the "great universal" religions such as Hinduism, Buddhism, Islam, Judaism, and Catholicism where all five dimensions are strongly elaborated and interwoven, the denominational religious forms have characteristically selected one, perhaps two, dimensions as their distinctive denominational emphasis. This selection is related historically to the fact that all our current mainline denominations were sect offshoots of universal Catholicism. As competing sects, each typically developed one motif as their organizing theme or ethos.

These five dimensions are, however, analytically insufficient when we turn to an analysis of sects and cults. The problem stems from the fact that our mainline denominations all accept a single major source for the construction of their cosmology, but sects and cults typically reject the extant culture as a source of cosmology. Thus when we examine sects, cults, and other equivalent forms we must add a variable indicative of the *source* of cosmology. In Figure 6 we describe a fourfold typology for sources of cosmology.

In the *"syncretistic"* orientation foreign and extant sources are integrated. A classic example occurred in postwar Japan, where traditional Shintoism, Buddhism, and newly introduced Christianity were concurrently adopted and practiced together.

In the *"innovative"* orientation, the known, extant culture is

Dimension	Defining Characteristics	Examples
Ideological	Religion is commitment to a group based on social history, devoid of content.	Unitarian Congregational Main Line Liberal Denominations
Intellectual	Religion is adherance to a set of beliefs, explanations, and cognitive structure of meaning.	Orthodox Presbyterians Dutch Reformed Weslyan Methodist "Evangelicalism"
Experiential	Religion is construed as specific, personal emotional experiences, either privately or in a group.	Charismatics Pentecostals "Holiness" Churches
Ritual	Religion is participation in symbolic rituals, with no necessary intellectual or emotional concomitant.	Lutheran Catholic Episcopal
Consequential	Religion is construed as manifest in behavioral conduct in accord with group morality.	"Fundamentalism" Mennonites Seventh Day Adventists

Figure 5. Five dimensions of the "ethos" of religion.

	KNOWN-EXTANT SOURCES	
	ACCEPT	**REJECT**
KNOWN — FOREIGN SOURCES **ACCEPT**	SYNCRETISTIC (Current Foreign Sources)	INNOVATIVE (Foreign Sources Only)
KNOWN — FOREIGN SOURCES **REJECT**	RECAPITULATIVE (Prior Extant Sources)	INTRUSIVE (New Alien Sources)

Figure 6. Four strategies for construction of a cosmology.

rejected as a source of cosmology and foreign cultural traditions are imported. Within the past 15 years we have seen, for example, the importation of cosmological shreds derivative from Hinduism, Buddhism, Islam, and so on.

The third orientation, *"recapitulative,"* draws upon past forms of the extant culture in order to fashion a meaningful cosmology by a recapitulation of the known past. The classic example is the formation of monastic communities to "recapture the form and substance of the pure first century Christian life." More recently, the Moral Majority is a "sect expression" of this orientation coupled, however, with an effort to live within our modern ethos, rather than withdrawing fully from it.

The final orientation, called the *"intrusive,"* indicates the effort by some groups to reject both extant and foreign sources of cosmology. Thus the source of cosmology is sought outside "known" human conventions. Conceptually, for example, cults of demonology, spiritualism, astrology, and flying saucers all rely on "alien spirits" to bring inspiration, orientation, and cosmology.

We conclude from this analysis that the "cosmological orientations" of current sects and cults are not new orientations, but rather they are enduring variations in the panhuman quest for cosmological constructions which will inspire, organize, and maintain human communions.

Toward a Taxonomy of Sects and Cults

Continuing our effort to bring analytical order to the vast array of sects and cults in America, it is useful to combine the four cosmological sources we have described above with the Glock-Stark typology of five ethos dimensions of religion, yielding the 20-cell taxonomy of sects and cults illustrated in Figure 7.

In order to emphasize the historical continuity of each form within Figure 7, we have listed both past and current examples. In addition to indicating how various groups are related to one another, Figure 7 enables us to anticipate the ideas and behavior of any given group within a specific cell. For example, in the "innovative-ideological" cell we expect to find groups that meet to discuss eclectic philosophical ideals. In contrast, within the "syncretistic-experiential" cell we anticipate groups that focus on multiple forms of emotional experience such as psycho-

Cosmological Source

Religious Dimensions

		Ideological	Intellectual	Experiential	Ritual	Consequential
Innovative	N	Apocalyptic "Watchtower"	"Irreligious" Groups	Holiness Churches	Esoteric	"Eastern Communes"
	O	Apocalyptic "Millerites"	Jehovah's Witnesses	Holiness Churches	Esoteric	Plymouth Brethren River Brethren
Intrusive	N	Flying Saucer U.F.O.	Astrology	Charismatic Pentecostal	Satanic Witch Covens	Possession/Exorcism Cults
	O	Occultism	Spiritualists	Charismatic Pentecostal	Satanic Witch Covens	Possession/Exorcism Cults
Syncretistic	N	Futurology	Christian Life Seminars	"Cursillo" Movement	Psychics	Wholistic Healing
	O	Utopianism	"New Thought" Movements	Mesmerism Magnetism	Psychics	Christian Science Scientology
Recapitulative	N	Antiquarianism	"Primitive" Baptists	"Tent" Revivalism	Immigrant Orthodox	Utopian Communes
	O	Antiquarianism	"Hard Shell" Baptists	Frontier Revivalism	Eastern Catholic Orthodox	Utopian Communes Agragrilan Communes

N = New, Current Examples   O = Old Historic Examples

Figure 7. A taxonomy of religious forms.

therapy cults that seek intense emotional encounters based upon various religious and psychotherapeutic traditions.

We suspect that the whole line of "consequential" groups are likely to be the most intense forms of communion formation because they attempt to construct a complete ethos and cosmos. It is within this sector that we find the isolationist, withdrawn, and self-encapsulated forms of cult-communes that have attracted so much media attention. It should be clear, however, that these particular forms represent only one variant within a wide panoply of communal forms. We must, therefore, be circumspect in our generalizations about "cults," recognizing the variety of distinctive forms and their varying relationships to society as a whole.

The Geographical Distribution of Sects and Cults in America

The variety of communion forms described above are distributed randomly in America. Rather, distribution is functionally related to the level of social organization most pervasive in the four major regions of our country.

1. In the *Northeast*, where the dominant social organization is the postmodern state, we expect a significant cult rate, but a low traditional sect rate. Cult forms are of the "innovative" cosmological orientation, while the ethos forms are "ideological" and "intellectual." Thus cults in this region do not greatly influence daily behavior; they are privatized cognitive cosmologies which permit people to continually participate in the secular ethos of the region.
2. In the *Midwest*, where the federalist form of social organization is prevalent, we anticipate few dissident cults and multiple sect forms reflecting variants of Christianity. Here the dominant source of cosmos is "recapitulative" and the ethos form tends to be "consequential": we see a variety of communal forms attempting to recreate traditional religious communities.
3. In the *Far West*, we discern a continuing ethos of tribalism and thus expect moderate sect growth in rural areas along with a very high cult rate in the postmodern cities. Reflecting the syncretistic nature of the Far West itself, we find "syncretism"

is a dominant source of cosmos, in conjunction with "consequential" ethos affecting daily life-styles in communelike settings.

4. In the *South*, the ethos of the monarchial state is latent, but pervasive. In this region we expect to find moderate sect rates as Christian variants, while low cult rates reflect the persecution of such religious dissidence. Throughout this region communal groups typically draw upon "intrusive" sources for cosmological construction, and develop ethos forms which are "experiential" or "ritualistic."

These social patterns in the four major regions of our country are compatible with some recently published empirical data reporting the rates of sect and cult membership in America (31, 34). These data, along with a summary of our regional analysis, are presented in Figure 8.

The data are clearly supportive of our theoretical formulation and predictions. Differential rates of sect and cult development in each geographical region are functionally related to varying sociocultural contexts. More specifically, the national characteristics of current communion forms reflects the historical distribution of levels of social organization in the four major regions of our country.

Concluding Observations on Religious Forms in America

We do not have the space here to fully discuss Figure 7, although we consider it central to our analysis; using an analogy from physics, the figure is a contribution toward a taxonomy of "atomic weights and masses" for religious forms in society. The figure has, in fact, generated a number of reflections for us which warrant further research.

1. The sociocultural characteristics of those who are attracted to different cell types in Figure 7 will vary. Recent studies, for example, of the so-called "new" sects and cults reveal that members were likely to be younger, unmarried, middle-class, college educated, and upwardly mobile (43). In contrast, the Christian Identity groups such as the Church of Jesus Christ Christians attract bankrupt farmers and the unemployed

Geographic Area	Historical Ethos of Social Organization	Dominant Religious Form	Cosmological Source Form	Ethos Pattern	Cults Per Million	Sects Per Million
Northeast	Post-Modern	Civil Religion	Innovative	Intellectual Ideological	1.9	0.25
Midwest	Federalism	Denomination Sect	Recapitulative	Consequential	1.5	2.46
Far West	Tribal	Sect Cult	Syncretistic	Consequential	6.9	1.42
South	Monarchial State	State-Church Cult	Intrusive	Experimental	0.9	3.19

Figure 8. Current sect/cult distribution in the United States.

(44). Thus *patterns of affiliation* within Figure 7 and their relationship to the social demography of our society are complex
and warrant further study.

2. The *degree of affiliation* also appears to vary with cell type. A
recent study, for example, of nine new religious groups in
Montreal, many of the "ideological" or "intellectual" type,
found that 95 percent of the 29,000 members were "loose
affiliates" (43). Moreover, the drop out rate was very high
(75.5 percent) and participants were likely to shop around,
moving from one group to another: 40 percent had tried three
groups. Hard-core adherence to these new religious groups
was low—in the range of 5 percent to 8 percent of all participants. In contrast, some communal groups with a "consequential" emphasis, such as the Amish or Jehovah's Witnesses may maintain a higher degree of congruence between
initial membership and long-term adherence.

3. The *process of affiliation* appears to be fundamentally structured by personal relationships and contact with friendship
networks. The adoption of a particular cosmological construction usually follows affiliation with a group (45). Thus social
bonding underlies the development and maintenance of cosmologically constituted communions. The process of "forced
membership" does not apply to most sects and cults.

4. Patterns of affiliation and participation are confounded further by the fact that people often participate in several groups
simultaneously. The American proliferation of "particularized communions" generates a series of interwoven
memberships that constrains the actual number of potential
members available for a "total communion." The degree of
overlapping memberships across cell-types in Figure 7, for
example, is not known and warrants further research.

5. A given "religion" may assume a different posture simultaneously in different social contexts. As an example, Mormonism assumes the form of a universal church cosmology in
Utah, but functions as a denomination in the democratic
pluralism of California. In the Midwest, Mormons exist in
tension with other competing Christian sects, while in the
South the Mormons are viewed as a dissident cult. The particular "posture" such a group assumes affects the pattern,
degree, and process of affiliation with the group.

6. Finally, we note that the cell-type (Figure 7) of a particular

group may transform over time. The tragic Jonestown saga illustrates the process whereby a typical Baptist denominational group retreated into an independent sectarian stance, and ultimately to a dissident revolutionary cult. Bainbridge has detailed a similar process in which a psychotherapy group developed into a satanic cult (19).

In conclusion, our cross-sectional survey of religious forms in America reveals a remarkable array of forms and functions. Contrary to conventional wisdom that America has become the epitome of the "secular society," we have documented how secularization creates new quests for cosmologically constituted communions. And we have demonstrated that the form of those communions is functionally related to the level of sociocultural organization within which they emerge. Thus, the publicized "innovative" and "intrusive" sects and cults were "solutions" for some to the "cosmological crisis" of our postmodern state during the 1960s. Currently, we see the reemergence of "syncretistic" and "recapitulative" forms of communion. The ebb and flow of these forms reflects the enduring quest for a "fit" between cosmos and ethos, meaning and behavior.

Social Interpretations of Religious Deviancy

Our examination of sects and cults would be incomplete without a careful appraisal of the relationship between religion and insanity. This theme must be explicitly analyzed because many cosmologically constituted groups today have been assessed in terms of their mental health effects.

Our concern here is the interpretation or labeling of religious beliefs and behavior as manifestations of psychopathology. That is, a particular style of being religious is interpreted as either evidence of mental illness or causing mental illness. We shall label this concept "religious insanity."

In the current psychiatric literature, there are a plethora of psychopathological interpretations of cults. Tseng and McDermott state, for example, that "cults are one of the dangers to mental health . . . the ultimate goal is, of course, to prevent young people from joining cults" (46). Other similar indictments are not difficult to find (47, 48).

It is certainly the case that some persons who join cults dem-

onstrate preexistent psychopathology, may join to meet psychopathological needs, and may experience adverse emotional effects from cult participation. Our concern, however, is the
concept of "religious insanity," namely, that the sole or primary
evaluation of cults is framed in terms of ipso facto psychopathology. We wish to explore here why a dominant, mainstream
profession such as psychiatry may contribute to such "anticult"
social interpretations and meanings.

Starting with our conclusion, we find that the social response
to cults as deviant religious movements which we observe today
is not unique, but exemplifies a general social process observed
throughout Western history. Horowitz has demonstrated, for
example, that all societies engage in the process of defining the
boundaries within which to define persons as mentally ill (49). In
the less complex, nonliterate societies such boundary control is
informal and even inchoate. As social organization becomes
increasingly complex, however, the boundary building and
maintaining become more formal and specialized. In a postmodern society we find the situation where mental health specialists play a key role in the social construction of the "boundaries" for mental illness. Of course, psychiatry never proceeds in
this process alone; it operates within a social matrix that may act
in concert with our opposition to psychiatric opinions and definitions.

Horowitz has further shown that a massive amount of social
research supports the general proposition that *the greater the
social distance between persons, the greater will be the tendency to
perceive unfamiliar beliefs and behaviors as abnormal and even pathologic* (49). Regardless of individual attributes, members of an
entire class or group are likely to be labeled as "mentally ill" if
the social distance is great.

Factors producing social distance include geographical distance, ethnic difference, social class distinctions, and cultural
differences. Within the latter category we believe that cosmological commitments, often expressed in religious terms, generate
social distance and associated class labeling in terms of "religious insanity."

A cosmology, maintained and elaborated by group process,
provides a social definition of "reality" and a source of intersubjective confirmation of that reality. But, as we examine the four
major religious forms we find increasing differentiation within

society and concomitantly, increasing social distance from other groups within society. This general proposition is diagrammed in Figure 9.

Briefly, we note that in the universal church form there is but one cosmology which is isomorphic with everyday behavior: cosmos and ethos approach veridicality.

In the denominational form of religion, there are a few large consanguineous forms—about 10 in the United States today. The denominations all accept the same cultural constitution of reality, supporting it in the form of "civil religion." There is, in other words, a shared intersubjectivity about "reality." There may be idiosyncratic, privatized perceptions, but these do not challenge, alter, or intrude upon the constitution of everyday definitions of society.

In the sect form there is substantial competition about the nature of the "true" cosmological construction of transcendental reality. Sect members, while seeking validation for their cosmology from only within the sect, also participate in the wider ethos relations of the wider society. As such, they are "socially accepted deviants" who move congruently in everyday affairs and embrace beliefs that appear odd, but do not threaten daily affairs.

In the cult form we move to a rejection of the social reality of ethos and cosmos. There is no shared reality between cult and dominant society. Cult members turn to their own group for intersubjective validation of their cosmology.

Since the dominant culture has no basis for validation of the "separate reality" of the cult, the beliefs and values of the cult become labeled as "irrational," "crazy," or "out of touch with reality." In a similar process, the behavior of cult members is labeled as "abnormal." The profession of psychiatry, as a representative of the dominant cultural construction of reality, often similarly perceives and labels these groups as ipso facto mentally ill.

Labeling of religious dissidence as mental illness becomes especially virulent under two very different circumstances: 1) when cults attempt to change the cosmos of America and 2) when a cult or sect makes explicit claims to change the ethos of America. In contrast, those religious, quasireligious, or equivalent communions that are insipid do not threaten the discourse about everyday life and therefore attract the attention of no one.

Religious Form	Number of Form/Type	Competition Among Types	Society/Religion Intersubjectivity	Social View of Religious Reality
Monopolistic Religion	One	None	"Isomorphic Reality"	Isomorphic
a) Village Cosmology	Informal	Individual Dissidence	"Experimental" Isomorphism	Isomorphic
b) Church-State	Official	(Cult Dissidence)	"Official" Isomorphism	(Denial of Cult Reality)
Denomination	Low (10 in U.S.)	Low Democratic Pluralism	High "Same Reality"	Acceptance Civil Religion Isomorphism Religion as Irrelevant
Sect	High (500 in U.S.)	High Competing Cosmos	Mixed Public Shared "Ethos" Private Religious "Cosmos" in Different "Realities"	Tolerance Private Belief is a Deviant Reality
Cult	Very High (5000? in U.S.) (Includes Cosmological Equivalents)	Very High Mutual Exclusion	Low-Absent No Shared Cosmos/Ethos "Separate Realities"	Total Rejection "Ethos" is Socially Deviant "Cosmos" is Irrational

Figure 9. Social reality differentiation in religious forms.

Thus the current blanket responses we observe from representatives of the dominant society are manifestations of ubiquitous
social process: the perception of "the other" as evil, bad, wrong,
or mentally ill when that "other" does not confirm and support
the extant social construction of reality. Thus, although our
political tradition of democratic pluralism has fostered high tolerance of religious dissidence, there is an implicit, not-so-latent
capacity in postmodern American society to respond with virulent labeling of religious dissidence as mental illness when sects
and cults threaten either our political stability or our ethos of
autonomous individualism.

Such "social threats" are thus explained away and rationalized; the dissenting groups and its members placed under the
social control of society's agents, the mental health professionals, whose task it is to "treat" the dissenters. The response of
psychiatry as a social institution may be considered in three
major categories. First, psychiatry may refuse to accept the social
judgment of society before conducting a technical examination
of particular patients. Based on this examination, psychiatry
concludes whether the dissident beliefs and behavior reflect
mental illness or rationally chosen dissidence. The early name
for psychiatrists—the "alienist"—reflects the task of examining
the person "alienated" from normal social discourse.

In a second type of response, psychiatry may support the
perspective of the dissident group and throw its professional
weight into the attack on the social status quo. This was the ethos
of the early days of psychoanalysis in Vienna, the ethos of Franz
Fanon and his revolutionary psychiatry, and the ethos of "radical
psychiatry" during the halcyon days of social psychiatry in the
1960s.

Finally, in the third case, psychiatry may join the dominant
conventional culture, labeling social and political dissidence as
mental illness and using the institutional social controls of the
profession to quell such dissidence. This response is seen today
in both the Soviet Union and in South America where psychiatrists label political dissidents as mentally ill.

Here we are concerned with the social circumstances within
which psychiatry chooses one of these three postures in relation
to religious expressions of dissent, which in the American milieu
is the dominant vehicle for social dissent. We therefore turn now
to briefly examine the interesting role psychiatry has played in

the historical unfolding of social response to deviance and dissidence.

We begin with a critical observation by the great medical historian George Rosen (50). Rosen notes that there has always been an implicit linking of mental illness with social deviance in general and deviant religious behavior in particular. These inchoate links are not, however, explicitly identified as codified in Western history until the Middle Ages.

In our earlier discussion we noted that, in the monarchial state, the universal cosmology linked with an oppressive social order and permitted no dissidence, but that it was in this very context that the dissident religious cults make their singular appearance. In such a context, Rosen notes, no one dare dissent from the truth of the universal cosmology "save madmen and angels," giving rise to the idea of "holy madness." It was in this outburst of cultic religion, with epidemics of frenzied deviancy and features such as possession by spiders in "tartantism," that such religious madness could give safe voice to social dissent. As this dissension increasingly threatened the social and moral order, "blasphemy, religious profanation, and witchcraft fell into the same category because they disturbed the religious and public order." Finally, in an attempt to solidify the official cosmology of the monarchial state, regulations were enacted which transformed dissent into illness, instituting class-labeling of dissident groups as mentally ill as a means of social control. The concept of "religious insanity" was born (50).

The concept of "religious insanity" was quickly adopted within the European psychiatric milieu. Historical illustrations include the following.

- Richard Burton in his *Anatomy of Melancholia* (1621) concluded that the Puritan cult members suffered from "religious melancholia," a severe mental illness (51).
- In eighteenth century England the dissident offshoot of Anglicanism (Methodism) was evaluated by British psychiatrists as a manifestation of a new form of religious insanity called "religion and Methodism" (51).
- In 1821, a British psychiatrist, Burrows, published an entire book on the theme of "religious insanity," linking mental illness with religious and political dissent (50).
- In 1849, the eminent Viennese physician, Rudolph Virchow,

published an influential book on epidemic diseases in which he claimed that all religious and political dissent movements were evidence of psychopathology in the participants and that the psychotic process was linked to the revolutionary dissident ideas of the religious (50).

- In 1851, a new form of epidemic, "whose virus has of late circulated throughout the Continental Nations," called the "democratic disease" was reported in the *American Journal of Insanity* as "A New Form of Insanity" (50).
- Benjamin Rush, signer of the Declaration of Independence and founding father of American psychiatry, argued that "individual and social health depended upon correct political principles." He argued that the Loyalists showed an increase in symptoms called "protection fever" which developed into a new disease called "Revolutiana." On the other hand, Rush the psychiatrist also found that some patriots had developed a new disease called "Anarchia" due to an excess concern for liberty (50).

We pause here to recall that the monarchial state level of social organization characterized the period in American history between 1776 and 1865. Cults erupted on the American scene as expressions of social and political dissent and American psychiatry labeled them as manifestations of group psychopathology. In 1835, for example, Amariah Bringham, a father of American psychiatry, declared such religious insanity "more dangerous than yellow fever or cholera to public health," and by 1840 religious insanity was the fourth or fifth most common mental illness diagnosis among 30 diagnoses in use at that time (51). The historian of this era, MacDonald, notes that this perspective had become conventional psychiatric wisdom in early nineteenth century America, where "the ruling elite used the concept of religious insanity to discredit socially disruptive religious dissidents" (51).

The transformation of the American social structure into a federalist structure following the Civil War led, as we might expect, to a decline in strident cults as the democratic pluralism of the times supported local dissent. As these groups were seen as less of a threat to the body politic, the social labeling of cults as manifestations of mental illness began to diminish. The 1850s was the last intense epoch of "religious causes" and John Gray at the Utica Asylum noted "a decrease in religious insanity as an attributed cause of insanity." By the time of the death of Thomas Kirkbride, superintendent of the Pennsylvania Hospital, in 1883, religious insanity had disappeared from the diagnosis list of the hospital (51).

Has the concept of "religious insanity" disappeared from the psychiatric armamentarium? In the last several decades we have observed the recrudescence of the notion of "religious insanity" on the American psychiatric scene. We find many psychiatrists joining the conventional culture to label new religious movements as evidence of "group psychopathology." Conway and Siegelman, for example, have called this contemporary form of religious insanity "the information disease" (52). They observe that psychiatrists perceive "a new form of mental illness attributed to alteration of brain pathways due to chronic bombardment by information experience in cults."

In contrast, we do have a substantial number of clinical accounts that reveal that some cult members do have obvious psychopathology—but certainly most are not chronically mentally ill. Other clinical reports indicated no mental illness and even improvement in mental well-being among cult adherents. To which psychiatric opinions should we give credence?

Evaluation of Sects and Cults

Our major premise in this section is that it is absolutely necessary to separate technical professional evaluation from ideological evaluation (53). In philosophical discourse, this is the familiar distinction between facts and values. We believe both to be important, but it is critical to avoid confusing the two.

During the past two centuries the philosophy of scientific naturalism has persistently conjoined fact and value into one "natural-empirical" method of assessment which has encouraged the symbolic disguise of ideological value judgments in the form of technical professional judgment. More specifically, scientific naturalism has obfuscated the process of evaluation on two counts: 1) it has made the evaluation of the mental health of persons dependent upon their conformity to the social order, and 2) it eliminates the moral evaluation of social behavior on any ground other than whether the behavior promotes individual good health.

We therefore explicitly discard the philosophical assumptions and consequences of scientific naturalism, striving instead to reinstate the distinction between fact and value, as two distinct domains which should be evaluated in their own right according to separate rules of the game.

First, fact evaluation of the mental health cult members can only be properly conducted as a clinical mental status evaluation of a specific person. Here, we explicitly reject ideological beliefs or social behaviors as relevant, unless they coexist with impairment in mental status.

The related task of evaluating the relationship between mental status and a cause-effect assessment of sect and cult participation is a precarious task if based solely on clinical psychiatric evaluations of individuals. Such a causal analysis requires population samples, and multifactorial, multimethod, quasiexperimental designs.

In contrast, our second evaluation, a social moral evaluation, cannot be achieved by the scientific method. This evaluation arises out of social discourse, political debate, and moral inquiry; it employs the analytic tools of philosophy, theology, and social and political theory. This form of evaluation involves ultimately philosophical choices and answers to the question: What is the good life? We believe psychiatry can and should contribute in this debate but not as scientific arbiters, rather as informed and interested participants in the larger social dialogue.

With these distinctions in mind we propose four major classes of evaluation of new religious movements in which we can compare the fact evaluation of mental health with the moral social evaluation as shown in Figure 10. Using the two-dimensional frame in this figure it would be possible to construct a multidimensional scaling distribution of sects and cults. We will consider here only a few polar examples to highlight the extremes of evaluation.

In the upper left quadrant, there are a wide variety of "cosmologically equivalent" groups that could be classified here. Politser and Pattison, for example, have evaluated over 60 different types of natural community groups and found that they generally benefit both individual members and society (54).

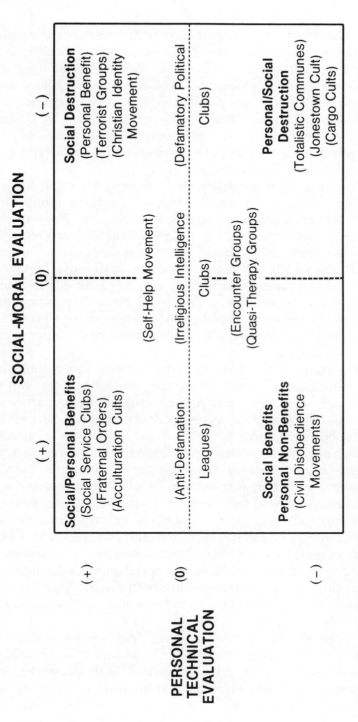

Figure 10. Two-dimensional evaluation criteria.

In the lower left quadrant, we classify groups that are socially beneficient although there may be personal mental health casualties: the French freedom fighters in World War II, religious groups in civil disobedience, and a variety of quasireligious and quasitherapeutic cults are possible examples. We explicitly include in this cell groups that are socially dissident. This is an explicit moral choice on our part congruent with those political philosophers who hold that the expression of dissidence is a positive moral value of our society.

In the upper right quadrant we include groups that have a negative and destructive social value, although the group may promote mental healthiness among its members. The terrorist Canadian Doukabors are a classic example (55). More recently Post has documented the mentally healthy comradeship of terrorist groups which are savagely socially destructive (56).

Our final cell consists of groups that are both socially and personally destructive. Here we would place "totalistic communes" that make no contribution to society in either a prosocial or dissenting form, and which also dehumanize or depersonalize their members.

Summarizing this section we would like to underscore the following points: 1) a given group may move from one cell to another over time thus limiting our evaluations to particular periods of time; 2) no global assessment of sect or cult can ever be set forth because it immediately conjoins fact and value assessments; 3) a negative or positive evaluation in one dimension does not necessarily covary with the other dimension; 4) the mental health status of participants can and should be evaluated where appropriate for clinical treatment, but such evaluation must be kept conceptually and methodologically separate from cause-and-effect interpretations; 5) mental health status should not be allowed to replace social moral evaluation, nor be used as a symbolic guise under which latent social moral evaluation is made; 6) the criteria for determining both mental health status and social moral evaluation should be explicit and available for public analysis.

We believe that adherence to these principles of evaluation may substantially clarify the proper boundaries within which evaluation can and should be conducted. Both fact and value evaluation are critically important, yet neither can take precedence over the other (57).

Comment

At the outset we defined the cult as a "culture writ small." Yet our pursuit of understanding these groups has led us to examine "culture writ large." We have thus endeavored to locate recognizable patterns in the larger social tapestry within which the reader can recognize the smaller threads and figures that constitute the tapestry details of sects, cults, and other cosmologically constituted communions. We have found that, upon close examination, the newer designs bear a close resemblance to the more ancient figures in the same tapestry.

References

1. Beckford JA: Cult Controversies: The Societal Response to the New Religious Movements. New York, Tavistock, 1985
2. Glock CY, Bellah RN (eds): The New Religious Consciousness. Berkeley, University of California Press, 1976
3. Robbins T: New religious movements, brainwashing, and deprogramming—the view from the law journals: a review essay and survey. Religious Studies Review 11:361–369, 1985
4. Needleman J, Baker G (eds): Understanding the New Religions. New York, Seabury Press, 1978
5. Richardson H (ed): New Religions and Mental Health: Understanding the Issues. New York, Edwin Mellen Press, 1980
6. Stark R, Bainbridge WS: The Future of Religion: Secularization, Revival and Cult Formation. Berkeley, University of California Press, 1985
7. Schwartz H: The end of the beginning: millenarian studies, 1969–1975. Religious Studies Review 2:1–15, 1976
8. Pattison EM, Ness RC: The social and historical analysis of cults and new religious movements. Unpublished manuscript.
9. Foucault M: The Order of Things: An Archaeology of the Human Science. New York, Random House, 1970
10. Chidester D: Michel Foucault and the Study of Religion. Religious Studies Review 12:1–9, 1986
11. Schmalenbach H: The sociological category of communion, in Theories of Society, vol 1. Edited by Parsons T, Shils E, Naegle K, et al. New York, Free Press of Glencoe, 1961
12. Pattison EM: A theoretical-empirical base for social systems therapy, in Current Perspectives in Cultural Psychiatry. Edited by Foulkes E. New York, Spectrum, 1977
13. Kluckhohn C: Introduction, in Reader in Comparative Religion: An Anthropological Approach. Edited by Less WA, Vogt EZ. New York, Harper & Row, 1966

14. Anderson RT: Voluntary Associations in History. Anthropologist 73:209–222, 1971
15. Smith C, Freedman A: Voluntary Associations: Perspectives on the Literature. Cambridge, MA, Harvard University Press, 1972
16. Lamert G: Toward a definition of religion. Religious Studies Review 12:273–281, 1978
17. Berger P, Luckman T: The Social Construction of Reality. Garden City, NY, Doubleday, 1966
18. Swatos WH Jr: Into Denominationalism. Storrs, CT, Society for the Scientific Study of Religion, 1979
19. Bainbridge WS: Satan's Power: A Deviant Psychotherapy Cult. Berkeley, University of California Press, 1978
20. Simmons L: The Role of the Aged in Primitive Society. New Haven, Yale University Press, 1945
21. Barrett DB: Schism and Renewal in Africa. Nairobi, Oxford University Press, 1968
22. Cohn N: The Pursuit of the Millennium (rev. ed.). New York, Oxford University Press, 1970
23. Garrett C: Respectable Folly: Millenarians and the French Revolution in France and England. Baltimore, Johns Hopkins University Press, 1975
24. Martin D: A General Theory of Secularization. New York, Harper & Row, 1978
25. Whorton JC: Crusades for Fitness: The History of American Health Reformers. Princeton, NJ, Princeton University Press, 1982
26. Fuller RC: Mesmerism and the American Cure of Souls. Philadelphia, University of Pennsylvania Press, 1982
27. Clark ET: The Small Sects in America. New York, Abingdon Press, 1937
28. Zaretsky I, Leone MP (eds): Contemporary Religious Movements in America. Princeton, NJ, Princeton University Press, 1974
29. Campbell C: Toward a Sociology of Irreligion. New York, Herder and Herder, 1972
30. Ahlstrom SE: A Religious History of the American People. New Haven, Yale University Press, 1972
31. Stark R, Bainbridge WS: American-born sects: individual findings. Journal for the Scientific Study of Religion 20:130–149, 1981
32. Noyes JH: Strange Cults and Utopias of 19th-Century America. New York, Dover Publications, 1966
33. Dieter ME: The Holiness Revival of the Nineteenth Century. Metuchen, NJ, Scarecrow Press, 1980
34. Stark R, Bainbridge WS, Doyle DP: Cults of America: a reconnaissance in space and time. Sociological Analysis 40:347–359, 1979
35. Warren R: The Community in America. Chicago, Rand McNally, 1963
36. Gehrig G: American Civil Religion: An Assessment. Storrs, CT, Society for the Scientific Study of Religion, 1979
37. Needleman J (1970): The New Religions. Garden City, NY, Doubleday, 1970

38. Veysey L: The Communal Experience: Anarchist and Mystical Communities in Twentieth-Century America. Chicago, University of Chicago Press, 1973
39. Judah JS: The Hare Krishna Movement, in Contemporary Religious Movements in America. Edited by Zaetsky I, Leone P. Princeton, NJ, Princeton University Press, 1974
40. Wilson J: Voluntary associations and civil religion: the case of Freemasonry. Review of Religious Research 22:125–136, 1980
41. Jolicoeur PM, Knowles LL: Fraternal associations and civil religion: Scottish Rite Freemasonry. Review of Religious Research 20:3–22, 1978
42. Glock CY, Stark R: Religion and Society in Tension. Chicago, Rand McNally, 1965
43. Bird F, Reimer B: Participation rates in new religious and para-religious movements. Journal for the Scientific Study of Religion 21:1–4, 1982
44. *Time*, October 20, 1986; p 74
45. Stark R, Bainbridge WS: Networks of faith: interpersonal bonds and recruitment to cults and sects. Am J Sociol 85:1376–1395, 1980
46. Tseng WS, McDermott JF: Culture, Mind, and Therapy. New York, Brunner/Mazel, 1981
47. Meissner WW: The cult phenomenon: psychoanalytic perspective, in The Psychoanalytic Study of Society, vol 10. Edited by Muensterberger W, Boyer LB, Grolnick SA. Hillsdale, NJ, Analytic Press, 1984
48. Kaslow F, Sussman MB (eds): Cults and the family. Marriage Family Rev 4:1–192, 1981
49. Horowitz AV: The social control of mental illness. New York, Academic Press, 1982
50. Rosen G: Madness in Society. Chicago, University of Chicago Press, 1968
51. Numbers RL, Numbers JS: Millerism and madness: a study of "religious insanity" in nineteenth-century America. Bull Menninger Clin 49:289–320, 1985
52. Conway F, Siegelman J: Snapping: America's Epidemic of Sudden Personality Change. New York, Delta Books, 1979
53. Wright W: The Social Logic of Health. New Brunswick, NJ, Rutgers University Press, 1982
54. Politser PE, Pattison EM: Social climates in community groups: toward a taxonomy. Community Mental Health J 16:187–200, 1980
55. Holt S: Terror in the Name of God. New York, Crown Publishers, 1964
56. Post JM: Hostilité, conformité, fraternité: the group dynamics of terrorist behavior. Int J Group Psychother 36:211–224, 1986
57. Robitscher J: The limits of psychiatric authority. Int J Law Psychiatry 1:183–204, 1978

Chapter 5

CONTEMPORARY YOUTH: THEIR PSYCHOLOGICAL NEEDS AND BELIEFS

Henry Work, M.D.

Young people to some extent have always been a source of concern for every society. Unique social customs and institutions have been erected to deal with these concerns. From the earliest writings in the Egyptian papyri it has been noted that youth, in each society, is going to the dogs. But somehow these individuals, unstable and often psychologically fragile, seem to survive, and most make it to adulthood.

Certain aspects of contemporary life make adolescence seem even more a period of turmoil in the process of growth than has been true in the past. It is apparent that many of the characteristics of adolescence seem to be occurring earlier in young people's lives, both in boys and girls, than previously. Furthermore, although it may be braggadocio in the face of history to say so, there seems to be an increase in the complexity of life and the pressures of life that surround these individuals at this more or less fragile stage in their progress. Characteristically, this group of young people has always been described as highly subject to peer pressure. To the peer pressures of the past have been added a whole host of new pressures manifested by newer vehicles of communication, ones that were unavailable 50 years ago. The mass media of radio and television have added a force that uses and abuses the vulnerability of this group (as well as affecting many younger children) and have added a new set of pressures. These pressures take advantage of the normal phenomena of growth during this period: the search for independence, identity, and conformity with the peer group. Equally, every psychological discovery of the scientific world has been utilized by societal forces trying to influence the activities, behavior, and life-styles of the preteenager, the teenager, and of older youth in this country and elsewhere.

The phenomenon of striving for independence because of new skills is not unique to the teenage individual. The first "adolescence" seems to occur during the second year of life when the availability of walking, talking, and independent activities puts the young individual in conflict with parental society and is often as frustrating as later adolescence is classically described. Just as small humans going through their second year of life bother their parents, so adolescents, striving also to establish themselves, trouble adults and stimulate societal worries as to the outcome of growth, development, and psychological formation during this decade of life. As a recent report of the Group for the Advancement of Psychiatry has pointed out, we are in need of strong individuals to take our place. Thus we try to foster self-esteem on the one hand and yet continue to offer psychological discipline on the other.

Just as the two-year-old has new capacities to move and to shake off the dependence of infancy, so the teenager is in the process of not only developing new physical strength, but also, and more importantly, developing sexual maturity at the same time. The exploratory curiosity of the teenager thus extends to curiosity about the use of his or her sexual apparatus and the interrelationship between the sexes.

Because of these contradictory forces we characteristically describe these adolescent periods as unstable. Young people manifest great potentials on the one hand but these are opposed by a lack of knowledge, experience, and judgment on the other. It is a shibboleth that this period is seen almost as a battleground between the values society places on adulthood and maturity versus the values that are inherent in the teenager's peer culture.

The values of society are also changing. Certain distinct themes are apparent with a host of variations. At times these changing themes seem to be in conflict and, certainly, different aspects of society are affected in different fashions. A notable example of this is the structure of the family itself. This century has seen great changes in the composition of the nuclear family which formerly provided support and guidance to the growth of children. This has led to a lessening within many families of the supports that previously were available to assist a young person to get comfortably through this stage of growth. By contrast, within some intact nuclear families and even within those where there is but a single parent, there has been an increasing attention to the intellectual and behavioral growth of the child over and above all other values. Thus we see, on the one hand, children developing more or less in a cultural vacuum, either fatherless or motherless and not fully understanding the supportive value that an intact family can convey. On the other hand, and in contrast, we see children growing up in a society which overly stresses the early attainment of adult knowledge, responsible behavior, and places an extraordinary emphasis on learning and performance to the point where childhood itself seems to be disappearing.

Thus, at the time of adolescence we have at least two groups of children, one of which has grown up without supports, without the base of the capacity to learn, and which flounders increasingly as education itself becomes more difficult. The other group, stressed and pushed from infancy, may often be burned out at adolescence or else has developed the characteristics of a mature individual at a point where maturity has not yet arrived. To take another example of the fashion in which society is pressuring the psychological development of children, one only has to look at sports activities, particularly in this country. There was a time when play was considered to be the normal experience of childhood and the concept of play as a preparation for future experience was thought to be most salutary. Children learned not only the physical activities of performance but the appropriate rules of competition. Over the last four or five decades, the push to get children involved earlier and earlier in organized sports has gradually increased. More Little Leagues have sprung up, adding to the stress on small children as well as on latency age and teenage individuals. So organized has this process become (often for the pleasure of adults running the sports far more than the children involved) that the progress through a sport often leaves children burned out even before they arrive at the teenage level. Once again children are subjected to a process of forced competition, valuable, perhaps, to only a relative few of the survivors. Others are exhausted by what once was considered "play."

A more sinister aspect of this phenomenon has been evidenced by what appears to be not only a commercialization of athletics but the attendant phenomenon of outright cheating practiced by those managing sports and athletic activities. While this was once more prevalent at the end of the adolescent period, as younger individuals went into the arena of college athletics, it has now penetrated downward into the teenage athletic scene.

What are the evidence of changes in the behavior of youth at this current stage of history? A cursory reading of the literature, both lay and scientific, would almost suggest that there are no normal or healthy individuals in this age period. If one begins to add up the totality of conditions that are indicators of ill health it is hard to find where normal youth exists. We see that a certain percentage of the youth population is retarded, another has developmental disabilities, while a third has major emotional disorders, a fourth has handicaps from earlier experiences, and so on. It would thus appear that the picture of childhood in America is indeed grim. It is obvious, however, that the literatures, both lay and scientific, tend to focus on the pathologic rather than the normal. The latter is often perceived as unexciting. One often has a sense that physicians see normality among youth not only as bizarre but also as dull. Yet the statistics relating to the increasing problems among children are real and overwhelming. It is evident that some of the "unhealthy habits" of adult life are appearing earlier and earlier in the developmental process.

We live in a strange era where alcoholic intake is not uncommon in children beginning in the seventh grade. Other behavioral problems are apparent in even younger children. Depression and suicide are increasingly commonly reported. Studies of high school and junior high school populations show that over half of the children have thought of taking their lives and that an increasing number of children at the 10-, 11-, and 12-year-old levels are doing so. The sale of drugs is so common among junior and high school children that the individual salesmen, peers of their customers, carry beepers in order to be in contact with their sources. All of this involves money and thus contributes to the economic woes that children perceive in their own changing families.

School is not only a place of learning but a focus for many of the changing pressures that impinge on the instability of teen-age individuals. Thus, the crisis of reading and writing disability has become evidence of the strains that are going on between the child's capacity to learn and the difficulties thereof. There is growing evidence that dyslexia among children is increasing. Whether this is a biologic phenomenon or a result of changes in patterns of earlier education is not clear. What is clear is that the inability to read and write affects every phase of the adolescent's school performance, and that the continuing pressure to excel in school activities results in increasing school failure. For 50 years this nation has struggled with the issue of "why can't Johnny read." The number of theories that surround this issue have increased progressively as time goes on, but it is evident that family, economic factors, and even racial factors strongly affect this issue. As noted above, we rely on an influx of strong, well-educated individuals into the mature population. If, instead, children drop out of school and thus fail to accomplish the task of learning to read and write, the nation will become more impoverished.

The evidence that adolescents are facing more difficulties is manifested in a variety of physical and psychological illnesses. We have already noted the great increase in suicide, and within recent years anorexia and bulimia have stood out as examples of the psychological frailty of the adolescent. Classically adolescence has been seen as highly subject to the fads of the peer group and of society in general. The pervasiveness of the mass media contributes to the spread of these fads, not only in this country but around the world, and has increased the striving for conformity among young people with a seemingly casual disregard of methods that might promote health. In recent years there has been a marked increase among younger children of the use of tobacco. Not only has there been an increase in smoking, but recently smokeless tobacco has become a psychological fad which carries its own hazards for the physical health of younger and younger children. The Surgeon General has noted a curious state in the apparel of youth, that of having a "white ring on the back pocket of a pair of jeans." The ring is produced by the user's snuff can which is stored in that pocket and wears an impression into the denim. Of such seemingly minor actions are behavioral trends constituted.

While some young people become depressed and think about suicide, others turn their increasing interest in sexuality into ever younger and active exploration with unfortunate consequences. Curiosity impels teenagers to look, to explore, and to act in ways that result in the currently exaggerated increase of pregnancy among teenagers. This phenomenon represents another phase of the misuse of the striving toward adulthood and independence on the one hand, and the lack of caution, maturity, and judgment on the other. The exaggerated expression of sexuality in the media not surprisingly makes an impression on this vulnerable age of childhood. The seeking after immediate gratification that is characteristic of this cultural period is also part of the mores of the current youth culture.

The world has become increasingly lacking in stability. Within the 2 months prior to this writing, terrorism has vastly increased and a major nuclear catastrophe has occurred which will affect not only the USSR but the entire world. It is not surprising then that children moving through their adolescence are greatly affected by the problems of environmental decay and commercialism that surround them. Should we be surprised when we read in the paper that John Smith, 16, *who displayed no emotion*, was convicted of sexually molesting a 12-year-old girl and given a prison term for life? Or should we be equally impressed with John Doe, also 16, *who also showed no emotion* when he was sent to prison for 40 years following the shooting of a peer in an exploit in school?

We know that there are normal and healthy children in our population in this decade. We are comforted when we see a high school band in a parade. We are reassured by the examples of young people participating in the Olympics. Offer has taught us something about normal and healthy children. The pattern of health he describes is similar to that postulated by many psychoanalytic thinkers. One outstanding criterion is that healthy young individuals are not afraid to look at themselves. They may worry about sex, religion, and money, but they are able to perceive their own role in society. The capacity to look at self, to be aware of self, and to understand it makes many healthy young individuals sexually conservative; and, even though they may perpetrate minor delinquencies, they have goals. Offer notes that in certain families, children emerge from adolescence with good health, high intelligence, and consistent behavior. These homes tend to be stable and offer consistent values. Parents in these homes allow independence with support, and respect the young people reciprocally so that the values are shared.

In particular, one of the primary needs of adolescents is the enjoyment of normal physical health. It is important, therefore, not to preach to young people about healthy living, nor to judge them harshly, but to openly help them to develop good health habits and adult values.

The British use of the concept of awkwardness in this period serves as an excellent description of the physical and emotional status of youth. Just as young people's bones are growing so rapidly that their muscles often become out-of-phase, they develop awkward gaits and characteristically become embarrassed and therefore, more awkward. This embarrassment carries over into their psychological processes. We have talked of the striving for independence and maturity, but such strivings are always accompanied by stresses that make the individual seem mature one day and immature the next. No one can watch a young teenager going through despair because of a minor bad grade and then becoming exhilarated following a call about a date, without noting how transitory are the psychological processes of the young teenager's mind. And yet it is the awkwardness of both the mind and body that seems to concern adults. We look at these young people, we set them apart as pariahs, and we make their lives more difficult by not accepting them as normal human beings going through an important struggle for which they are not always equipped.

It is difficult to know whether we as adults should continue to participate in the 5,000-year-old tradition of concern about the distressing state of adolescent behavior, thought, and action. We as adults have speeded up our own activities and forced children to act and seem more mature than sometimes they are capable of being. The media have pushed children endlessly to be more adult. The entertainment world has offered spectacles to children that were never offered before. Newer and louder noises and newer and stranger idols crowd upon them. Small wonder that the normal faddism of adolescence is an exaggerated phenomenon at the present time. It does no good to blame adoles-

cents for being members of the teenage decade. Rather, it becomes critical not only to understand the phenomenon of
growth and development within the individual but also to look
more clearly and more extensively on the pressures of society
that surround this age period.

THE IMPACT OF MEMBERSHIP

Chapter 6

LIFE IN THE CULTS

Saul V. Levine, M.D., C.M., F.R.C.P.(C)

Readers of this volume and other literature on the subject (1–6) might conclude that all cults are particularly bizarre and oppressive. They might also assume that these terrible groups have typical life-styles which defy imagination, and which are obviously weird, unique, and novel. The truth is that these groups did not invent the wheel; just about every ritual or practice, good or bad, which I have seen in the various groups deemed by the public as cults, has had precedence in other settings, perpetrated by individuals, families, and "acceptable" religions as well as businesses, political movements, and other closed social systems.

There is no prototypic "Day in the Life of . . . " in these groups, any more than there is a uniform pattern for all families. But there are similarities of process, as opposed to content. All the intense group belief systems (a far less lilting but more accurate depiction than that pejorative, four-letter "cult") have overriding characteristics that account for their hold on their members.

Let us examine some common features of all the groups that society as a whole calls cults. We must bear in mind, however, that the label cult is partly in the eye of the beholder, and that a remarkable array of groups has had that eponym applied to them. Groups that this author has heard called cults by concerned relatives of members have included Catholics, Mormons,

Orthodox Jewry, Born Again Christians, Bahai, IBM, est, and
Gestalt, to name but a few. For purposes of this chapter, however, we will use as examples groups about which there appears
to be considerable external unanimity. That is, these four—Hare
Krishna, the Unification Church, Children of God, and the Divine Light Mission—have probably been held in less esteem by
more people than most of the other groups combined (other
similarly vilified groups models which have inspired widespread fear and loathing include Scientology, The Way International, Bagwan Rajneesh, Jews for Jesus, Synanon, and others).

Common Characteristics

Belief System

Each group has a written tome which is supposed to be the
ultimate font of resident knowledge accumulated over the mil-
lennia (or months!) and passed down from the deceased or very
much alive and deified guru to the common membership. The
theology may seem illogical or incomprehensible to an outsider,
but this is of little consequence. They can and do level the same
charges against our own beliefs. As a matter of fact, this "not
understanding" is sometimes comforting to novices, as it suggests an exalted level of comprehension among the leadership,
and something to aspire to. The tome, in the form of papers or
books, tracts or treatises, or magazines, is used in recruitment
and often sold in order to raise money for the group. The magazine of the Hare Krishna, *Back to Godhead,* is often disseminated
freely, while the "Mo Letter" written by the leader of the Children of God (Rev. Moses Berg) is used as a tract to guide behavior. The Moonie bible, called *The Divine Principle,* is written by the
Unification Church's Rev. Sun Myung Moon, and is sold in
many parts of the world. The magazines of the Divine Light
Mission, a Hindu-derived religion with Guru Maharaj Ji at the
helm (deposed in 1977), are called *And It Is Divine* and *Love Song*
and are sold extensively on the streets of North America.
    The Belief System provides an overriding raison d'être, a
seemingly new system of values, an external focus of attention
(7, 8). It is furthermore "sanctified," or given a lofty level of

spiritual and worldly significance. The members feel that instead of being preoccupied with materialism, competition, and acquisitiveness, or contemplating their navels in philosophical and existential dilemmas, they are now involved in something which is not only captivating but of vital importance to the group, and by extention, to the world. When one reads between the lines, however, and observes closely, the "new" values are not only not radically different, but in fact often approximate the very practices (especially accumulation of wealth) which they avowedly deride.

Belonging

It may sound silly, but one cannot be a cult unto oneself. It takes numbers of people acting in a concerted, shared, cohesive effort to produce the phenomenal elevation of the group in importance and the subjugation of the self, which we see so regularly. The group's beliefs, activities, members, and leaders become all-encompassing and embracing. The members feel that they are unequivocally accepted, and integrated into this special social system. They are vital cogs in a wheel of vast significance. The sense of belonging cannot be overemphasized. It creates an inner "specialness" (some might call it "preciousness"), and a united feeling of "us (inside) against them (outside)." The more the perceived outside antagonism or even persecution, the greater the sense of justification of the group cause. Everything is done by everyone: there are shared emotions, catharses, and experiences. Even in groups with few demands, an implicit and powerful group pressure is engendered; a centripetal force which involves group cohesion and unwavering commitment. There are two levels of group: one is the greater membership throughout the country and world. The other is the particular and relatively small congregation or temple, ashram, or commune. Even if a large religious organization is "known" to be dangerous, it is more important to look at the local representation, because there are often vast differences in attitudes, relationships, and treatment of members. The feeling of belonging to an important group with a shared belief system is considerably enhancing to the individual; as time goes on the smaller group becomes the top priority to the members, superseding the larger religion (9, 10). With the passage of a few months, the relationships formed in the small group become paramount, as vital, or, moreso, as the belief system.

Leadership

Virtually all the groups are rigidly structured, hierarchically and pyramidally. That is, there is no disputing that there is a single, overall leader, who is usually imbued by the group with super-human and mystical powers. At times he is formally deified, as with the Divine Light Mission's Maharaj Ji—"The Perfect Master"—or the Unification Church's Rev. Moon—"Messiah." But even if the leader does not make claims to having a direct pipeline to God, it is obviously a need among the membership to ascribe special personal characteristics to these exalted individuals.

These ultimate leaders can be young (Maharaj Ji was 15 at the height of his dominance) or old (Moon is in his 60s), male or female (e.g., Elizabeth Clare Prophet of the Church Universal and Triumphant), alive or deceased (the Hare Krishna follow the teachings of the late A.C. Bhaktivedanta Swami Prabhupada), and present or absent (the Church of God's Moses Berg has been missing for a few years, as was L. Ron Hubbard of Scientology). Charisma, contrary to popular misconception, is an unnecessary ingredient in the leader. However, the groups are in themselves intrinsically charismatic, demanding, proselytizing, and evangelical.

The senior members just "below" the top, the designated "lieutenants," have always struck me as being the obsessional enforcers of rigid dogma. The guru or reverend at the apex may have more flexibility, imagination, and creativity, but those on the rung below are the epitome of true believers—unwavering, inflexible, even intolerant. As time goes on, the local leaders become dominant in importance in the lives of members. It becomes very difficult to evaluate the life of a member merely on the basis of being a member of "a" group. I have seen loving, gentle members and local leaders in groups which are intrusive and exploitative, like the Children of God. Conversely, there have been groups not known for these coercive tactics that have had regional representatives who in fact subvert the ideology and life-style of the group.

Meeting Places

All the intense group belief systems have meeting places which, over a period of time, take on a decidedly uniform internal appearance, no matter where in the world they are located. This should not be surprising to anyone familiar with churches, synagogues, or mosques. Similarly, Hare Krishna temples and Divine Light Mission ashrams are largely replicated from city to city. These prayer centers are usually located in urban environments, in converted mansions, churches, or institutions. But this is the case even in groups which have not got formula or prescribed external and internal architecture and design. Common pictures (usually photographs of the leaders), statues, arrangement of seating, group literature, printed prayers or exhortations, ornaments, and a central focus (lectern) or podium of some sort, are de rigueur. Group activities of various sorts ensure that the space is utilized functionally as often as possible. That is, the meeting place "becomes" part of the daily rituals (see below). But, as with all aspects of group functioning, there is a unique atmosphere and culture, chemistry, and "vibes" which is almost palpable and varies from center to center, even within the same group. The members' coalesced personalities and backgrounds certainly play a role in determining the prevailing ambience, but the most important determinant is the local leader (mahatma—Divine Light Mission; president—Hare Krishna).

The majority of the meeting places are in urban areas, but most of these groups have rural retreats which serve multiple purposes. At times they are used as vacation centers which senior members utilize for rest, recreation, and rejuvenation. More commonly, they serve as initial recruiting centers, in the preliminary screening and indoctrination phases—certainly the Moonie rural retreats (camps) are commonly used in this way. Some of the groups live in rural communes, supporting themselves via farming or cottage industries, in addition to selling their religious wares (Children of God).

Rules and Regulations

Each of the intense group belief systems I have studied has had a set of precepts and rules, which are designed to regulate and control behavior. The various aspects of life so governed range from dress to diet, to sex, drugs, or social demeanor. The extent of control varies from moderate influence all the way to totalistic determinism.

For example, in the Hare Krishna movement, the bright saffron robes and shaven heads of the young men are not uncommon sights (although common civilian appearance is now acceptable); diet is strictly vegetarian, no meat, fish, or eggs; no intoxicants (including tea or coffee) are allowed; no gambling is permitted, including participating in "frivolous" sports or games; no illicit (i.e., premarital) sex, including dating or courtship. Similarly, in the Divine Light Mission, members are expected to turn over all material possessions and earnings to the religion and to abstain from alcohol, tobacco, meat, and sex. In both cases, total devotion and constant preoccupation with the teachings of the group are demanded. The young members of the Unification Church and the Children of God are indoctrinated into following the teachings of Rev. Moon and Rev. Berg, respectively, but the prime rules and regulations are designed to ensure successful fundraising.

There are implicit rewards for obeying and clearly living up to the letter and intent of the rules. In addition to explicit social reinforcement like smiles, congratulations, and compliments, there are implicit feelings of pleasure at fulfilling the precepts of the leader and the religion. It is also the only way to rise in the hierarchy. The "better" one does in more than meeting the demands of the group, the greater the chances for being selected as a shining light. Commonly, the extent to which one does not approximate the rules, or worse, breaks the rules, will determine a relatively short stay in the group. In these instances extrusion by directive or ostracism is guaranteed.

Members

With few exceptions, the members are young (median age 22), white, middle-class, relatively well educated, and from intact families. There are equal numbers of men and women in most groups. There is no evidence to suggest that the various memberships are any more "pathologic" than any other comparable cohort of nonmember peers. Because like members tend to attract each other, one finds subtle differences in group identities from center to center, even within the same religion. For example, some might be more intellectual; others are openly affectionate; others from more affluent backgrounds.

The new members might be called premies (Divine Light Mission), or novices, or trainees, and they come across as eager, closed-minded, happy true believers (see below). They join because of a confluence of factors. They are at that time in what I call a "critical period"—a state of alienation (feeling out of the mainstream, separate, powerless to affect their lives significantly), demoralization (dispirited, lack of enthusiasm, no raison d'être), low self-esteem, and some problems in separating from their families. During that critical period, an individual has a void to fill, manifesting itself in an emotional and ideological hunger. He is suggestible, with a need for stability and goals, support and structure. He is in a state that I call autohypnosis, that is, self-programmed to succumb. If during that particular period, a group makes itself available, a group that is clean-cut, seductive, and attractive, from the same social milieu, and is not threatening (drugs, sex, violence, etc.), then a small percentage (perhaps fewer than 1 in 200) will succumb to their warm invitation and overtures.

During the period of ultimate commitment to the group, they are often alienated or estranged from their parents. They are suffused with self-righteousness and justification. They feel especially sanctified and enhanced. Not only are their earlier feelings of alienation, demoralization, and low self-esteem overcome, but they feel "wonderful" in all respects. They experience happiness, clarity of thought, and high motivation. They feel healthier and want to share their sense of self-improvement; they proselytize, they propound, they bore. Their bliss and happiness are, however, not contagious. Their simplistic reasoning, their overriding commitment, their narrowed focus, their suspension of critical judgment—all of these offend and concern us, but they are hallmarks of fundamental true believers (11), of any ilk.

Miscellaneous Characteristics

Money.   It is extraordinary that a commodity that plays no role whatsoever in the theology of the groups except as a decidedly materialistic concern, should be such a dominant aspect of the total operation of these intense groups. Not only are selling, earning, and soliciting part and parcel of the daily operation, but taking and turning over personal savings are either encouraged, expected, or demanded. Furthermore, from the perspective of outsiders, especially parents, the perception that their children are being financially exploited is seen as one of the most pernicious and malevolent aspects of the group. This is particularly of concern when the leader (Moon, Majaraj Ji, Bagwan Rajneesh, Hubbard, and so on) lives in ostentation and offensive opulence, while the members may be at the subsistence level. In the state of ultimate commitment, a true believer feels better for having raised and or given money to the cause. It also aids in overcoming cognitive dissonance (the cause "must be" worthwhile to have attracted these funds). All kinds of rationales are given and accepted for the displayed wealth of the leaders, but it is fascinating to see the blind acceptance being replaced by questioning and scorn as the hypocrisies and double standards begin to make themselves felt.

Language. In any closed group, language takes on a particularly significant dimension. It becomes part of the uniqueness and cultish identity, a source of pride in being privy to special meanings, new words, or old words used in new ways. For example, in the Divine Light Mission, words like "knowledge" (a kind of revelation or insight to the Perfect Master), "beauty" (everything is "beautiful"), "divine," and "love" are used respectively during indoctrination and in everyday discourse. A new word like "satsang" (spiritual discourses in the Divine Light Mission), "darsheen" (seeing the Master), "litnessing" (witnessing in the Church of God), or "systemite" (evil, devil-influenced individual) can give the members the added sense of being part of a loftier, more esoteric and complex—and important—mission.

Pay-off. There is an implicit premise of a personal reward for wholly dedicating oneself to the group. That is, in addition to the altruistic creation of "a better world," the explicit goal (in so many words) of all the groups, there is the expectation of achieving personal salvation, eternal exalted life in the hereafter, reincarnation as an enriched being, or even great rewards, material as well as spiritual, while still in this world. This is frequently broadly alluded to or hinted at, but not to the extent that narcissism or selfishness can be attributed to members as a conscious motive.

The other payoff is in the here-and-now. Anyone studying these groups is struck by the happiness of the members. One might attribute this to "programmed bliss," but this does not do justice to the phenomenon. The members actually feel exceptionally well, physically and emotionally. Any symptoms of anxiety, somatic distress, mundane or existential preoccupations, simply melt away. The outer-directed, focused ideology, the overriding commitment, the intensity of the group, and the Answers enable imagined and real distress to dissipate.

A Day in the Life of . . .

Just like most families, these groups have set routines and rituals which become part of the everyday process of living. And, as with families, these vary widely in terms of schedule, rigidity, expectations, participation, and so on. There is no doubt, however, that the groups most universally condemned and labeled as cults are the ones that are the most demanding of rigid adherence to schedules, duties, and rituals.

In the Hare Krishna movement, the core daily behavior involves chanting and singing on sidewalks (sankirtana). By this means they spread their message, recruit, and raise funds by selling their magazine. But the day begins well before this activity, usually between 3:00 and 4:00 A.M. Showers are taken immediately, followed by dressing in clean clothes (saris for women, dhotis for men). At this point, chanting and prayers (from the *Bhagavad Gita,* a Hindu prayer book) would occur in a relatively formalized service. Between 6:00 and 7:00 A.M. there are classes, in which Sanskrit scriptures are read, translated, and discussed. Chanting is interspersed throughout and between these activities. Breakfast is taken at 7:30 A.M. followed by cleanup and chores. The sexes are fairly well segregated. The women are expected to do more of the "domestic" chores, and generally have less of a prominent decision-making role (some would say more of a servile position). By about 10:00 A.M., the group is ready to leave the temple to begin the sankirtana, and continue in this activity throughout the day, with some breaks for lunch and chanting. They return around 6:00 P.M., shower, and after a vegetarian repast, the sequence chanting of classes and prayer and study would recommence, ending at about 9:30 P.M., followed by bedtime (around 10:00 P.M.).

In the Children of God, wake-up is around 6:30 A.M. After wash-up, there follows a sequence of prayer (7:30 A.M. to 8:30 A.M.) and memorization and review (8:00 A.M. to 8:30 A.M.) of scripture (New Testament) and Mo quotes, and reading Mo letters (8:30 A.M. to 10:00 A.M.). At 10:00 A.M. the members have a communal breakfast, followed by Bible study until 11:00 A.M. Clean-up and chores ensue, and by noon, the group is ready to "hit the streets" with literature and motivation for proselytization and sales (of Mo letters). They return at 6:00 P.M., to have dinner at 7:00 P.M., and begin another hour and a half of prayers, classes, and reciting. This schedule is rigidly imposed six days out of seven; on a "free day," members are often expected to do work for the religion, and are seldom, if ever, alone.

The Divine Light Mission makes similar demands on its members, but the daily routine varies considerably depending on whether the Premie is living in an Ashram or on the outside. In the former, a fairly regimented, totalistic life-style is demanded, with the day's programs filled from the 5:00 A.M. awakening with meditation, prayers, selling magazines, proselytizing, and service. This last term refers to any activity enhancing the image of the Maharaj Ji but it often takes the form of working in a Divine Light Mission–run business (aside from selling *And It Is Divine*) like a restaurant, second-hand shop, or drug rehabilitation center. Those who live outside are expected to devote as much of their time as possible to the repetitive program, but it cannot be controlled as assiduously.

In the Unification Church, a comparable daily program is imposed on the trainees in the rural retreats. In contrast, however, interspersed throughout the day are dedicated opportunities for physical exertion—volleyball, calisthenics, fitness classes, and the like. There is also a seemingly jovial laissez-faire period of joking and singing songs. But ex-members describe these as equally well organized, programmed, and repetitive, all in the service of indoctrination and control.

Specific knowledge, doctrine, the musings of the master, the particular theology, and a rationale to translate these teachings into marketable entities, especially sales and recruitment, form the basis of the daily functioning of these groups. Nothing else is as important. While I have been seen to be somewhat sympathetic to the groups for their cries of persecution, and outside attacks of ignorance, there is no doubt that the so-called cults have these as their central raison d'être. The lyrics (content) change, but the melodies (process) are identical.

In all of these groups, deviations from the norm are seen as heretical, undermining, and even dangerous. In the stage of ultimate commitment (true believers), it is highly unusual for members to choose to buck the phenomenal group pressure in order to pursue independent or different activities. But true believership is in by far the majority of instances a temporary phenomenon. It is followed, inexorably and almost inevitably, by a stage I call "seeds of doubt." This is typified by the member seemingly suddenly being aware of two major issues which had for many months (usually) or years been buried. The first is the apparent inconsistencies and hypocrisies in the group itself: for example, living at a subsistence level in the Divine Light Mission while the Maharaj Ji lived in ostentatious opulence. The second is the upsurging of longing and homesickness. Birthdays, anniversaries, parents, friends, lovers, pets, and so on, are increasingly missed. The armor of total belief and belonging is pierced. Once that happens, the individual will leave no matter what the group may decide to do to counter the sensed withdrawal. The first external signs are an apparent diminishment in zeal, followed by demonstrated fluctuations in participation in routines and ritual. The group might attempt overt pressure, confrontation, reasoning, ostracism, or a number of other ploys, but never to any avail. But observers looking at groups over a period of time will be able to pick out members who change in their dedication to the cause. They smile less, struggle more, ask for leaves, and do not engage in all the group activities. They are the ones on their way out, and out they will undoubtedly go.

Comment

Having been involved in clinical work and research on intense-believing groups and their members (9, 10, 12–17) for a few years, I have become both sanguine and cynical about global pronouncements and generalizations. I have seen terrible deeds perpetrated in cults (and in families and other groups), and I have seen benevolent and uplifting experiences. Most, however, fall in between, being for the most part pedestrian and unimpressive. But the rhetoric among family members, true believers, and involved clinicians and others is deafening, and at times vicious. The vast majority of members go through these experiences relatively unscathed, have a tough time after they (almost inevitably) come out (usually in under two years), and gradually reconstitute and reintegrate. For most of the youthful members, the radical departure ends up as an intense life experience which few people would have recommended or prescribed, but which manages to serve a developmental purpose. They were undoubtedly jolted by the events and in retrospect, have difficulty comprehending how they could have gone that route. Once out, if "allowed" to leave by the "natural" processes of disillusionment (rather than extrusion or kidnapping), their feelings about the group are mixed, and almost never totally condemnatory.

Finally, if we have doubts as to the illegal or criminal intent or practices of particular groups, then prosecution and even persecution are in order. If not, in a democratic society, all manner of intense group belief systems have to be tolerated, as long as the laws are not broken. We can even learn from some of the groups about how to stimulate and captivate the energy and idealism of our normal youth, and about how to help or rehabilitate drifting or deviant young people.

References

1. Enroth R: Youth, Brainwashing and the Extremist Cults. Grand Rapids, MI, Zondervan Press, 1977
2. Needleman J, Baker G (eds): Understanding the New Religions. New York, Seabury Press, 1978
3. Stoner C, Parke J: All God's Children: The Cult Experience: Salvation or Slavery? Radnor, PA, Chilton Book Co., 1977
4. West LJ: Contemporary cults—utopian image, infernal reality. The Center Magazine 15:2, 1982
5. Zaretsky I, Leone M: Religious Movements in Contemporary America. Princeton, NJ, Princeton University Press, 1974
6. Singer M: Coming out of cults. Psychology Today, 1979
7. Frank JD: Sources and functions of belief systems, in Psychotherapy and the Human Predicament. Edited by Dietz PE. New York, Schocken, 1978, pp 260–269

8. Levine SV: Belief and belonging in adult behavior. Perspectives in Psychiatry 3:1, 1984
9. Levine SV: Fringe religions: data and dilemmas. Ann Soc Adolescent Psychiatry 6:75–89, 1978
10. Levine SV, Salter NE: Youth and contemporary religious movements: psychosocial findings. Can J Psychiatry 21:411, 1976
11. Hoffer E: The True Believer. New York, Harper & Row, 1951
12. Levine SV: Adolescents, believing and belonging. Ann Soc Adolescent Psychiatry 7:41–53, 1979
13. Levine SV: The role of psychiatry in the phenomenon of cults. Canadian Psychiatric Association Journal 24:593–603, 1979
14. Levine SV: Report on physical and mental health aspects of religious cults and mind expansion groups, in Study of Mind Development Groups. Ontario, Government of Ontario, 1980, pp 665–738
15. Levine SV: Cults and mental health: clinical conclusions. Canadian Journal of Psychiatry 26:534–539, 1981
16. Levine SV: Radical Departures: Desperate Detours to Growing Up. San Diego, CA, Harcourt Brace Jovanovich, 1984
17. Levine SV: Alienated Jewish youth and religious seminaries—an alternative to cults? Adolescence 29:73, 1984

Chapter 7

FAMILIES OF CULT MEMBERS: CONSULTATION AND TREATMENT

David A. Halperin, M.D.

Cult affiliation is an extraordinarily dramatic action within the family setting. It is frequently so wrenching and stressful an act because through the act of affiliation, a family member declares in a profound manner that he or she does not share his family's spiritual or material values. It cuts across generational continuities. In a stroke, cult affiliation relegates to the realm of frustrated expectations all past plans. It indicates that henceforth a family member will be marching to the tune of a decidedly different drummer. Cult affiliation elicits a plethora of intense responses from family members ranging from profound soul-searching to more pragmatic concern. This chapter examines the role of the psychiatrist in the consultation with and the treatment of the family of the cult member.

The term *cult* cannot be defined with mathematical precision. West and Singer (1) have advanced 10 criteria as guidelines. Ultilizing these criteria, cults may be defined as authoritarian organizations headed by a self-proclaimed leader with messianic religious or political pretensions. Cult leaders exercise total-itarian control over the cult's organization and arrogate to themselves totalistic control over almost every aspect of the cult member's life. While cult leaders may live in a style of extraordinary luxury, they demand from their members a degree of emotional and financial commitment that leaves members in a state of economic and emotional penury, and without any significant financial, social, or emotional resources should they choose to leave the organization.

The family's initial responses to cult affiliation may range from shock and surprise to calm acceptance. The very intensity of the familial responses reflects the fear and the appropriate concern of the family that their child, sibling, or parent may become unable to function autonomously and regress to a quasi-infantile dependency. Not surprisingly, families become very concerned when a family member changes previously held goals and plans with a startling rapidity or dissipates vast material resources in the service of a "higher" cause. Whatever the nature of their previous relationship with the cult member, cult affiliation rapidly assumes the status of a focus for all the members of the family. For the family of the cult member, cult membership presents a clear and present danger to a family member. However, the very intensity of the familial response may be disconcerting to the psychiatrist who finds it difficult to appreciate the extent to which cult affiliation presents a crisis to the family system. Moreover, the family's exaggerated demands for the psychiatrist's total involvement may elicit an equally intense countertransference in which withdrawal is rationalized as a judgment that the family's concern is either exaggerated or the product of narcissistic injury to the parents' amour propre (2). Cult affiliation, like other crises in the family system, demands and deserves careful evaluation. However, it is exceedingly important for the psychiatrist even in this initial phase of consultation to set limits on the professional relationship.

Psychiatric Consultation During the Early Phases

The role(s) that the psychiatrist plays in consultation with the family of cult members changes with the duration of cult affiliation. During the initial phase of affiliation, the psychiatrist works with a family as they respond on an acute basis to the problems posed by a recent cult affiliation. The psychiatrist's role changes when he or she is consulted by a family, one of whose members has been established within a cult group over an extended time. Finally, the psychiatrist's role changes as he or she works with an individual who has left the cult group. The goals of consultation change with the chronological context. Also, the goals of consultation vary with the individual at risk. The majority of consultations are sought by the parents of cult members, but consultation may be sought when the question of custody arises, particularly when one of a child's parents has left a cult group. Psychiatric consultation may even be sought by grandparents concerned over the welfare of grandchildren. Finally, children may seek psychiatric consultation in order to protect their parents from emotional and financial exploitation by cult groups [some cults have begun to actively recruit the elderly (3)].

The family's insight into the precult life of the new cult member is often very limited. Some may appreciate that the cult member was isolated and alienated prior to cult affiliation. They may even appreciate that the cult member was seemingly searching for a transcendent experience via drugs, causes, or religious enthusiasm. Nonetheless, the majority of family members present an idealized picture of the individual's functioning and of the family's relationship with the cult member prior to affiliation. Typically, they regard the cult as an alien excrescence, simplistically assuming that when the individual has severed the connection with the group, both the individual and the family will return to the status quo antebellum. Families relatively rarely seek psychiatric consultation with the goal of preparing the ground for further psychiatric treatment (even when they recognize that the individual did join the group because the group provided some measure of support). The family agenda tends to be limited to seeking assistance in casting out the evil (cult) and reinstituting the good (anticult) (4).

Cult affiliation comes, in almost all cases, as a profound shock to the family of the cult member. Even though they may have been subliminally aware that their child or sibling has been developing a new set of friends, that his or her life-style had been radically changing, that he seemed to be increasingly preoccupied with novel, eccentric, or esoterically religious ideas, the reality of cult affiliation still comes as a shock to other family members. Their surprise may reflect their need to deny the obvious, as well as a familial pattern of obtuseness and indirection. Their shock and surprise and their fears that the cult group will exploit their child and destroy their relationship with their child are very much in evidence when they attend their first meeting of a parent self-help group for the parents of cult members. (Self-help groups have been extremely helpful in working with parents of cult members.) However, their surprise may also reflect the cult's having encouraged the new member to adopt a vague or deceptive attitude vis-à-vis the family during the early period of affiliation. Cults encourage this vagueness and may discourage new members from presenting a realistic picture of the member's actual degree of involvement because they fear (and rightly so) that the family would become concerned and mobilized by the cult member's new interests and possible commitments. At this early stage, psychiatrists should encourage parents to contact knowledgeable parties, for example, mental health professionals, self-help groups such as the Cult Awareness Network, the American Family Foundation, or the Cult Hotline and Clinic of the Jewish Board of Family and Children's Services of New York City, when they suspect that changes in conduct or interests represent more than the normal turmoil of adolescence. When parents do contact these resources they may be reassured that the group is unusual but not cultic—that it simply reflects the American traditions of diversity and nonconformity. Or, they may be alerted to the cultic nature of the Group. At this very early stage of affiliation, family intervention is often extremely helpful.

The psychiatrist's primary role at this very early point is to support the family in their approach to the "identified" patient. Intervention at an early stage is often particularly effective because many cult organizations operate through a wide variety of front organizations—for example, the Collegiate Association for the Research of Principles is actually the collegiate affiliate of the Unification Church—and if the family can approach the "identified patient" in a calm, nonjudgmental manner they can provide the prospective cult member with information which enables them to consider the realistic implications of the step they are about to undertake. However, psychiatric consultation should not be simply an educational process in which the psychiatrist informs the family of the pathologic nature of the "cult group." During these initial consultations, despite the fact that they are being conducted at a remove, the psychiatrist attempts to assess the ego strengths and deficits of the individual who is the object of concern.

In developing this assessment, the psychiatrist examines the context in which the individual's cult affiliation has occurred. A history of recent losses and disappointments, or a history of impending transitions, separations and departures is significant. Likewise, a family genogram of religious and political enthusiasm may point to a familial pattern of communication around areas of political or religious concern (5). In longitudinal terms, a past history of intense spiritual questioning or short-lived enthusiasm is of particular interest. The families of cult members often scrutinize the cult member's past life for evidence of previously ignored eccentric belief or exotic religious interests. Many cult members do, in fact, present with a past history of spiritual, religious, or mystical concerns. A significant number of cult members are "seekers" with a history of multiple or serial affiliations (6). However, this past history may be easily exaggerated in importance, because of concerns over separation and individuation (7). However, the psychiatrist can be of immediate assistance to the concerned family by forestalling the splitting and mutual recrimination—the massive burden of self-condemnation that many families feel because they did not intervene at an earlier time.

In the initial contacts with the family of the cult member, the psychiatrist attempts to assess both the ego strengths and deficits of the "identified patient." The psychiatrist also considers the family's strengths and weaknesses, and the pattern of communication within the total familial context. Cult members usually experience severe depression during the period prior to affiliation. The act of cult affiliation is, above all else, an attempt to deal with the intense depression whose source lies in the cult member's difficulty in separating from the original family and attempting to forge a more individuated persona during the transition to adulthood. Indeed, in the act of affiliation, the cult member joins a new community and acquires a new support system which will presumably enable him to deal with the process of separation. (Many cult groups recognize this and refer to themselves as The Family, and so on.) Indeed, cult members appear to have relatively limited resources to deal with the normal if traumatic process of separation, and their sense of depression often appears to have been unusually severe. Their paucity of internal resources may reflect a familial pattern of enmeshment which has given the cult member the message that separation poses an unendurable threat to his survival. During this early stage of consultation, the psychiatrist must differentiate between the family's expression of a concern which is appropriate, as opposed to their need to perpetuate a pattern of enmeshment. When confronted by a histrionic, demanding family in crisis, this may be an exceedingly difficult task.

The assessment of the individual's strengths and weaknesses is often very difficult because the family may have seen the individual cult member as being less capable of functioning autonomously than their other children. The parental assessment may represent a perpetuation of a preexisting pathologic pattern of enmeshment and infantilization. However, the family's assessment may have been astute and their concern may be well placed. Thus, during the initial phase of consultation, the psychiatrist may help family members clarify the intense feelings about the cult member that they bring to the consultation, particularly the extent to which their assessment of the cult member's strengths and weaknesses reflects their own ambivalence toward the cult member.

Families may respond with relief at their child's having joined a group which offers a sense of direction and a place where their child can deposit his or her intense dependency needs. The psychiatrist must respond on a nonjudgmental basis to the father whose initial response to his daughter's joining a group was, "Well, at least there won't be any more frantic 2 A.M. phone calls." Likewise, he must appreciate the sense of hopelessness that pervaded the family who welcomed the support their son initially appeared to receive from his group (particularly as their own sense of futility mounted with their son's being fired from yet another of many positions). But the families' initial acceptance turns to fury as they begin to appreciate the full implications of cult affiliation (particularly as the cult's financial demands intensify). During the initial consultation, they may express to the psychiatrist all their fury at the group's betrayal of their trust.

Many families regard group affiliation as a plausible if eccentric means of obtaining support. (The parents matured, themselves, during the 1960s.) However, as they see their children becoming totally enmeshed within the cultic environment, their anger intensifies, along with their sense of their basic trust having been violated.

The family of the cult member often experiences cult affiliation as a rejection of their value system as well as of their religious or ethnic identity. Their sense of narcissistic injury may be particularly profound when the parents, themselves, have made sacrifices in the service of preserving that identity, for example, if the family are Holocaust survivors. But it is the totality of the lifestyle changes—for example, altering educational goals and severing ties with family members—that provoke concern and an appropriate, understandable consternation. Likewise, the rapidity of change and the family's sense that the change occurred (or at the very least was accelerated) under dubious and deceptive auspices elicits parental interest in providing the child with a setting in which these changes can be examined at leisure and with objectivity. In this context, we can appreciate the profound dilemma of the family of the young woman who went to Stanford University to study communications, but who joined instead upon arrival a fundamentalist group that attributes to its prayers the prevention of a collision between the earth and Halley's comet. They were further taken aback by the fact that the group's leader is a former prostitute with no formal religious credentials. But they were particularly conflicted because of their feelings that their child was exceedingly needy. This family's dilemma arose out of their sense that the "identified patient" had significant pre-existing pathology and their fear of further decompensation should their child exit from the group. Thus, the family's sense that the "identified patient" has significant preexisting psychopathology may exacerbate the difficulties inherent in the psychiatrist's task of working with a family and of helping them to achieve a consensus over what action, if any, should be undertaken.

Whatever action is taken should unite rather than divide the family. A wide variety of approaches are available. The family's choices are not limited to involuntary deprogramming (a costly and exceedingly problematic venture) or passive acquiescence. Yet, whatever action is undertaken should be the product of a familial consensus and not subject to mutual recrimination. The families of cult members have been described as overinvested in their children and showing a lack of flexibility in problem-solving (8). However, enmeshment and rigidity are not universally characteristic of either families or individual family members. Indeed, many families appear to respect the individual's boundaries even when such a course clearly pushes beyond the limits of prudence, as the case of Frederick E. illustrates.

> Frederick E. was the middle child of a wealthy German-Jewish family. His family identified themselves as Jews primarily through their active participation in a wide variety of philanthropic activities. His family entrusted him with the management of his substantial estate at a very youthful age. Frederick pursued a wide variety of personal options. He sought the guidance and direction of older women. Eventually he married a woman some years his senior. She was employed in the media. During his wife's absence on an assignment, he met members of an authoritarian fundamentalistic, cultlike organization headed by a female "prophet." Initially, his wife and family did not object to his involvement in the group's activities. They sought psychiatric consultation after Frederick had taken steps to give the group leader control over his entire fortune and she began to openly interfere in his marriage.

In their initial consultation, Frederick's family were extremely troubled by their son's plans. As the psychiatrist suggested a variety of therapeutic and legal avenues available to them, he realized that in his urging this family to take a consistent position with their son, he was urging them to act contrary to the past history of their interaction. They were very concerned that they were able to decide, in conjunction with her, to confront Frederick about his actions. They met with Frederick in a series of meetings, chaired by a former member of Frederick's group. As a result of this voluntary, noncoercive process, Frederick reevaluated his emotional and financial commitments. He is currently engaged in a tedious legal proceeding to recover his "gifts." During the course of consultation the psychiatrist enabled the family to explore their fear that Frederick might be totally alienated from them if they even questioned his activity (and his wife's fear that if she joined with his family in confronting him that he might divorce her in favor of the cult leader).

Cult affiliation frequently occurs at a time of crisis, transition, or loss of significant object. Frederick E. felt quite overwhelmed by his wife's absence, particularly as it placed the entire burden of rearing their children on his shoulders. In other cases, the family of the cult member has suffered a significant reversal, for example, the severe or crippling illness of a parent, decreased financial security, or business reversal. Or the loss of emotional security may result from the individual's having left home for college or having left college for graduate school. In general, the prospective cult member appears to be less capable of dealing with this loss of accessibility to significant family members than other youth. For the prospective cult member, these periods of separation create an intense depression which leads them on a fervid search for a new support system. Parenthetically, it must be noted that colleges and graduate schools themselves have become settings for greater anomie because of increased student population, their neglecting to create physical structures like quadrangles which foster a sense of community, and decreased participation of students in fraternal organizations. Morever, exaggerated familial expectations may direct a vulnerable youth toward competitive and relatively impersonal universities which do not suit the particular individual's need for support. Thus, it is not surprising that groups that appear to promise the missing support and extol a simpler world of faith appeal to students caught in the throes of their resentment toward a family who urged them toward a place that is currently creating their anxiety. Cult groups appeal because they offer a return to the simplicities of the grandparental generation, in attitude, if not in specific religious doctrine. (Note, however, the increasing vigor of traditional religious groups within both Jewish and Christian religious communities.)

During the initial consultation the family's expectations confer an exaggerated power on the psychiatrist. The psychiatrist is transformed into an individual capable of raising the dead or resurrecting the moribund—and restoring their child. The family of the cult member is often disappointed when the psychiatrist is not a deprogrammer cautioning them about using the "magic bullet," or emphasizes in a noncharismatic manner the importance of maintaining communication with the cult member. The question of communication with the new cult member is of primary importance. While some cultlike groups do restrict with considerable effectiveness any contact between the new cult member and the family of origin, most new members do have the opportunity to maintain contact with their family. This contact often has a routinized, rotelike quality to it (and is frequently related to demands for financial assistance). Nonetheless, when contact is possible, the psychiatrist can be extremely helpful to the family in supporting their efforts to maintain an open, nonjudgmental, nondefensive, and positive mode of interaction (some families have previously interacted primarily around difficulties). The psychiatrist should encourage the family to meet with cult members to discuss their recent differences. This can be extremely helpful in clarifying issues. In a surprising number of cases, the cult member may then be willing to meet with mental health professionals either in psychiatric consultation or in an outpatient setting such as the Cult Hotline and Clinic of the Jewish Board of Family and Children's Services of New York City.

During the contact with the cult member and the family of the cult member, of great importance are the psychiatrist's calm and reasoned emphasis that the family's concerns are not simply a product of their desire to prevent the cult member from exploring new religious systems but are the product of their concern over the epiphenomena of cult life, for example, exploitative working conditions and the context in which a profound and novel commitment was made. During these sessions, the psychiatrist does not assume the mantle of "deprogrammer." Rather, he remains a mental health professional whose role is limited to helping the cult member appreciate the context (emotional, social, and cultural) in which the commitment was made. While the psychiatrist may share the family's skepticism about the cult member's new vocation (and the psychiatrist's actions may indeed encourage the cult member to reconsider the decision), the psychiatrist may significantly help improve the individual's social and vocational functioning even though the individual's personal faith remains essentially unchanged.

Psychiatric Consultation During the Later Phases

The families of cult members share a pervasive fear that their child's new religious affiliation will sever all contact. While many cultlike groups are quite absorbing in their demands, and individual cult members often become quite preoccupied with their "mission," a total preoccupation is by no means universal. Even in groups that are pervasive in their demands, the individual often retains considerable latitude for contact with the family. Contact may be shadowed by cultic rhetoric, ideology, and ritual. Nonetheless, families often can maintain a reasonable relationship with their children if they receive psychiatric support which enables them to deal with their children in a nonprovocative manner and to avoid responding to their children's often provocative behavior in kind. But eliminating contact may be used by the cult member as a threat in interactions with the family. The cult member may blackmail the family to give him or the cult money and to stop confronting him or her about any aspect of his behavior. The existence of this sword of Damocles often pervades the contact between the cult member and the family and may limit any real relatedness in interactions. The psychiatrist does serve to help the family to confront this controlling behavior. The threat of severance is almost always manipulative in character, and is rarely carried out in practice.

A factor creating additional parental anxiety which may shadow the relationship with the cult member is the parents' fear that the "contagion" of cult affiliation will afflict their other children. This is not wholly groundless. There are families in which the cult member has induced his or her siblings to join the cult group. This is rare. Indeed, the contact between the cult member and his or her siblings is often very productive and may be extremely helpful in maintaining his relationship with the noncult world, as the following case illustrates.

> Quincy T., a 26-year-old man, was an almost identical twin. However, he had always been in his brother's shadow (actually, he was two inches shorter than his brother!). His career as an actor had been faltering and despite his significant talents, he did not meet with significant recognition. Eventually, he was recruited by an Eastern-style group which emphasized that a number of its members were celebrities in show business. In rapid succession, Quincy stopped auditioning for roles and began to spend his time chanting a mantra over and over again in front of a scroll which he placed in an altar on his wall. He withdrew socially. He continued to share an apartment with his brother and, at times, shared with his brother his doubts about his new commitment. Nonetheless his commitment to the group intensified. The group contacted him on a very frequent basis to ensure his adherence, and finally his brother and the rest of the family became extremely concerned over his change in religious orientation. His family sought and was seen in psychiatric consultation over his impending departure to the group's residence.

Quincy's father was unable to attend either consultation. During the consultation, Quincy's brother, Quentin, was the family spokesman. He described his brother as having had a long-term history of excessive, sudden enthusiasm for individuals and causes. Quincy's cult affiliation had occurred in the aftermath of the breakup of a relationship with a woman friend. His relationship with his parents had always been very problematic (his father was usually absent and his mother had focused her energies on his brother). Yet, he was able to share with his brother his feeling of having reached an impasse in his career and his hope that the cult group might offer a way out of his career failure and his social isolation. Quentin responded with alacrity to the psychiatrist's observation that his brother was in a crisis. He was able to work with the other family members to help them provide Quincy with a supportive, accessible network. Within a week, Quincy reconsidered his decision to live with the group and had ended his contact with it. Quincy's history of sudden enthusiasms and disengagements was suggestive of borderline personality disorder. He seemed unable to tolerate either separation or isolation. Further psychiatric consultation was suggested, but efforts to involve Quincy in any therapeutic process were unavailing. Soon thereafter, the family discontinued contact.

Quincy's case illustrates the role that a sibling may play in helping the cult member reconsider his commitment. It also illustrates a number of other aspects of working with cult members and their families. Quincy was clearly the "identified patient" within the family. Both his parents and siblings had considered him to be the vulnerable child. Despite his past history of career failure and personal indecisiveness, neither he nor his family considered his difficulties to be sufficiently great to warrant any psychiatric consultation except around the limited issue of cult affiliation. When the emergency presented by his cult affiliation arose, their response was to place almost exclusive responsibility for his behavior at the door of the cult, even while superficially acknowledging that Quincy did have "problems." The refusal to follow through with treatment plans conforms to a pattern of reliance upon "deprogramming" [noted elsewhere (2, 4)]. Fortunately, "deprogrammers," many of whom are being replaced by exit counselors, have received formal training as mental health professionals. For example, many are certified social workers, so that the gap in perspective between the psychiatrist and the informal exit counseling network is decreasing. Psychiatrists, as a matter of principle, should not participate in any involuntary action directed toward changing a person's religious or political orientation when it is conducted under coercive circumstances.

Similar issues arose in the case of Kevin C., which illustrates other aspects of the interface between the family of the cult member and the individual's psychopathology.

> Kevin C. was referred for psychiatric evaluation and consultation from the inpatient service of a community hospital. Kevin's adolescence had been tumultuous. A period of intense drug use had ended when he discovered Jesus. At age 16, he left his home to participate in the fund-raising campaigns of an eccentric fundamentalist group. He remained with them for the next 10 years. He did not return to attend his father's funeral. Eventually, his behavior became so disorganized that the group considered him to be a liability. They sent him home with a plane ticket and five dollars. On his return home, he was extremely disorganized, grandiose, and was having auditory hallucinations. The diagnosis of bipolar disorder, manic phase was made. Kevin was placed on lithium and halperidol. He responded well, remained in his home and was able to work for about a year. During this time, he remained in contact with a similar group and spent all his free time distributing literature with this group. However, after a year he became increasingly disorganized and left in company of his friends on a "mission to Mexico." His behavior became increasingly bizarre and he was again returned home in a state of extreme agitation and required rehospitalization.

When Kevin was first seen in outpatient consultation, he was extremely suspicious and expressed fear of his being "deprogrammed." He had periods of absences although he denied having auditory hallucinations. Since his group had excommunicated him after his second psychotic episode, he recognized (unhappily) that his future lay with his family. He had been placed on halperidol during his second hospitalization, and on this medication he began to reintegrate. After discharge from the hospital, however, Kevin remained preoccupied with his having been placed on psychotropic medication. He gradually became totally resistant to using any psychotropic medication. He discontinued it against medical advice. He did continue episodically in psychiatric consultation. At last report, he had started to work at an entry-level position. Kevin's family was seen in consultation throughout this period. They recognized that Kevin was a severely dysfunctional young man. Yet, they continued to see his difficulties as primarily cult induced, wondering if a "deprogrammer" might not solve his difficulties!

Kevin's history illustrates the problems in working with the family and with an individual who has had a prolonged period of cult affiliation. Kevin's rehabilitation was exceedingly problematic because during the period of cult affiliation he had not developed the academic, vocational, or social skills which would normally be present in a middle-class youth of his age. He could obtain only menial, entry-level positions which were hardly consistent with the grandiose self-image perpetuated by the cult's description of itself as an elite organizing a "new world." Nor was this reality consistent with his parents' previous grandiose expectations. The paucity of vocational and social opportunities open to Kevin made his rejoining the group have a certain momentary plausibility (the destructive nature of the group and its callous disregard for Kevin did not make this a serious possibility). Yet, despite the difficulties inherent in Kevin's case, consultation with his family and a supportive reality-oriented approach was able to provide sufficient support to enable Kevin to move toward the noncult world.

While many cult members lose academic or vocational skills during the period of cult affiliation, this is not inevitable. Parents may even need psychiatric consultation because of difficulties that arise when a child receives advancement within the cult group because this may require increased commitment. Relatively few long-term members leave but some do "burn out" and like many others who are not cult members begin to reassess during their late thirties the idealistic commitments of their youth. Parents and siblings can be of considerable assistance to them if this period of reassessment occurs, as the following case illustrates.

> Norman G. started psychotherapy in 1975 with a psychoanalyst at a recognized credentialed psychoanalytic institute. His psychoanalyst was an extremely charismatic figure, whose grandiosity eventually led him to form his own "institute." Norman followed his psychoanalyst into this new institute. The "institute" became an increasingly incestuous setting in which psychoanalysts and psychoanalysands developed social and professional relationships in which all professional and social boundaries were blurred. The group's ideology

emphasized the destructive nature of the biologic family. Eventually, Norman moved into the group's communal apartments and totally severed all his ties with his family. He did not contact his family for nine years. In 1985, Norman met and married a fellow group member. They had a child. Norman became an appropriately involved and doting parent. His wife's "analyst" then told her that the child was becoming too "focused" on Norman, that is, that his close relationship with the child would "destroy" the child. Norman was peremptorily barred from any contact with his child. The "analyst's" arbitrary dictate precipitated within Norman a period of intense soul-searching. Norman's entire personal life centered around the group. He had virtually no savings because all of his substantial income had been donated to the group or been used to pay for "psychoanalysis." Nonetheless, Norman was able to discover the strength within himself to reestablish himself as an autonomous adult. He contacted his family and with their support was able to resume a non-group-centered social and professional life. Eventually with his family's support, he pursued appropriate legal action to obtain joint custody and has been able to play a significant role in his child's life.

Norman's history illustrates that beneath the facade of cultic rhetoric, the individual remains and evolves even if that evolution may not be superficially apparent. The family of the long-term cult member frequently disengage from the cult member. However, the psychiatrist can still play a significant role in enabling them to remain accessible even if superficially detached. This accessibility can foster the process of reconciliation when the opportunity arises.

As Norman's case illustrates, with long-term cult affiliation, other issues arise. Cult members have children. Questions of child abuse and the adequacy of child care may arise, particularly when the cult member adheres to a group which adopts a punitive and destructive disciplinary regimen. As has been noted elsewhere (3, 9), the resolution of the issues of custody, custodial arrangements, child neglect and abuse, and grandparenting rights are extraordinarily complex. Psychiatrists may be consulted either by concerned grandparents or by parents who are former cult members. While child abuse or neglect is not always present when a child is raised within a cult, it should be noted at the very least that children may be relegated to a very secondary position in the cult's agenda for world renewal. Given the cult's messianic pretensions, parents are often absent for extended missions and children may be raised with minimal contact with biologic parents. Childcare may be considered a low-status activity within the group. The group itself may have extremely idiosyncratic ideas about education. Within the I.S.K.O.N. (Hare Krishna) girls are considered intellectually inferior to boys and given only a minimal education. In other groups, church schools provide an extremely limited or eccentric curriculum which does not equip children for life outside the group. In still other groups, children routinely arise at 4 A.M. for three hours of meditation. Or, children may be denied minimal medical care and parents are advised to substitute prayer or "holistic" approaches for legitimate medical care. Noncult members are appropriately concerned about the implications of these practices.

The parent who has left the group is regarded as a traitor for having betrayed the group's "sacred" mission so that the parent's concern for a child's physical well-being is doubly suspect. Moreover, the group may support the parent who remains within it in any efforts to evade usual custodial or visitation arrangements. Thus, the normal complexities and acrimony of divorce may be exacerbated by the cult member's sense that he or she has a sacred mission to evade court jurisdiction in order to ensure that the children are given a proper "orientation." Unfortunately, the courts may not be aware of the cult's arrogant attitude and willingness to evade the judicial process. The courts may award joint custody without being aware of how unrealistic this decision may prove to be when one parent remains an active member of a cult. Psychiatrists who participate as experts for the court in custody proceedings should carefully evaluate the realistic potential for the parties to form a workable custodial relationship when one parent remains an active cult member.

Cults encourage their members to make major and frequently excessive financial commitments to the cult group. These demands may create conflict between parents and children. The family of the cult member may seek psychiatric consultation because of their ambivalence at leaving monies to their children or making other testamentary dispositions, particularly when they are reasonably certain that their child may donate the estate to a cult. Or, parents may seek psychiatric consultation when it appears that a child is stripping himself or herself of financial assets through unwise loans to a cult-sponsored organization even if the money is not formally donated. Parents may initially seek consultation in order to improve their communication with the cult member to avert impending damage. Or, they may be referred by an attorney who recognizes that the courts have recognized that cult members, because they are subject to coercive group pressure, may make loans that reflect a vulnerability to this species of pressure, and in exceptional cases have been willing to establish conservatorships in order to protect the vulnerable individual. When psychiatrists are involved in this legal process, their role extends beyond that of simply being an expert witness at court. Parents who participate in these legal proceedings usually do so only with the greatest reluctance. The possibility of establishing a conservatorship is problematic. The adversarial nature of the court proceeding may damage whatever relationship between family members that remains. Thus, while the psychiatrist may be called upon to act primarily as an expert in formal court proceedings, his or her actual role extends to providing support to a family in anguish over having to pursue so formidable a proceeding in the service of protecting a child from behavior that is as obstinate as it is self-destructive.

Summary

The psychiatrist's role in working with the families of cult members is extremely complex. In the protophase or in the very early stages of cult affiliation, the psychiatrist's support and guidance may enable the family to mobilize itself. At this stage, the family's efforts to maintain an open, nonjudgmental channel of communication with the cult member may be sufficient to enable the cult member to reconsider his or her affiliation. At later stages, the psychiatrist's support may allow the family to maintain the semblance of a reasonable relationship with their children. The family's accessibility may foster the process of maturation which will ultimately allow the member to reconsider his or her affiliation or to establish a relatively nonexploitive relationship with the group. However, the cult member may act in an inappropriate and self-destructive manner by allowing his or her children to be harshly and inappropriately disciplined, or denied appropriate medical care or otherwise abused and neglected. In these situations, the psychiatrist functions both as a support to those family members who seek to provide appropriate care and in the role of an expert witness to any court proceedings. In other instances, families may seek psychiatric consultation to prevent a cult member from dissipating their assets and to establish a conservatorship. Even when acting as an expert witness in an adversarial proceeding, psychiatrists should recognize their responsibility in fostering any potential for reconciliation.

References

1. West LJ, Singer MT: Cults, quacks and nonprofessional psychotherapies, in Comprehensive Textbook of Psychiatry III. Edited by Kaplan H, Freedman A, Sadock B. Baltimore, Williams & Wilkins, 1980
2. Halperin DA: Self-help groups for parents of cult members: agenda, issues and the role of the group leader, in Psychodynamic Perspectives on Religion, Sect and Cult. Edited by Halperin DA. Littleton, MA, John Wright-PSG, 1983
3. Rudin M: Women, elderly and children in religious cults. Cultic Studies Journal 1:8–27, 1984
4. Maleson FG: Dilemmas in evaluation and management of religious cultists. Am J Psychiatry 136:925–929, 1981
5. Halperin DA: Psychiatric consultation and supervision in the treatment of cult members, in Psychodynamic Perspectives on Religion, Sect and Cult. Edited by Halperin DA. Littleton, MA, John Wright—PSG, 1983
6. Galanter M, Rabkin R, Rabkin J, et al: The "Moonies"—a psychological study of conversion and membership in a contemporary religious sect. Am J Psychiatry 136:165–170, 1979
7. Blos P: The generation gap, in The Adolescent Passage. New York, International Universities Press, 1976
8. Markowitz A: The role of family therapy in the treatment of symptoms associated with cult affiliation, in Psychodynamic Perspectives on Religion, Sect and Cult. Edited by Halperin DA. Littleton, MA, John Wright-PSG, 1983
9. Halperin DA: Psychiatric approaches to cults: therapeutic and legal parameters, in Emerging Issues in Child Psychiatry and the Law. Edited by Schetky DH, Benedek EP. New York, Brunner-Mazel, 1985

Chapter 8

PSYCHOTHERAPEUTIC IMPLICATIONS OF NEW RELIGIOUS AFFILIATION

Brock K. Kilbourne, Ph.D.

In any discussion of new religions, the question of the normality of new religious preference is almost inevitably raised. This is most apparent in the psychiatric literature. Psychiatric researchers and practitioners alike debate the adherent's motivations and the consequences of new religious affiliation to the individual. Usually this takes the form of either a pathologic or nonpathologic perspective. The pathologic perspective contends that new religious adherents indicate some psychiatric condition prior to joining the group or are psychiatrically impaired by their experiences in the group. The nonpathologic perspective, on the other hand, contends that new religions attract members from the ranks of the middle class and any occurrence of psychopathology is generally no greater than in other groups in contemporary American society. A third perspective, however, has emerged in recent years. That view focuses on the psychotherapeutic effects sometimes associated with new religious affiliation.

Interestingly, and little appreciated, each of the three perspectives probably holds some grain of truth depending upon the individual, his or her life circumstances, and the particular new religion. A tremendous diversity exists in the members, goals,

The author thanks Janet Dileonardo for her helpful comments and suggestions.

beliefs, values, indoctrination procedures, support methods, developmental stages, and structure of such groups (1, 2).

The purpose of this chapter is to offer a body of evidence which indicates that psychotherapeutic effects are sometimes associated with new religious affiliation. This report attempts to explain these effects as well as to provide a cogent explanation of "why" these effects have not been appreciated by psychologists and psychiatrists.

Psychotherapeutic Effects in New Religions

Over the years, researchers of different perspectives have collected evidence indicating the integrative role of new religious affiliation. Studies indicating psychological and social integration resulting from religious experiences are not uncommon, and frequently focus on the adherent's enhanced sense of self, improved familial relationships, or new community involvements. Robbins and Anthony (3) have perhaps best summarized the psychotherapeutic effects of new religious or quasireligious affiliation. They are 1) termination of illicit drug use, 2) renewed vocational motivation, 3) mitigation of neurotic distress, 4) suicide prevention, 5) decrease in anomie and moral confusion, 6) increase in social compassion or social responsibility, 7) self-actualization, 8) decrease in psychosomatic symptoms, 9) clarification of ego identity, and 10) general positive therapeutic and problem-solving assistance. More recently, Kilbourne and Richardson (4) have compared psychotherapy and new religions and have examined the research indicating psychotherapeutic effects associated with new religious affiliation. Some of the more pertinent studies discussed by Kilbourne and Richardson are presented below.

Galanter and Buckley (5) used data from a random sample of 119 "premies" attending a national Divine Light Mission (DLM) festival. Participants were asked to fill out a 170-item questionnaire, which included questions about group functions, psychiatric symptoms, drug use, and meditation. The DLM members were typically white, single, in their twenties, and, on the average, had been members for about two years. They also indicated a high incidence of prior drug use. Members displayed a "strong sense of cohesiveness and communal sharing" (p. 687) and expressed strong feelings of trust toward each other. Adherents' transcendental experiences predicted symptomatic relief and, in general, membership in the DLM facilitated both psychological and social integration. Galanter and Buckley concluded the following in relation to their findings:

> The diversity of specific psychological symptoms alleviated here is notable. A decline was reported in symptoms affected by behavioral norms, such as drug taking and job trouble; it was also found in subjectively experienced symptoms, such as anxiety, not readily regulated. (p. 690)

Another study by Galanter et al. (6) provides an excellent example of how new religious affiliation facilitates psychological and social integration. In a study of the Unification Church (UC), which compared a sample of 237 members to a comparison group of 305 people, Galanter and associates found a marked incidence of prior drug use among members, a factor related to high neurotic distress scores for the period prior to joining the group. Of those sampled, 25 percent reported serious drug problems before joining, 30 percent had required professional care, and 6% had been hospitalized. These findings suggested that the population from which the members were drawn had a higher likelihood of psychiatric illness than the general population. Galanter et al. (6) concluded the following:

> Affiliation with the Unification Church apparently provided considerable and sustained relief from neurotic distress. Although improvement was ubiquitous, a greater religious commitment was reported by those who indicated the most improvement. (p. 168)

A study by another psychiatrist (7) presents additional evidence of integration effects from a sample of Harvard and Radcliffe students who did not belong to a "cult," but who were apparently normal college students who had recently experienced conversion to a biblical faith and who had participated in a campus group involved in Bible studies. Nicholi gave these young people (17 in all) intensive interviews covering a number of subjects. They minimized their parents' influence over their spiritual interests and emphasized that peers had interested them in religion. These students had also used drugs, although not to the extent previously described for the DLM or the UC. The subjects seemed interested in filling a spiritual void left by little religious instruction at all during their early years. They expressed concern in the area of personal and sexual relations, and they suffered from what Nicholi called "existential despair." After joining the Bible study group the subjects stopped using drugs, cigarettes, and alcohol. They generally expressed higher self-esteem and a greater concern for others. Their relationships were improved, including those with their parents. Chastity became the rule for sexual matters, "general affect" was positive, performance at studies was higher, and the students expressed less fear of death. Also, a number of them made career plan changes involving a move into the helping professions. Nicholi summarized his findings by saying that conversion resulted in "a marked improvement in ego functioning" (p. 400).

Similar findings for one of the largest Jesus Movement groups have been reported by Richardson et al. (8). In this study, heavy involvement with drug use, alcohol, and tobacco and various deviant behavior patterns was overcome in large part through participation in this nationwide communal organization. Social integration was also evident as a result of participation because many youths otherwise estranged from society were taught useful occupational skills while in the group.

Mauss and Petersen (9), in an article that characterized participants in the Jesus Movement as "prodigals," have argued that the major function of the movement on the individual level was to provide a "way station to respectability" for a cohort or generation of stigmatized youth. Although the style of life of such youths often remained considerably different from that of conventional society, the youths' values and behaviors generally shifted toward those of the dominant society. Of particular importance was the sizable proportion of movement members who returned to their families after and in part as a result of participation in the movement. Others returned to school, took jobs in normal society, and engaged in traditional forms of family life and sexual expression. Thus, Mauss and Peterson concluded that the major effect of the Jesus Movement may have been to socialize participants in the dominant values of society and to ultimately convert youngsters from lives of crime, sex, and drug use.

Downton's in-depth study (10) of some members of the DLM

leads one to similar conclusions about the functions of participation. He says:

> There is little doubt in my mind that these premies have changed in a positive way. Today they seem less alienated, aimless, worried, afraid, and more peaceful, loving, confident, and appreciative of life. We could attribute those changes to surrender, devotion, and their involvement in premie community. Each of these undoubtedly had a positive impact, but, if we accept what premies say, none were as critical as their experience of [meditation]. . . . They report having more positive attitudes about themselves. (p. 210)

Ironically, even in those studies attempting to demonstrate the psychopathologic effects of new religious affiliation, a contrary pattern of psychotherapeutic benefits has sometimes been uncovered. Kilbourne's analysis and reanalysis (11) of the Conway and Siegelman study of five major cults—Unification Church, Hare Krishna, Scientology, Divine Light, and The Way—makes this point. Using two computer programs (i.e., SAS and SPSS) and exact statistical tests, Kilbourne demonstrated that there was no support for the Conway and Siegelman "information disease" hypothesis and found, instead, a pattern of results suggesting positive and therapeutic effects. Kilbourne found: 1) a negative correlation between "average hours per day in ritual process" and "hallucinations and delusions," 2) a negative correlation between "total hours per week in ritual and indoctrination" and "hallucinations and delusions," and 3) a negative correlation between "hallucinations and delusions" and "inability to break mental rhythms of chanting." While these data clearly leave much to be desired, they still remain consistent with other studies indicating psychotherapeutic effects of new religious affiliation.

Explanation of Psychotherapeutic Effects

Two explanations have emerged concerning the psychotherapeutic effects sometimes associated with new religious affiliation. Not too surprisingly, these two explanations—"underlying deep structure" and "the relief effect"—tend to rely on psychological concepts and principles. They are, moreover, complementary rather than competing explanations which differ in focus. The "underlying deep structure" (4) hypothesis is a largely structural explanation and concerns itself with the common structure of healing relationships in general, although an implicit mechanism is assumed. The "relief effect" (12) hypothesis, on the other hand, focuses on the intraindividual processes that are presumably related to psychological well-being and the reduction of distress. Taken together, both hypotheses offer a plausible explanation of the psychotherapeutic effects sometimes associated with new religious affiliation.

According to the "underlying deep structure" hypothesis, the effectiveness of both psychotherapy and religious conversion depends on a common structure by which the therapist or religious group counteracts the individual's sense of demoralization (13). That structure is indicated by the following: 1) a special supportive, empathic, and confiding relationship between the client and therapist or religious adherent and the religious group; 2) a special setting imbued with powerful symbols of expertise, help, hope, and healing; 3) a special rationale, ideology, or indisputable myth that explains normality and abnormality and renders sensible the individual's self-preoccupations and inexplicable feelings; and 4) a special set of rituals and practices that confirms the individual's assumptive world.

Successful treatments and successful conversions function, then, to counteract debilitating feelings of demoralization with positive expectations of hope, help, healing, and feelings of self-mastery. Corrective experiences and direct feedback in therapy or religious settings (14) (e.g., new learning experiences, successful outcomes, self-monitoring, and positive self-attributions, and so on) come to be associated with a general increase in psychological well-being.

Galanter's 1980 study (15) of the large-group-induction techniques used by the Unification Church provides a good example of these common structural elements in many new religious settings. In his examination of three workshop periods, Galanter found support for 1) *a special relationship between the novitiate and the religious group*—a strong sense of cohesiveness developed during the workshops, especially in the close relationship between the novitiate and the group (e.g., constant supervision, group discussions, shared reflections and insights); 2) *a special setting*—the workshop center was located in a secluded, rustic setting and was imbued with powerful symbols of hope, healing, and spiritual growth; 3) *a special rationale*—the novitiate was encouraged to learn the group's creed and religious beliefs, which were offered to explain past, present, and future experiences; and 4) *a special set of rituals*—the workshops were structured around a number of activities (e.g., lectures, group discussion, recreational activities, and meditation/reflection periods) that confirmed the group's world view and indicated the way an individual should go about converting himself or herself.

At present, support for the above line of theorizing is largely indirect. It seems to be a plausible account of what happens in psychotherapy and new religious conversion. The paradox of nonequivalent psychotherapy content and equivalent psychotherapy outcomes, for example, has led some researchers (16) to give psychotherapists the "dodo bird" verdict (one form of psychotherapy is as good as the next and, therefore, all deserve prizes). The same can be said of some new religious and quasi-religious groups as well, given a growing body of evidence of the same common structural elements and nonspecific effects (4). Indeed, similar effects have been demonstrated with individuals from different backgrounds (7), in a variety of different religious groups and movements (17), just by attending a series of religious seminars (18), and even in one of the more totalistic communal groups (6).

Alternatively, the "relief effect" hypothesis (12) emerged from studies that indicated that the perceived life disruption of some new religious adherents was relieved by their affiliation with the group. Generally, the relief from distress correlated with the intensity of continued new religious affiliation. Galanter (19) has subsequently proposed several possible processes to account for this phenomenon: 1) *operant conditioning*—closeness and conformity to the group's beliefs and practices leads to the reduction of distress and vulnerability to disruptive life events; 2) *cognitive dissonance or self-perception*—individuals in new religions may become aware of inconsistent thoughts and behaviors, particularly in relation to their sense of self, and reduce such dissonance by increasing their affiliation and attraction to the group. Or, they may believe that they have freely chosen to engage in new religious activities and infer, with the help of the provided religious perspective, that they are a certain kind of person; and 3) *genetic programming* (a sociobiologic perspective)—social affiliation in nonhuman primates and hominids ensures adaptation and species survival. Affiliation based on relief has evolutionary significance because it facilitates group cohesion and cooperation.

Notwithstanding, there are more parsimonious explanations than the "underlying deep structure" and "relief effect" hypotheses to explain psychotherapeutic effects in new religions. Such explanations come from the literature on psychotherapy effectiveness and social psychology. Concerning the former, there is a substantial body of evidence and theorizing on placebo effects and waiting list studies. Gross (20), for example, has summarized some of the research comparing placebo-takers and psychotherapy recipients. Often placebo-takers show positive improvement (even when the patient knows that he is being fooled), and sometimes as much improvement as those receiving psychotherapy. Placebo gains, moreover, have stood up well against minor medications. Gross has further summarized waiting list studies which have demonstrated the spontaneous remissions of individuals waiting to receive psychotherapy. These latter studies suggest that at least some nonpsychotic complaints might be self-limiting, and time, alone, may be a splendid healer.

Ullmann and Krasner (21) have discussed the special characteristics of the placebo administrator. They claim that the healer should be dignified and efficient, provide services in impressive surroundings, and manipulate symbols of healing and ritualistic paraphernalia, some of which might include mysterious charts and long waiting lists. From this perspective, expectations of help, hope, and healing are elicited in any healing relationship, whether or not a placebo pill or a waiting list is provided to the patient.

Similarly, social psychological studies on social comparison processes seem germane in explaining the nonspecific "relief effect" in some new religions. Schacter (22) found, for example, that individuals under stress seek out others with similar stress experiences. Affiliation enables individuals to make social comparisons in order to obtain information from similar others as to how to interpret a stressful situation. Affiliation can also result in assurance and fear reduction, a finding compatible with Galanter's (19) discussion of a nonspecific "relief effect" in some new religions.

Other research by Schacter and Singer (23) on emotion has shown that in unfamiliar or ambiguous situations individuals who experience physiologic arousal are likely to interpret their emotions based on the information cues provided to them by others. Interpreting one's emotions in terms of social comparison might explain why some new religious adherents label their physiologic arousal as elation and bliss, and subsequently report feelings of psychological well-being and relief.

Additionally, social psychological studies on conformity must be considered an important aspect of any explanation of psychotherapeutic effects in new religions. Some of the factors found to influence conformity behavior—ambiguity, low self-confidence and esteem, goal interdependence and reinforcement, social support and high cohesiveness—are readily apparent in some new religious settings (24). But more importantly, the establishment of norms in a group context is a generally powerful means by which to induce conformity behavior (25, 26), whether such behavior is linked to task goals or affective states. For example, some new religions use group norms and social support to regulate behaviors related to psychological well-being. They may also use group norms, explicitly or implicitly, to induce adherents to report psychological well-being to outsiders. Distinguishing between the experience of psychological well-being and the verbal account of psychological well-being in new religions is conceptually analogous to Asch's (27) early distinction between public compliance and private disagreement. Thus, researchers investigating psychotherapeutic effects in new religions need to ascertain whether adherents are reporting therapeutic effects because they actually experience them or because group norms encourage adherents to do so.

In sum, a number of plausible processes can explicate the psychotherapeutic effects sometimes reported in new religions. These are an underlying deep structure, a relief effect, a placebo effect, the self-limiting nature of nonpsychotic reactions, stress-motivated affiliation, the attribution of emotion, and conformity. The specific mechanism or mechanisms have not yet been ascertained.

Why Psychotherapeutic Effects in New Religions Have Not Been Appreciated

Despite the aforementioned body of evidence of psychotherapeutic effects sometimes associated with new religions, many psychologists and psychiatrists remain unaware of these findings. The reasons for this are varied, though in general, they can be attributed to the objective and subjective criteria used by psychologists and psychiatrists to assess the impact of new religious affiliation.

When we think of objective criteria, we are most likely to consider the problems of definition, methodology, and psychiatric diagnosis. For example, psychologists and psychiatrists are often reluctant to consider psychotherapeutic effects of any kind apart from the definition of psychotherapy. Psychotherapy entails "the informed and deliberate application of established psychological principles by trained and experienced specialists. The therapist's knowledge and skills are addressed to specific emotional, attitudinal and behavioral problems of the clients" (28, p. 308). It follows from this definition that psychotherapeutic effects only result when a psychologist or psychiatrist systematically applies psychological principles to specific emotional, attitudinal, and behavioral problems. By definition then, anything short of this does not constitute psychotherapy or psychotherapeutic effects. Nevertheless, some psychologists and psychiatrists are willing to consider salutary effects resulting from alternative healing relationships as analogous to the benefits of psychotherapy (13, 29).

Another objective stumbling block for some psychologists and psychiatrists concerns the methodology employed to ascertain psychotherapeutic effects in new religions. Most of the evidence mustered together in support of psychotherapeutic effects comes from case and field studies of nonrandom samples of new religious adherents or quasi-experimental studies of the same. These studies usually employ impressionistic or correlation assessment techniques and use measures that are global and intuitive rather than standardized and specific.

On the other hand, in recent years psychotherapy researchers have grown accustomed to a particular methodology to assess the effects of psychotherapy (28). While by no means always the case, the recommended method to obtain dependable data on the effects of psychotherapy is to carefully measure the status of patients before and after therapy. Ideally, the progress of a treated group is compared to an untreated control group who are matched on all important characteristics except treatment. Measurements are specified in advance and are objectively recorded before or after an established time period. Some attempts have been made to standardize treatment techniques in order to ensure comparability across different therapists and studies. This experimental approach obviously permits the researcher to make causal statements about the efficacy of psychotherapy in general and different forms of psychotherapy in particular.

Clearly, controlled experimental studies designed to assess psychotherapeutic effects associated with new religious affiliation are absent in the literature. Subsequently, anyone subscribing to this methodology is unlikely to be swayed by the evidence for psychotherapeutic effects in new religions. The basic problem concerns whether or not it would be possible or feasible to implement the simplest controlled experimental design comparing matched individuals among new religious adherents and psychotherapy recipients. And the problems naturally magnify, certainly from an ethical point of view, if we entertain randomly assigning individuals to psychotherapy, a new religion, an established religion, or to a no-treatment control. In short, not all research questions can be addressed by an experimental approach, and the ideal experimental methodology is not likely to be implemented in the study of new religions. Research on new religions will continue to be dominated by case and field studies and quasi-experimental designs that rely on impressionistic and correlational techniques of assessment.

Case studies and quasi-experimental designs limit the researchers' control and ability to make casual statements. Yet they still permit the researcher to ascertain relationships between theoretically relevant variables and to approach the issue of generalization from the standpoint of replication across studies using different subjects, measures, settings and times. We should, therefore, learn to qualify the limitations of our data without losing sight of what can reasonably be said.

The third objective criterion that interferes with an appreciation of psychotherapeutic effects in new religions concerns certain diagnostic disorders in the Diagnostic and Statistical Manual of Mental Disorders, 3rd ed. (DSM-III) and their selective application by some psychologists and psychiatrists. Two diagnostic disorders in the DSM-III—atypical dissociative disorder and post-traumatic stress disorder—have been applied to new religious adherents (30, 31). While the application of these two DSM-III disorders appears to have resulted from the clinical impressions and intuitions of a handful of clinicians, that usage unfortunately preempts, ipso facto, most psychologists and psychiatrists who are unfamiliar with new religions from considering anything other than a psychiatric label. For most, it becomes a simple question of choosing between normality and abnormality, without considering the complexities of life in the group. Diagnostic short-changing occurs and increases the likelihood of misdiagnosis.

The application of these two DSM-III diagnostic disorders to new religious adherents can be criticized on the following grounds: 1) atypical dissociative disorder is vague and incomplete in diagnostic information, lacking in established reliability and validity, confused conceptually with brainwashing and terrorism, and does not specify how new religious affiliation results in dissociated states; and 2) post-traumatic stress disorder was never intended to be used to diagnose new religious adherents, although it is, and, as such, is being used by some to equate new religious adherents with victims of natural and manmade disasters. This usage lacks any empirical support, fails to specify a priori why new religious affiliation is inherently stressful or what the specific stressors are, ignores inconsistencies in new religious experiences and criteria symptoms, fails to separate the multiple influences impacting on adherents, and overlooks the sociological evidence questioning a common disaster syndrome among natural disaster victims (32).

Added to the above, there are several subjective criteria used by psychologists and psychiatrists to assess new religious preference that interfere with an appreciation of psychotherapeutic effects. One of the most striking of these is a general bias or professional ethnocentricity of clinicians. That is, while a recommended methodology has emerged to assess the effects of psychotherapy, most practicing clinicians, nonetheless, express antiempirical, even antiresearch (33), attitudes toward psychotherapy. For example, private practitioners do little research (34), rarely publish (35), are often unwilling to participate in research (36), and generally have a negative attitude toward research and research training (35). Moreover, theoretical orientation tends to bias the appraisal of the methodological adequacy of psychotherapy outcome studies (37), and clinical decision-making is most often influenced by practical experience with clients and advice from colleagues (33). These just-cited findings are by no means less relevant to the investigation of psychotherapeutic effects associated with new religions, especially in relation to certain alleged critiques of research on new religions. Indeed, the antiresearch bias of many practicing clinicians precludes the possibility that they will investigate psychotherapeutic effects associated with new religions or ever be convinced by the research of others.

Another subjective criterion used by psychologists and psychiatrists pertains to their use of group stereotypes, personal biases, and value preferences to assess new religions. Misconceptions about new religions are fairly widespread in contemporary American society and are often perpetuated in the mass media. In this regard, Richardson and Kilbourne (38) have identified the following "cult" stereotype: 1) individuals who join new religions or cults suffer from some prior personal vulnerability, 2) new religions or cults use powerful and sophisticated recruitment techniques to manipulate and exploit their members, and 3) new religions or cult membership results in some kind of personal incapacitation or psychiatric disability. Such negative social labeling, of course, mistakenly equates all new religions or cults and ignores important differences between individuals within the same group. Consequently, there is a tendency for those who operate on such assumptions to think that the expected cult behavior has been confirmed or to perceive only the behavior that was expected. Negative stereotyping and personal biases can cause one to misconstrue contrary evidence as consistent with the cult stereotype as well as to explain how the same cult behavior can be interpreted in diametrically opposed ways. The extreme example, of course, occurs in those instances of cultphobia (39).

Value conflicts over the nature of society, personal freedom and autonomy, human relationships, development, and the family can similarly bias one's perceptions of life in new religions. For example, Kilbourne and Richardson (4) have discussed two levels of conflict between the new religions and the psychotherapies. At one level, there is the specific "guildlike" conflict that exists between the two groups over the competition for clients, conceptual territory, status, wealth, and influence. At still another level, there is the conflict of values and models of reality that each group symbolizes to other individuals and groups in society. New religions and psychotherapies compete on their own behalf and on behalf of other individuals and groups in society (e.g., the family, established religions, the educational system, the state). Competition develops on several levels and is quite vigorous as psychotherapists defend their ascendant role in society against the claims of new religions. In any case, what we should recognize is that stereotypes, personal biases, and values can function as a master criterion and color all other considerations, objective and subjective.

Conclusions

In this chapter I have reviewed some of the research indicating psychotherapeutic effects in new religions. Additionally, the viable explanations of this phenomenon—underlying deep structure, relief effect, placebo effects, self-limiting nature of certain disorders, social comparison and conformity—as well as the objective and subjective criteria used by psychologists and psychiatrists to assess new religions have been discussed. Concerning the latter, problems of definition, methodology, diagnosis, antiresearch attitudes, and value biases have often impeded efforts to ascertain the reliability and validity of psychotherapeutic effects in new religions.

Two implications of the preceding analysis are apparent. The first implication concerns the delivery of psychiatric services. As Galanter (19) has previously suggested, the investigation of psychotherapeutic effects in new religions may facilitate our understanding of the dynamics of large-group therapy and help us to identify those psychiatric problems most likely to respond to such an approach (e.g., alcohol and drug abuse). We might simply call this effective case management. On the other hand, as a comparative strategy, the investigation of new religions might also help psychologists and psychiatrists to better understand the nonspecific effects associated with any healing relationship, in order that a better understanding of the psychotherapeutic process might be achieved.

In this latter regard, a chief purpose of the professions of psychiatry and psychology is to profess (i.e., to claim to have knowledge and skill not shared by other individuals and groups in society). Psychiatrists and psychologists are concerned with the general welfare and have developed a body of scientific knowledge and ethical principles to safeguard the rights of consumers. Both professions have a responsibility, then, to ascertain the mechanisms of self-change in diverse social contexts and to provide that knowledge in their respective professional capacities. In other words, psychiatry and psychology have a scientific and ethical responsibility to understand psychotherapeutic or quasipsychotherapeutic effects in other healing relationships and to apply that understanding when feasible to their own clientele. Our clientele should expect, in turn, services based on the most advanced scientific findings and certain ethical safeguards not afforded to them in other healing relationships.

A second implication of studying psychotherapeutic effects in new religions pertains to psychological assessment. Psychiatrists and psychologists have the responsibility to promote the best interests of the client, regardless of race, creed, sex, level of functioning, or religious preference. This is obviously the case, for example, in the administration, scoring, analysis, and interpretation of test results in a scientific manner. But it is no less true when we consider the sensitivities or insensitivities of the clinician to the value differences between himself or herself and a new religious adherent. In relation to the diagnosis of new religious adherents who come to the attention of the clinician, Kilbourne (2) has specifically recommended the use of objective and standardized testing procedures in conjunction with a case history. Clinicians should make every effort to obtain multiple sources of information (e.g., family, friends, work associates, professional colleagues, and other new religious adherents) in determining a diagnosis of a new religious adherent. They should, moreover, self-consciously seek out evidence at variance with their preconceived ideas and value biases. Seeking consultation from a professional colleague with a different perspective should be actively encouraged.

In summary, it is clear that new religions or cults are complex and controversial, and that no systematic pattern has emerged to date that would permit gross generalizations across all new religions or all new religious adherents. Psychiatrists and psychologists should proceed, therefore, with caution and treat each case on an individual basis. A case-by-case strategy permits the clinician to fully appreciate the complexity of new religious affiliation and to avoid reflexively assigning new religious adherents to gray boxes in the DSM-III without due consideration to all relevant factors. Some people are no doubt hurt by new religions and some people benefit in many ways. Probably most individuals, however, are unaffected one way or the other and simply go their various ways after a short period of social experimentation. It is the responsibility of professional psychiatry and psychology to know the difference, by no means a simple task, and to act in such a way as to ensure the welfare and basic human rights of all members of a pluralistic and democratic society.

References

1. Stark R, Bainbridge WS, Doyle DP: Cults of America: a reconnaissance in space and time. Sociological Analysis 40:347–359, 1979
2. Kilbourne BK: Standardized procedures, psychological norms, and new religious affiliation, in Scientific Research and New Religions: Divergent Perspectives. Edited by Kilbourne BK. San Francisco, Pacific Division, American Association for the Advancement of Science, 1985
3. Robbins T, Anthony D: Deprogramming, brainwashing and the medicalization of deviant religious groups. Social Problems 29:283–297, 1982
4. Kilbourne BK, Richardson JT: Psychotherapy and new religions in a pluralistic society. American Psychol 39:237–251, 1984
5. Galanter M, Buckley P: Evangelical religion and meditation: psychotherapeutic effects. J Nerv Ment Dis 166:685–691, 1978
6. Galanter M, Rabkin R, Rabkin F, et al: The "Moonies": a psychological study of conversion and membership in a contemporary religious sect. Am J Psychiatry 136:165–169, 1979
7. Nicholi AM: A new dimension of the youth culture. Am J Psychiatry 131:396–401, 1974
8. Richardson JT, Stewart M, Simmonds R: Organized Miracles. New Brunswick, NJ, Transaction Books, 1979
9. Mauss A, Petersen D: Les Jesus Freaks et la retour à la respectibilité. Social Compass 21:283–301, 1974
10. Downton JV: Sacred Journeys: The Conversion of Young Americans to Divine Light Mission. New York, Columbia University Press, 1979
11. Kilbourne BK: A reply to Maher and Langone's statistical critique of Kilbourne. Journal for the Scientific Study of Religion 25:116–123, 1986
12. Galanter M: The "relief effect": a sociobiological model for neurotic distress and large-group therapy. Am J Psychiatry 135:588–591, 1978
13. Frank J: Persuasion and Healing: A Comparative Study of Psychotherapy (rev ed). New York, Schocken Books, 1974

14. Goldfried MR: Toward the delineation of therapeutic change principles. Am Psychol 35:991–999, 1980
15. Galanter M: Psychological induction into the large-group: findings from a modern religious sect. Am J Psychiatry 137:1574–1579, 1980
16. Stiles WB, Shapiro DA, Elliot R: "Are all psychotherapies equivalent?" Am Psychol 41:165–180, 1986
17. Ungerleider JT, Wellisch KK: Coercive persuasion (brainwashing), religious cults, and deprogramming. Am J Psychiatry 136:279–282, 1979
18. Lovekin A, Maloney HN: Religious glossolalia: a longitudinal study of personality changes. Journal for the Scientific Study of Religion 16:383–393, 1977
19. Galanter M: New religious movements and large-group psychology, in Scientific Research and New Religions: Divergent Perspectives. Edited by Kilbourne BK. San Francisco, Pacific Division, American Association for the Advancement of Science, 1985
20. Gross ML: The Psychological Society. New York, Random House, 1978
21. Ullmann LP, Krasner L: A Psychological Approach to Abnormal Behavior. Englewood Cliffs, NJ, Prentice-Hall, 1969
22. Schacter S: The Psychology of Affiliation. Stanford, CA, Stanford University Press, 1959
23. Schacter S, Singer JE: Cognitive, social, and physiological determinants of emotional state. Psychol Rev 69:379–399, 1962
24. Raven BH, Ruben JZ: Social Psychology, 2nd ed. New York, John Wiley & Sons, 1983
25. French JRP, Raven BH: The bases of social power, in Studies in Social Power. Edited by Cartwright D. Ann Arbor, Institute for Social Research, University of Michigan, 1959
26. Secord PF, Backman CW: Social Psychology, 2nd ed. New York, McGraw-Hill
27. Asch SE: Effects of group pressure upon the modification and distortion of judgment, in Groups, Leadership, and Men. Edited by Guptzkow H. Pittsburgh, PA, Carnegie, 1951
28. Meltzoff J, Kornreich M: It works. Psychology Today, 1971
29. Rappaport H, Rappaport M: The integration of scientific and traditional healing: a proposed model. Am Psychol 36:774–781, 1981
30. Zerin MF: The pied piper phenomenon and the processing of victims: the transactional analysis perspective re-examined. Transactional Analysis Journal 13:172–177, 1983
31. Schwartz LL: Viewing the cults: differences of opinion, in Scientific Research and New Religions: Divergent Perspectives. Edited by Kilbourne BK. San Francisco, Pacific Division, American Association for the Advancement of Science, 1985
32. Quarantelli EL, Dynes RR: Organizational and group behaviors in disasters. American Behavioral Scientist 13:325–426, 1970
33. Cohen LH, Sargent MM, Sechrest LB: Use of psychotherapy research by psychologists. Am Psychol 41:198–206, 1986

34. Prochaska JO, Norcross JC: Contemporary psychotherapists: a national survey of characteristics, practices, orientations, and attitudes. Psychotherapy Theory Res Pract 20:161–173, 1983
35. Kelly EL, Goldberg LR, Fiske DW, et al: Twenty-five years later: a follow-up study of the graduate students in clinical psychology assessed in the VA selection research project. Am Psychol 33:746–755, 1978
36. Bednar RL, Shapiro JG: Professional research commitment: a symptom or a syndrome. Journal of Consulting and Clinical Psychology 34:323–326, 1970
37. Cohen LH: Methodological prerequisites for psychotherapy outcome research. Knowledge Creation Diffusion Utilization 2:263–272, 1980
38. Richardson JT, Kilbourne BK: Classical and contemporary brainwashing models: a comparison and critique, in The Brainwashing/Deprogramming Controversy: Sociological, Psychological, Legal, and Historical Perspectives. Edited by Bromley D, Richardson JT. New York and Toronto, Edwin Mellen Press, 1983
39. Kilbourne BK, Richardson JT. Cultphobia. Thought 61:258–266, 1986

GROUP FUNCTION AND SOCIAL CONTROL

Chapter 9

PSYCHOLOGICAL PERSPECTIVES ON CULT LEADERSHIP

Alexander Deutsch, M.D.

> And if thou say in thy heart: How shall we know the word the Lord hath not spoken? When a prophet speaks in the name of the Lord, if the things follow not, nor come to pass, that is the thing the Lord hath not spoken, the prophet hath spoken it presumptuously, thou shalt not be afraid of him. (1)

The quotation from Deuteronomy suggests that problems created by deviant and charismatic religious leaders date back to the beginnings of organized religion. The contemporary religious cult leader, claiming a special revelation, presents himself or herself as a modern-day prophet (2). While ignored by most people, such a leader develops a following over whom he or she exerts enormous influence.

In this chapter, which focuses on three contemporary religious groups, I will attempt to explain the power and attraction of the cult leader. I will describe and analyze the paradoxical adherence of certain devotees to their leaders in the face of facts which should logically lead to disillusionment. In the last section, I will describe how devotees of a psychotic leader can become pawns for the acting out of the leader's bizarre inner conflicts. The groups to be focused on include the Unification Church, led by the Korean evangelist, Reverend Sun Myung Moon; the American following of the Indian holy man and miracle worker, Satya Sai Baba; and a small Hindu-style group called "The Family" led by Jeff, an American guru. In the first section of the paper, I will describe the supernatural experiences of each of these leaders which stimulated them to spread their religious teachings.

The "Call to Prophecy"

Many cult leaders report miraculous mystical and conversion experiences which start them on their road to religious leadership. These stories become part of the legend surrounding them and contribute immensely to their charisma. Present-day cultists have a strong leaning toward occult and magical-mystical beliefs (3–5) and many report visions or other supernatural experiences themselves (6–8). They are thus particularly prone to idealize the grandiose mystical experiences of their leaders. For a number of cultists an avenue to "reality" opened up by psychedelic drugs becomes validated by their leaders' legendary experiences (6).

Reverend Moon reports that on an Easter morning when he was 16, he had a visitation from Jesus who informed him that he was chosen to try to complete Christ's mission. Moon struggled with this burden for many years. Through research and prayer he discovered the truths which were incorporated in the Unification Church holy book, the *Divine Principle*. Twenty years after his first miraculous revelation, Reverend Moon began his public religious mission (9).

Satya Sai Baba is the leader of a large and controversial Indian sect which, over the years, has developed a substantial but unpublicized Western following (10). Sai Baba's miraculous inner change, which took place when he was 14, is detailed in a devotional biography (11). Following an apparent scorpion bite, the young man had a personality change, alternating between periods of silence and bursts into song and poetry. Exorcists and physicians were brought in by the youth's parents to no avail. Gradually the young man's declaration that he was a reincarnation of a legendary Indian Saint, Sai Baba of Shirdi, and ultimately of the Hindu God Krishna, was accepted by those around him and by other Indians.

Jeff, the American guru, was a leader of a small cult which I followed for a number of years. His miraculous call to spiritual leadership was inextricably tied to his relationship with Sai Baba.

In his mid-thirties, Jeff regarded his life as unhappy and empty. He met a group of Sai Baba devotees and saw a film in which the holy man's miraculous powers were demonstrated. That night he had a vision of Sai Baba's eyes which was both frightening and exalting. He traveled to the Hindu leader's ashram in India in order to find "release and freedom" (6).

> I finally had eye contact with Swami and something happened . . . there was a spiritual circuit of some kind, something that passed from his body to mine and . . . I received some occult powers in the exchange. After that, I was aware of future events to a certain extent. It satisfied a small part of me but still there was discomfort. (12)

An ambivalent, argumentative relationship with the holy man ensued which resulted in Jeff's expulsion from the ashram. He went to an isolated beach where he meditated and chanted and "opened himself up to spiritual powers." Becoming increasingly despondent, he decided to commit suicide but before doing so, recited the mantra which Sai Baba had given him. Suddenly, two people appeared to engage him in conversation. Jeff turned his head for a moment and his visitors disappeared but so did his suicidal feelings. He states that Sai Baba subsequently let him know that it was he who had miraculously appeared to him on the beach to prevent his suicide (12, 13). Jeff's eventual cult leadership appeared to be based on a primitive identification with Sai Baba (13, 14).

While miraculous experiences and calls to prophecy are very impressive to members of cults or sects, they do present problems to those of a more naturalistic bent, whether layperson or psychiatrist. The following exchanges which took place during a trial which followed a lawsuit brought against a deprogrammer by a Unification Church member, point up some of the difficulties.

> The [defense attorney] sought to question Mr. Moon about what he said was his first conversation with Jesus . . .
> [Mr. Moon's attorney] leaped to his feet protesting the line of questioning, "This is an American courtroom . . . I must protect my client's rights."
> [The judge] interjected: "I have heard testimony during this trial from college graduates who said they spent two to three years fund-raising on the streets, who have been told that the

witness is their personal Messiah and that he is responsible for
their well-being on this earth and the hereafter."

"It is on the basis of this that these young people follow him
doing incredible acts of almost self-slavery . . . [the de-
programmer] has been charged with trying to interrupt this life
and so we want to know whether this is a bona fide religion or
not."

[The judge] said that one reason so many young people are
joining the Unification Church was that they believed in Mr.
Moon's conversations with Moses and Buddha. If these conversations did not take place, the judge said, that was important to know.

Mr. Moon said, "I am ready to answer. I met Jesus Christ."

"How did you know it was Jesus Christ?"

"I remember him from his holy picture," Mr. Moon answered. "He said he was the Jesus Christ." Mr. Moon said he
still spoke with Jesus, "whenever I pray." (15)

Does Reverend Moon's testimony under oath about his meeting with Jesus make him the founder of a bona fide religion? Is he
lying? Did he have a hallucination based on a psychotic disorder? Is his vision a product of a deep spiritual wish perhaps
helped along by an altered state due to prolonged prayer or
fasting? Can his vision be distinguished from the founders of the
great religions and the prophets of the past? (16, 17)

I do not propose, for the most part, to grapple with these kinds
of questions and their broad implications in this chapter. I will,
however, present data later that show a relationship between
hallucinatory psychosis and religious experience in Jeff, the cult
leader with whom I was most familiar.

Power and Attraction of the Cult Leader

I have indicated that the central figures of certain cults claim a
special relationship to a higher power. Something akin to supernatural powers is often attributed to the leader himself (2, 18).
Thus, Jeff's followers believed that their leader knew who was
coming to see him if the person thought of the guru during his
trip (6). Reverend Moon was sometimes credited with divine
intuition in his ability to match up marital partners and, indeed,
many believe him to be the Messiah.

My visit to Sai Baba's ashram in the mid-1970s left an indelible
impression of the enormous attraction certain Westerners had

toward the supernatural and miraculous. In Indian culture, where a claim to divinity does not have the ring of bizarreness that it does in our own, Sai Baba's use of "miracles" was central to his identity and power. His daily "materialization" of sacred ash (*vibhuti*) or other objects from the air, his purported ability to be in two places at one time, the alleged production of *vibhuti* by some of his pictures, all were accepted, almost without question, by his Western devotees. In the magical atmosphere that permeated the ashram there was a pervasive belief that nothing took place without Swami's knowledge or direction (Deutsch A: unpublished manuscript).

While Jeff and Reverend Moon make no claims to divinity, they are perceived, by virtue of their special experiences, revelations, and powers as being close to God. By joining groups headed by them or similar leaders, members have direct contact with God's representative (2, 6, 18). This has an obvious appeal for those who consciously seek spiritual enightenment or transcendence but it is also a powerful magnet to the individual who might join a cult for a variety of other conscious or unconscious purposes. This includes those seeking guidance, nurture, love, purpose, affiliation, alleviation of conflict, self-control, or self-esteem. Studies have shown that the individuals with all these needs and tendencies are well represented among cult joiners (6, 8, 19–22). The bolstering of self-esteem can be conceptualized along Kohut's lines as the mirroring entailed in receiving recognition or approbation from the grandiose leader, or more regularly through the "merger" with the idealized figure (6, 23).

Like most religious doctrines, the teachings of the cult leaders tend to be all-embracing with prescriptions for beliefs and daily behaviors, for permitted acts and proscribed acts. The fact that these rules come from a grandiose religious figure helps provide a powerful auxiliary superego for individual joiners who may otherwise have difficulty dealing with sexual and aggressive drives or with cravings for illicit drugs (6, 21, 24).

The Movement

The movement, which is initiated by a cult leader or by a devoted follower, can be seen as an extension of the leader's personality and teachings. The movement encompasses the leader's following, the organization that is set up, its formal doctrines, and its sacred text. The grandeur and the association with divinity that is attributed to the leader are easily transferred to the movement. An intense feeling of specialness and importance is attained by those who belong. In a large, geographically dispersed movement such as the Unification Church, this transfer has advantages in that it obviates the need for frequent contact with the leader. Often, charismatic lieutenants can fill in quite well, at least temporarily, for the leader. The appearances of the leader may become all the more exciting because of their infrequency (8).

Groups as different as Reverend Moon's and Charles Manson's can strike similar chords in conferring on their members a sense of transcendent specialness. For example, members of both groups were led to believe that they were the vanguard of the 144,000 converts (Revelation 7:4–5) who would transform the world (7, 25).

Large organized groups such as the Unification Church are obviously different from small cults with a primitive organization such as Jeff's Family in that they are set up to publicize, to recruit, to invest in business, to publish newspapers, and to raise funds. From the point of view of the psychology of the members there is another important difference. In the larger organized group, an ambivalent or disillusioned member can readily "split" his or her feelings and direct anger or disappointment toward a lieutenant while preserving adoration toward the central figure. In the smaller group, this is less readily done and there may be a correspondingly greater use of other defense mechanisms to deal with the anxiety created by potential disillusionment.

The Cult as a Vehicle for Rebellion

In addition to the above "benefits," joining a fringe movement centered around an unorthodox religious leader might help express a latent rebellious attitude against one's family or the dominant culture (6, 21). I've observed several variations on this theme. For example, Jeff seemed to embody an anarchical ego ideal (26) which was most attractive to his followers. They felt that Jeff received direction directly from God and thus was totally free from conventional restraint. They were delighted when he confused and outsmarted "authority figures" like the police (27).

Highly rigid behavior may also express latent rebellion [as in the fringe Catholic group led by a priest characterized as being "more Catholic than the Pope" (28)].

> A Unification Church member, Jean, had powerful sexual inhibitions which appeared to be related to her strict Catholic upbringing and a punitive maternal introject. By joining the Unification Church she could rebel against her mother and her religion of origin, experience a loving union with female leaders in the organization, and at the same time, reduce conflict by accepting a sexual morality stricter than the one she was brought up with. (13)

An even more paradoxical example of rebelliousness in cult members was observable in a substantial number of Western followers of Sai Baba (Deutsch A: unpublished manuscript). Emerging from the hippie counterculture, they appeared to project their anarchic and rebellious trends on their leader and distorted his teachings which were actually quite conservative. His playfulness, seductiveness, and magic and his controversial and unorthodox position within his own culture facilitated the projection and distortion. The holy man angrily recounted for me, in an interview, the misdeeds of the Westerners: they illegally overextended their visas; the men and women were too close to each other; they embarrassed him in front of his Indian devotees; they followed behind him in a car when he left the ashram; some women touched him; and so on. The misreading of Swami by the Western devotees is discussed further in the following section.

When Prophecy Fails

In their classic study of an apocalyptic cult the social psychologists Festinger et al. (29) tested and verified their hypothesis that commitment to the cult as judged by proselytizing activity would increase when the prophecy of the cult leader regarding world cataclysm and the landing of a rescuing spaceship did not materialize. Their prediction was contrary to the commonsense point of view that disconfirmation of a prophecy would lead to disillusionment and the breaking away from the cult. Group support appeared to be a factor in the maintenance of belief by cult members, and the increased proselytization was seen as a way of increasing group support in the face of potential disillusionment.

If the concept of the failure of prophecy is expanded from the notion of the failure of a specific prediction to any disappointment in the idealized leader, be it in his or her kindness, judgment, fairness, morality, or rationality, we will be confronted with a paradoxical dynamic which is apparently inherent in cults, that is, in the face of disconfirming evidence relating to the idealized central figure, cult members frequently remain steadfast in their belief.

An instructive historical example is provided by the movement surrounding Sabbatai Zevi, the seventeenth century Jewish kabbalist and false messiah. An apparent sufferer from manic-depressive disease, Zevi so impressed Nathan of Gaza by his periods of "illumination" that Nathan proclaimed him the Messiah. Zevi had a vast following while Nathan and other kabbalists provided intellectual justifications for his lapses into depression and for his various antinomian practices. Zevi's ultimate conversion to Islam under threat of execution by the Sultan should rationally have provided overwhelming evidence as to the "failure of prophecy." In fact, a substantial number of Zevi's followers maintained their belief in his messianic role and some even converted to Islam themselves. Using kabbalistic and biblical texts, they found ingenious rationalizations not only to justify but to claim the historical necessity of Zevi's apostasy (30, 31).

Jeff and The Family provide some interesting parallels to the Sabbatian movement. While Jeff's illness appeared to be schizophrenic rather than manic-depressive, he nonetheless also went through periods of mood and behavioral swings, at times seeming benign and loving and at other times cruel and punishing. His followers were able to maintain their prophetic image of him by conceiving of each phase as a revelation of a different Hindu divinity. The good phase was a manifestation of the Hindu god of love, Krishna, while the cruel behavior belonged to his Shiva phase, patterned after the Hindu god of destruction. His "craziness" and antinomian behavior were idealized as demonstrations of freedom from societal restraints (27). Jeff's "discovery" following a period of hallucinatory self-destructiveness, that his idol and mentor, Sai Baba, was the Devil, and his conversion to Christianity split The Family. (When he gave permission to publish material about him, Jeff asked me to mention that he eventually returned to Judaism, his religion of origin.) Some remained true to their Hindu ideals while others followed their leader and became born-again Christians (24).

At Sai Baba's ashram, as I indicated above, the Western devotees flagrantly denied the holy man's growing disenchantment with them, which was clearly shown by his not granting them personal interviews and other indications of unfriendliness. When I told the devotees what Sai Baba had told me about his negative feelings toward them, the characteristic response was that the holy man didn't really mean what he told me, that he was telling me, a Western doctor, just what I wanted to hear, and that the whole episode was meant as a test of their faith in him. (The notion that a disconfirming event is engineered by the leader as a test of faith seems common in cult thinking.) A theological justification for their thinking was readily available here too. Did not Sai Baba proclaim himself as an incarnation of Krishna and did not Krishna play tricks (*leela*) on his devoted followers? (Deutsch A: unpublished manuscript.)

Reverend Moon's followers likewise experienced disappointing evidence relating to his power and beneficence. For example, some Moonies developed skin eruptions following avid cleansing of a newly purchased but filthy building, notwithstanding reassurances that Reverend Moon had purified each room with "holy salt." When a few complained about Moon's inability to protect them, they were told "don't be like Satan, don't be an accuser." On a more serious level, many Unification Church members had moral questions about fund-raising techniques which often involved deception of potential customers. As indicated above, in a large organization such as the Unification Church, the leader can be spared criticism while others (ambitious American or rigid Japanese team leaders) can be blamed for excesses. In addition, the techniques were rationalized under the rubric of "holy deception."

We may conclude, based on material presented above and in an earlier publication (27), that when belief in an idealized cult leader and his mission is met by disconfirming evidence, the anxiety that arises is frequently warded off by defenses among which denial is primary. The denial is buttressed by group support and may be enhanced by regressive processes inherent in an authoritarian group (27). Denial is further supplemented by rationalization, magical thinking (27), and displacement of hostility from the leader. The angry reaction caused by disappointment in the leader may be turned toward the self, resulting in abject submission, while preserving the image of the leader as benevolent, powerful, and godly (27). It can be projected on the outside world, and thus intensify paranoid strains within the cult (21). The vulnerable ego of a cult member is further weakened by these reality-distorting defenses, sometimes leading, in a vicious spiral, to ever-increasing reliance on the guidance of the leader (27). The end result can be a cult member in virtual bondage to a leader who may be unconscionably exploitative, violent, or even psychotic.

In spite of the above, some people do decide to leave cults and studies have indicated some individual and social psychological factors which may differentiate those who leave from those who remain (21, 22, 29). My impression is that a highly charged disappointment or a sense of personal victimization may influence some devotees who have relatively strong personalities to break their ties to their groups. Thus, Jeff's sexual approach to an Indian follower who had taken a vow of chastity led to the defection of the woman, her brother, and her brother's girlfriend. Others, however, rationalized the episode as "Jeff's wish to teach the devotee to 'let go.' " One moonie became distraught when the man she was in love with was matched by Reverend Moon with a Korean bride. Finding it difficult to accept that Reverend Moon could be guilty of such a lack of empathy toward her, she sought to penetrate the upper layers of the organization to find out directly from the leader the reasons for his decision. Upon not receiving satisfaction she turned to psychiatric consultation which eventuated in her leaving the movement. Others in the organization felt that she was too willful and lacked faith.

The Psychotic Cult Leader

A "worst case" example of blind obedience of cult members is provided by the mass suicide and murder in Jonestown, Guyana, in 1978. Jim Jones, the leader, in a state of paranoid deterioration, instigated the apocalyptic ending of the People's Temple. For many years prior to the massacre, while doing "good deeds" like helping the poor and preaching interracial harmony, there were signs of megalomania and paranoia in the leader. He performed "miracles," claimed Father Divine was reincarnated in him, and had extreme fears of nuclear holocaust. Accounts of his final years stress the leader's need for total control and domination over his subjects, along with paranoid fears of betrayal (32, 33).

While we have outlined some mechanisms to account for the attachment of devotees to a deranged cult leader, a complementary question asserts itself. What benefits accrue to a psychotic or prepsychotic leader from having a devoted following? What are the bonds that tie such an individual to his or her group?

Edith Jacobson has provided some useful formulations of the ties of the prepsychotic (or psychotic) individual to external objects. Due to the narcissistic nature of his or her relationships, and to the permeability of the ego boundaries, external objects may be experienced and dealt with by the prepsychotic (or psychotic) individual as part of the self to a much greater extent than in the neurotic (projective identification). These objects may represent or contain representations of unacceptable parts of the self; controlling them can be equated with controlling the self and changing them with changing the self. The ability to externalize in this way may save a patient from intolerable internal conflict and ward off a psychotic break. Admiration or tribute from external objects can also mitigate a dangerous lowering of the disturbed individual's self-esteem (34).

I have previously suggested that Jeff's becoming a guru resulted from a magical identification with Sai Baba, and was a regressive alternative to an ambivalent, frustrating object relationship with the holy man (13, 14). A central figure of Jeff's teachings was the idea of "letting go," an apparent amalgam of Hindu, Zen, and hippie philosophy (6). It involved a passive, detached surrender to inner experience and to the outer world, watching life go by "as if a movie." At first preaching in a benign and supportive manner, Jeff paradoxically became progressively more forceful in drumming this lesson into his devotees (27). In the latter days of the cult's history, a flicker of tension in a devotee could provoke a sudden physical attack from the guru. As mentioned above, a sexual approach to a devotee was explained as Jeff's attempt to teach her to "let go" (27). Apparently for similar reasons, Jeff once even tried to get me to disrobe in the temple.

Fortunately we have information about Jeff's inner life from material he later gave to an author who wrote a history of the cult (12). While Jeff in an increasingly bizarre and cruel manner was attempting to force others to let go and surrender, he was trying to deal with similar pressures within himself. Does he surrender to his "spirits," and let go, or does he fight them (13)?

> From the first time I started to spin, I was moved about by energy and spirits, not by my own will. I gave up my own desire and let the spirits move me where they would. Very often, they'd fling me into walls, bang me against buildings, and cause me bodily hurt. I sincerely thought it was from God, and that, by surrendering more and more to it, I was getting closer to God. (12)

That the spirits represented the incorporated image of Sai Baba seems clear from Jeff's account of his conversion to Christianity (13).

> I listened to the 700 Club every time it was on. . . . I heard Pat Robertson talk about the power of Jesus' name. . . . Shortly after . . . the demons were tormenting me badly . . . I called out "Jesus help me" and the spirit left me in peace for a short while. . . . I wondered . . . could it be that Jesus was more powerful than Sai Baba, more powerful than the spirits who controlled my body. . . . (12)

Jeff's conversion to Christianity was preceded by multiple exorcisms of his spirits and the burning of all pictures and relics of Sai Baba that were at the commune (13).

It appeared that Jeff was trying regressively to solve a desperate love-hate conflict toward Sai Baba by completely surrendering himself up to Swami's introjected image (the spirits). As this defense was failing (whether because of Jeff's anger projected on to the spirits or homosexual anxieties) (14) he tried to externalize the conflict by making The Family surrender to him while he took on the role of the tormenting guru. With the help of Christian teachings he could define his spirits as demons, exorcise them, give up his philosophy of letting go, and abdicate cult leadership (13).

Further indication of the psychotic guru's attempt to deal with inner conflict by projective identification and the associated control of his followers is seen in the following example which relates to sexual conflict.

One day in the final year of the commune, I saw Jeff at the temple service banging his thigh near his groin in a ferocious and fearsome, and, to me, incomprehensible manner. The devotees generally understood him to be criticizing them and warning them against sexual indulgence, and a few of them became very guilty and fearful because of their sexual habits.

Jeff later talked about his private fantasies which took place around this time.

> I sat twenty hours a day, stretched out in my chair, my torture rack. There were visions of sexual perversion which came straight from hell. I'd see visions of murders and horrible cruelty, and always the voices talking to me telling me to do things. . . . (12)

The permeability of ego boundaries is a two-way situation, facilitating not only projection, but also introjection. Jeff became extremely sensitive to his devotees, and it appeared that it was only by completely dehumanizing them that he could maintain control over them. On one occasion, I saw him move them around the temple in totally inexplicable fashion as if they were pieces of furniture. He later stated:

> I had to walk backwards into temple. Otherwise I'd feel all the bad vibes which brought me down very low. I'd feel what everybody else was feeling. I'd take on his vibes, his spirit. Others were held to go into bliss when I held my hand to them in a blessing, but I'd take on their bad experiences, I was the Family laundromat. They left [temple] feeling light and clean. . . . I took on . . . dark spirits. Many times I'd take on the attributes of another person. . . . I'd go back to my room and have hellish experiences. If a woman was afraid of mice, I'd take on her fear. The whole room would be crawling with mice, attacking me, climbing up my chair. I'd feel them clawing my skin, biting me. . . . (12)

Jeff's sensitivities and the taking on of sufferings of others was seen as self-sacrificial and sometimes Christ-like by his devotees, a theological rationalization that occurs in other cults, too. And in some ways, Jeff perhaps could be seen as a victim of his own cult members as their idealizations probably stimulated his megalomania, while their submissiveness and regressive defenses may have facilitated his distortions of reality.

There was no theology of violence or suicide in Jeff's Family and in this way it contrasts strongly with Jim Jones's People's Temple (32, 33). While both leaders had overwhelming needs to control their followers, Jeff's need was very concrete, and appeared limited to the people he was with at any given time. Jones, on the other hand, could not tolerate the loss of followers, and defections appeared to have led to "white nights" (mass rehearsals for suicide) (32, 33). Indeed, one of the things that makes Jeff's group interesting is that a substantial number of devotees remained loyal in spite of the absence of pressure from the leader for them to stay in The Family (27).

Comment

In this chapter, I have emphasized some of the psychological interplay between the cult leader and his followers. I have described the appeal to cult members of the grandiose unorthodox religious leader with his all-embracing doctrines; the need of the cultist to adhere to the idealized image of the leader and the defenses used to maintain belief; and how a seriously disturbed leader may project on to his or her followers aspects of himself or herself that he or she needs to control, while serving simultaneously as a repository for their idealizations.

To what degree are cult leaders motivated by the need for power, for self-aggrandizement, by greed, by rebellion, by regressive needs for control of others, by psychopathy, by self-delusion, or by genuine wishes to share spiritual insights? A number of factors hamper broader discussion of the motivation and psychological dynamics of the cult leader. One is that the leaders are generally unavailable for interview and study. A second factor is the undoubted differences among various leaders in personality, motivation, and pathology. Another problem is the lack of clear differentiation in current psychiatric thought between the mystical and various psychopathologic states (17). We are fortunate to have one ex-cult leader, Jeff, who gave a retrospective account of his thoughts and behavior, and a retrospective interpretation of his sense of being directed by God. His testimony may help us understand other highly disturbed cult leaders.

The types of phenomena described in this chapter are not necessarily limited to today's "new religions." Charismatic leaders within organized religion may have similar interplay with their followers. The accusation made by a Jewish leader that a particular Hasidic sect is a cult, and the questions raised recently concerning the probity of the founder of Mormonism attest to this possibility. In addition, messianic-type political leadership probably stirs up forces within followers similar to those in cult members (35). Indeed, the maintenance of faith in Soviet Communism by some left-wing Americans after the Hitler-Stalin pact (36) is reminiscent of the reaction of cult members following a disconfirming event. This compulsion to keep the faith, rooted in the universal childhood need for idealizations (14, 23), may have its most sublime manifestation in the phenomenon of theodicy.

References

1. Deuteronomy, 18:21–22
2. Appel W: Cults in America. New York, Holt, Rinehart and Winston, 1983
3. Marty M: The occult establishment. Social Research 37:212–230, 1970
4. Werman DS: Chance, ambiguity and psychological mindedness. Psychoanal Q 48:107–115, 1979
5. Singer B, Benassi VA: Occult beliefs. American Scientist 69:49–55, 1981
6. Deutsch A: Observations on a sidewalk ashram. Arch Gen Psychiatry 32:166–175, 1975
7. Lofland J: Doomsday Cult. New York, Irvington, 1981
8. Deutsch A: A clinical study of four Unification Church Members. Am J Psychiatry 140:767–770, 1983
9. Sontag F: Sun Myung Moon and the Unification Church. Nashville, TN, Abingdon, 1977
10. Schulman A: Baba. New York, Viking Press, 1971
11. Kasturi N: The Life of Bhagavan Sri Sathya Sai Baba, American ed. Bombay, Dolton Printers, 1969
12. Pakkala L: Yea-God. Trumansburg, NY, Crossing Press, 1980
13. Deutsch A: Psychiatric perspectives on an Eastern-style cult, part

II—A guru's psychosis, in Psychodynamic Perspectives on Religion, Sect and Cult. Edited by Halperin DA. Littleton, MA, John Wright-PSG, 1983

14. Jacobson E: Psychotic identifications, in Depression, Comparative Studies of Normal, Neurotic, and Psychotic Conditions. New York, International Universities Press, 1971
15. Moon, on stand, tells of his religious beliefs. New York Times, May 28, 1982, p 1
16. James W: The Varieties of Religious Experience. New York, New American Library, 1958
17. Committee on Psychiatry and Religion: Mysticism: Spiritual Quest or Psychic Disorder. GAP Publication No. 97. New York, Group for the Advancement of Psychiatry, 1976
18. Isolated, strongly led sects growing in U.S. New York Times, June 22, 1986, p 1
19. Levine SV, Salter NE: Youth and contemporary religious movements: psychosocial findings. Canadian Psychiatric Association Journal 21:411–420, 1976
20. Galanter M, Rabkin R, Rabkin J, et al: The "Moonies": a psychological study of conversion and membership in a contemporary religious sect. Am J Psychiatry 136:165–170, 1979
21. Ungerleider JT, Wellisch DK: Coercive persuasion (brainwashing), religious cults, and deprogramming. Am J Psychiatry 136:279–282, 1979
22. Maleson FG: Dilemmas in the evaluation and management of religious cultists. Am J Psychiatry 138:925–929, 1981
23. Kohut H: The Analysis of the Self. New York, International Universities Press, 1971
24. Deutsch A, Miller MJ: Conflict, character and conversion: study of a "new-religion" member, in Adolescent Psychiatry: Developmental and Clinical Studies, vol 7. Edited by Feinstein SC, Giovacchini P. Chicago, University of Chicago Press, 1979
25. Bugliosi V, Gentry C: Helter Skelter: The True Story of the Manson Murders. New York, WW Norton, 1974
26. Redl F: Group emotion and leadership. Psychiatry 5:573–596, 1942
27. Deutsch A: Tenacity of attachment to a cult leader: a psychiatric perspective. Am J Psychiatry 137:1569–1573, 1980
28. Scavullo FM: Leonard Feeney: the priest who was more Catholic than the Pope, in Psychodynamic Perspectives on Religion, Sect and Cult. Edited by Halperin DA. Littleton, MA, John Wright-PSG, 1983
29. Festinger L, Riecken HW, Schachter S: When Prophecy Fails. New York, Harper & Row, 1964
30. Scholem G: Sabbatai Sevi, the Mystical Messiah. Princeton, NJ, Princeton University Press, 1973
31. Yerushalmi YH: From Spanish Court to Italian Ghetto. Seattle, University of Washington Press, 1981

32. Levi K, ed: Violence and Religious Commitment. University Park, PA, and London, Pennsylvania State University Press, 1982
33. Weightman JM: Making Sense of the Jonestown Suicides. Lewiston, NY, Edwin Mellen Press, 1983
34. Jacobson E: Psychotic Conflict and Reality. New York, International Universities Press, 1967
35. Bychowski G: Dictators and Disciples. New York, International Universities Press, 1948
36. Klehr H: The Heyday of American Communism. New York, Basic Books, 1984

Chapter 10

PERSUASIVE TECHNIQUES IN CONTEMPORARY CULTS: A PUBLIC HEALTH APPROACH

Louis Jolyon West, M.D.

There are two very different public images of contemporary organizations which for the purposes of this essay I shall call "cults" (see discussion of definition, below), especially those cults to which the adjective "religious" is usually applied. The first image might be called utopian. It suggests the emergence of a healthy, new spiritual sectarianism, a flowering of "new religions" (a term held preferable to "cults" by their supporters). This image portrays congregations of pilgrims who, after a search for truth, self-fulfillment, or the meaning of life, have found a band of kindred spirits under the benign guidance of a divinely inspired prophet, guru, master, or paterfamilias, with whom they are now living happily. Their bliss is rarely troubled by memories of the rejected—perhaps doomed—society left behind, or by the attempted intrusions or "rescue" efforts of unenlightened, misguided family members or their agents. Fortunately, the wealth and strength of the cult is usually sufficient to foil the schemes of these outsiders. Against such schemes can

Portions of this material were presented at the International Conference on the Effects of New Totalitarian Religious and Pseudo-Religious Movements on Society and Health, 20–22 November, 1981, Bonn, Federal Republic of Germany, and published in the conference proceedings, *Destruktive Kulte*: Edited by Karbe KG, Müller-Küppers, M. Göttingen, Federal Republic of Germany, Verlag für Medizinische Psychologie, 1983. The valuable assistance of Marsha Addis and Deborah Ackerman is gratefully acknowledged.

be arrayed the power of the group, of its well-supported attorneys citing various laws including those that protect freedom of religion, and of numerous friendly organizations and sympathetic individuals in all walks of life.

The opposite image might be called infernal. This invokes the spirit of Dante Alighieri and his fourteenth century vision of hell. Through Dante's eyes we see a place where men, women, and children are bound to a satanic master. They trusted him in the beginning and believed his promises, but now they are sinking deeper and deeper into his power, surrendering their possessions, their bodies, their children, their very souls to his mysterious purpose. With Dante we follow them to a distant place, where "sighs, lamentations, and loud wailings resound through the starless air," making us weep in sympathy. We hear "words of pain, tones of anger, voices loud and hoarse, and with these the sound of hands, (making) a tumult which is whirling through that air forever, as sand eddies in a whirlwind." Above the cries of the damned, we might hear a single child's voice calling out, "I'd die for *you*, Dad." These were the tape-recorded words of a boy just before he took the fatal poison at the command of Jim Jones: Guyana's twentieth-century echo from Dante's Inferno.

These public images are mirrored by the propositions and publications of two groups of behavioral scientists and health professionals, using more technical terminology but with similar general orientations to the "utopian" versus the "infernal" (i.e., those "sympathetic" toward "new religions" versus those "critical" toward "cults"). Because there are relatively few scholars in this field, the players on the two sides are fairly well known—at least by name—to each other and to those who for one reason or another have a stake in the contest. Unfortunately (but perhaps inevitably) these scholars have become increasingly polarized and, as the public debates over cult-related matters multiply, have been pitted against each other as expert witnesses in lawsuits and in other arenas as well. The characteristics of these opposed groups, their allies, shibboleths, self-images, and perspectives about each other, comprise a topic of great interest in its own right, but about which space does not permit discussion here.

I have been following the phenomena of cults in America since 1950 when Dianetics burst upon the scene, originally as a psychotherapy cult, later to become the Church of Scientology. However, my continuing interest in these groups represents the confluence of several lines of inquiry. One has to do with studies of hypnosis and dissociative phenomena (1). The second has to do with coercive persuasion and the techniques employed in the Korean War by communist captors to induce a number of American prisoners to behave in ways deemed improper, or even treasonous (2, 3). The third relates to abuse by youth of alcohol and drugs (especially hallucinogens) and the flight by many young people from the drug abuse subculture into communes and (later) cults (4). The fourth is that of a clinical psychiatrist who must evaluate the psychopathology of patients who happen to be cult victims, specify their diagnoses, undertake treatments, evaluate therapeutic outcomes, and teach others to do the same (5).

The perspective on cults that I have developed is neither utopian nor infernal. It is, I hope, objective and scientific. However, I must admit that on occasion, when faced with some particularly shocking example of abuse of a cult member (especially a child) by the group or its leaders, to remain objective I have had to employ all the training and experience accumulated during nearly 40 years in the practice of medicine. I have learned so much about the suffering of cult victims and their families that I have come to regard cults as a public health hazard, and thus find myself in the camp of the critics. (The reader should understand that the opposing viewpoint is well represented elsewhere in this book.)

There are many religious sects, new and old, that I would not classify as cults. Cults are best identified by the authoritarian fashion in which they actually function rather than by their benign public image; by their de facto value systems largely based on power, money, and aggrandizement of the leaders rather than their alleged humane concerns, charitable practices, or spiritual enrichment of the followers; by their secretive practices, jealously guarded boundaries, and tough rules about the flow of information rather than their outward pretenses of openness, candor, and honesty.

Most cults undoubtedly are neither utopian nor infernal. At any given time, a number may be relatively harmless. But most—if not all—have the potentiality of becoming deadly, as the People's Temple of Jim Jones did. Some cults that currently may appear harmless are in fact already doing serious damage to members and their families, damage about which the general public knows nothing, damage that cult leaders cover up and deny, damage that apologists for cults consistently refuse to admit or inspect.

Some of the larger, more powerful cults have branches in many countries, extensive property holdings, subsidiary organizations with special names for special purposes, and a growing degree of influence. International concerns about the detrimental effects of certain cults on the well-being of their members, members' families, and society in general have led to such varied actions as a national conference on the problem in West Germany in 1981, resolutions against cults by the American Parent-Teacher Association (PTA) in 1982 and by the European Parliament in 1984 (see below), a nationally televised debate in Spain in 1984, the international Wingspread Conference on Cultism (Johnson Foundation Wingspread Conference Center, Racine, Wisconsin, 1985), the Vatican Report of 1986 (6), and an Israeli interministerial report in 1987. (The Israeli report denounced 10 cults [including Divine Light Mission, Church of Scientology, Unification Church, and the Hare Krishnas] as causing "a form of dependence, bondage, self-enslavement" and loss of property. After receipt of this report the Education Ministry warned that such cults promote rifts between their members and society that "can significantly affect the individual's judgment, autonomy and ability to make a choice.") Other governmental investigative reports have been carried out in Australia, Canada, France, and elsewhere.

Definition

The word *cult* is given several definitions by the dictionary (7). These definitions include the following.

4. A religion regarded as unorthodox or spurious (the exuberant growth of fantastic cults); also, a minority religious group holding beliefs regarded as unorthodox or spurious.
5. A system for the cure of disease based on the dogma, tenets, or principles set forth by its promulgator to the exclusion of scientific experience or demonstration.

6a. Great or excessive devotion or dedication to some person, idea, or thing.
b. The object of such devotion.
c(1): A body of persons characterized by such devotion (America's growing cult of home fixer uppers—Wall Street Journal).

Some of Webster's other definitions are even broader or more benign.

Needless to say, my concerns are not about cults of "home fixer uppers." Rather, I am concerned about fanatical groups capable of exploiting or harming their own members, disrupting or destroying members' families, and threatening or even attacking critics, former members now defined as traitors or renegades, or any person or group seen as opposed to their activities—not excluding government agencies, university scholars, or entire professional entities (e.g., psychiatry).

In this chapter, I use the term "cult" to describe groups that satisfy one or another of Webster's definitions but that also can properly be described as *totalist*, after Lifton (8). Lifton derived his concept of totalism from Erik Erikson's contribution to *Totalitarianism* (9). *Totalism* describes a tendency to "all-or-nothing emotional alignment" which can be exploited by "those ideologies which are most sweeping in content and most ambitious—or Messianic—in their claims, whether religious, political, or scientific. And where totalism exists, a religion, or political movement, or even a scientific organization becomes little more than an exclusive cult" (p. 429). In a later work, Lifton explicates "a dangerous four-step sequence from dislocation to totalism to victimization to violence" (10).

The following definition (similar to the one employed in the Wingspread Conference report) is provided for the reader of this chapter to understand my meaning as clearly as possible.

Cult (totalist type): a group or movement exhibiting a great or excessive devotion or dedication to some person, idea, or thing, and employing unethical, manipulative or coercive techniques of persuasion and control (e.g., isolation from former friends and family, debilitation, use of special methods to heighten suggestibility and subservience, powerful group pressures, information management, promotion of total dependency on the group and fear of leaving it, suspension of individuality and critical judgment, and so on, designed to advance the goals of the group's leaders, to the possible or actual detriment of members, their families, or the community.

Totalist cults are likely to exhibit three characteristics: 1) excessively zealous, unquestioning commitment to the group and its leadership by the members, 2) manipulation and exploitation of members, and 3) harm or the danger of harm. It should be noted that many groups do not fit neatly into a category of sect, commune, or cult. Furthermore, groups may change their characters over time, becoming more or less like cults, totalist or otherwise.

Terms such as "new religious movement" have been used by some to describe certain cultic groups. A problem with this approach is that it may lend unwarranted respectability to a less-than-respectable enterprise. Jim Jones's People's Temple was once considered a new religious movement. The term is also inappropriate to describe cultlike groups that are not religious; or groups of devotees that form around charismatic healers who then exploit their patients and followers in various ways; or nonprofessional psychotherapies, even if they convert themselves to "religions" in order to obtain various tax benefits and legal protections; or cabals of Satan worshipers which, while perhaps qualifying as "religious," could hardly qualify as "new."

Henceforth the reader should understand that in this essay I use the word "cult" to mean "totalist cult" as defined above.

The Scope of the Problem

The old and the young may be involved in cults, as demonstrated by the membership of the People's Temple and demography of the dead at Jonestown. However, persons between the ages of 18 and 30 are especially subject to cult recruitment. A recent study of students in San Francisco found that half were open to accepting an invitation to attend a cult meeting; approximately 3 percent reported that they already belonged to cultic groups (11).

My own observations, and those of colleagues whose judgment I respect, have led me to believe that no single personality profile characterizes those who join cults. Many well-adjusted, high-achieving persons from intact families have been successfully recruited by cults. So have individuals with varying degrees of psychological impairment. However, to the extent that predisposing factors exist, they may include one or more of the following: naive idealism, situational stress (frequently related to normal crises of adolescence and young adulthood, such as romantic disappointment or school problems), dependency, disillusionment, or an excessively trusting nature. Ignorance of the ways in which groups can manipulate individuals is a relatively general characteristic of cult victims—until it is too late.

From a public health perspective, we are presently dealing with an epidemic of cult-related damage. It has been estimated that there are now more than 2,500 cults in the United States. The majority of these are religious and, of course, they are not all alike. Some are very small—15, 30, or 50 people, and resemble communes. By my criteria (5), cults and communes differ in three main respects:

1. Cults nearly always have a strong, charismatic leader with a power structure of some kind; communes generally do not.
2. Cults are likely to have a manifesto—a book, a doctrine, a code—which, as interpreted by the leader, governs the behavior of the members through various rules and regulations; in communes one is more likely to find tracts on astrology or organic gardening.
3. Cults are surrounded by a tough boundary that clearly defines who is in, who is out, and who may pass in either direction; communes, on the other hand, are generally open to people coming and going, often from one communal setting to another.

As noted previously, many cults pose significant threats to the personal freedom and well-being of their members. Nevertheless, despite all the evidence of misdeeds perpetrated in the name of religion, these threats are, to a considerable degree, covered up, minimized, and obscured. This covering-up process is part of the condition that has enabled the epidemic to spread.

Much information has accumulated from various cult-related scandals—from cult refugees; from families, relatives, and friends of cult victims; and from a few studies. However, it is very difficult to obtain accurate data by direct investigations of cults because the cults systematically deceive the public. They conceal information; they harass their critics; they intimidate and dominate their members. All of this is designed to prevent a free flow of information.

Sometimes I am astonished to hear a colleague report that he or she has visited a certain cult and been persuaded that the people there are happy and content, or that he or she has distributed questionnaires to cult members and drawn similar conclusions from the results. Naive visitors may not see through the choreographed presentation regularly provided by cults to deal with outsiders, but scientists should not be so easily deceived. Former cult members have come forward to say, "But look, I was there! I took part in the deception! It is a well-practiced act that we always put on to deceive outsiders!" The investigator who is sympathetic to the cult may retort, "You are not a good reporter because, as a former member, your account is prejudiced. Even if you did live six or seven years in the cult, the very fact that you left proves that you are now biased and, therefore, your testimony is worthless."

It is hard to carry out good scientific research under conditions where genuine direct access to—or truly unrestricted observation of—the phenomena or subject material is forbidden, and where the cult leadership controls or can influence the circumstances of scrutiny, the choice of subjects, or the nature of the responses. Even so, existing data now suffice to convince any reasonable person that the claims of harm done by cults are bona fide. There are a good many people already dead or dying, ill or malfunctioning, crippled or developing improperly as a result of their involvement in cults. They are exploited; they are used and misused; their health suffers; they are made to commit improprieties ranging from lying ("heavenly deception") to murder. Their lives are being gobbled up by days, months, and years. Their families are often devastated.

For at least two decades the situation has been growing steadily worse. We do not know how many people are affected. I have seen estimates that as many as 10 million Americans have been at least briefly involved with cultic groups during the past 20 years. But even if it were only a million, the situation should be considered grave. Suppose a million people in the United States were afflicted with some mysterious infection about which many victims did not complain, but which caused considerable suffering in others and, while only a small percentage died, that was affecting a steadily increasing number of people. Would we not consider that an epidemic? I submit that we would, and that a public health approach would be considered an appropriate response by those responsible for public policy.

In spite of such evidence, however, there are many apologists for the cults. These individuals and organizations undoubtedly contribute to the cults' veneers of respectability behind which strange and ugly things are happening. Some of the apologists appear to be romantics. They project into the cults some of their own hopes for religious reform, spiritual rebirth, rejection of materialism, or even escape from the dangers of the thermonuclear age. Other apologists, including some civil libertarians, take a more seemingly pragmatic stand, shrugging off whatever abuses the cults may perpetrate, and pointing out that any countermeasures would be unacceptable because they might violate freedom of religion as guaranteed by the First Amendment to the Constitution of the United States.

A number of apologists appear to have been successfully deceived by charismatic cult leaders or their representatives. Certain politicians fall into this category, in some cases after the cult has contributed money to their election campaigns. There are even some armchair philosophers who have either never seen the destructive effects of cults or prefer to deny their reality, but who happily discuss cults (perhaps using another definition) at great length and in the most elaborate terms as an interesting new ferment in contemporary society, or in some other uncritical way. If the apologists are church officials, physicians, or behavioral scientists, the grateful cults have been known to reward them with grants, awards, published praise and even "research" opportunities.

Cult-Related Harms

The Wingspread Conference (12) pointed out that cults arouse concern because of their unethical or manipulative practices together with their lack of consideration for the individual's needs, goals, and social attachments. Of even graver concern is that these practices often result in harm to persons, families, and society at large. The harms outlined in the Wingspread Conference report appear below. All can be documented.

Individuals and Families

1. Mental or emotional illness, impaired psychological development, physical disease, injury, or death of cult members.
2. Fragmentation of families.
3. Financial exploitation of members and their families.
4. Neglect and abuse of children, including deaths resulting from physical violence, profound neglect, or the denial of medical treatment.

Government and Law

1. Infiltration of government agencies, political parties, community groups, and military organizations for the purpose of obtaining classified or private information, gaining economic advantage, or influencing the infiltrated organizations to serve the ends of the cult.
2. Tax evasion.
3. Fraudulent acquisition and illegal disposition of public assistance and social security funds.
4. Violation of immigration laws.
5. Abuse of the legal system through spurious lawsuits, groundless complaints to licensing and regulatory bodies, or extravagant demands for services (such as those provided by the Freedom of Information Act) as part of "fishing expeditions" against their enemies.
6. Pursuit of political goals while operating under the rubric of a nonpolitical, charitable, or religious organization.

Business

1. Deceptive fund-raising and selling practices.
2. Organizational and individual stress resulting from pressuring employees to participate in cultic "management training" and "growth seminars."
3. Misuse of charitable status in order to secure money for business and other noncharitable purposes.

4. Unfair competition through the use of underpaid labor or "recycled salaries" by cult-operated enterprises.

Education

1. Denial of, or interference with, legally required education of children in cults.
2. Misuse of school or college facilities, or misrepresentation of the cult's purposes, in order to gain respectability.
3. Recruitment of college students through violation of their privacy or deception, often with subsequent disruption of such students' educational programs or goals.

Religion

1. Attempts to gain the support of established religions by presenting a deceptive picture of the cult's goals, beliefs, and practices; and seeking to make "common cause" on various issues.
2. Infiltration of established religious groups in order to recruit members into the cult.

Although the Wingspread outline of harms is fairly comprehensive, it does not include a classification for certain major crimes, such as fraud, rape, battery, and murder, which have been committed at the instigation of cult leaders or in cult settings.

It should be understood that the Wingspread Conference was by no means the first review of cult-related public hazards, nor the first aegis under which recommendations were made for a realistic public response. For example, the following resolution was adopted by the 1982 National PTA Convention delegates.

Cults:

Whereas, various cults often recruit members by deceptive means; and

Whereas, cults often keep their members by using mind control and by alienating the members from their families; and

Whereas, many families have deep emotional scars caused by their children's dependence on cults; and

Whereas, an awareness of the recruitment and retention techniques of cults could help prevent a young person's entry into cults; therefore be it

Resolved

That the national PTA urge state PTAs/PTSAs and their units to hold education programs to inform families and youth about methods of recruitment, and techniques used to exercise control over members' thoughts and actions by cults; and be it further

Resolved

That the national PTA provide a list of available resources to assist state PTAs/PTSAs and their local units in planning such programs.

Two years later, on May 22, 1984, the European Parliament adopted a Resolution entitled *New Organizations Operating Under the Protection Afforded to Religious Bodies*. The Resolution expresses the Parliament's concern about the recruitment and treatment of members of the organizations in question and calls for an exchange of information among member states on problems arising from the activities of these groups with particular reference to charity status and tax exemption; labor and social security laws; missing persons; infringement of personal freedoms; existence of legal loopholes which enable proscribed activities to be pursued from one country to another; and creation of centers to provide those who leave the organizations in question with legal aid, assistance with social reintegration, and help in finding employment.

The Resolution states that "the validity of religious beliefs is not in question, but rather the lawfulness of the practices used to recruit new members and the treatment they receive." It goes on to call upon member states to pool their information about the "new organizations" as a prelude to developing "ways of ensuring the effective protection of (European) Community citizens." To achieve this, the Resolution "recommends that the following criteria be applied in investigating, reviewing, and assessing the activities of the above-mentioned organizations.

(a) Persons under the age of majority should not be forced, on becoming a member of an organization, to make a solemn, long-term commitment that will determine the course of their lives;

(b) There should be an adequate period of reflection on the financial or personal commitment involved;

(c) After joining an organization, contacts must be allowed with family and friends;

(d) Members who have already commenced a course of education should not be prevented from completing it;

(e) The following rights to the individual must be respected;
- The right to leave an organization unhindered;
- The right to contact family and friends in person or by letter and telephone;
- The right to seek independent advice, legal or otherwise;
- The right to seek medical attention at any time;

(f) No one may be incited to break any law, particularly with regard to fund-raising, for example, by begging or prostitution;

(g) Organizations may not extract permanent commitments from potential recruits, for example, students or tourists, who are visitors to a country in which they are not resident;

(h) During recruitment, the name and principles of the organization should always be made immediately clear;

(i) Such organizations must inform the competent authorities on request of the address or whereabouts of individual members;

(j) The above-mentioned organizations must ensure that individuals dependent on them and working on their behalf receive the social security benefits provided in the Member States in which they live or work;

(k) If a member travels abroad in . . . the interest of an organization, it must accept responsibility for bringing the individual home, especially in the event of illness;

(l) Telephone calls and letters from members' families must be immediately passed on to them;

(m) Where recruits have children, organizations must do their utmost to further their education and health, and avoid any circumstances in which the children's well-being might be at risk."

The Resolution of the European Parliament concludes by stating that it is desirable to develop "a common approach within the context of the Council of Europe," and "calls, therefore, on the governments of the Member States to press for appropriate agreements to be drawn by the Council of Europe which will guarantee the individual effective protection from possible machinations by those organizations and their physical or mental coercion." The provisions of the Resolution clearly reflect the experience of harm suffered by thousands of cult victims and their families in the European community.

Persuasive Techniques

The scholars who prepared the 1986 Vatican Report (6) summarized their findings in a list of such methods that is similar to listings by others (5, 13), but perhaps should be reproduced here because it comes from a clerical source outside the ongoing debate.

> Some recruitment, training techniques, and indoctrination procedures practiced by a number of sects and cults, which often are highly sophisticated, partly account for their success. Those most often attracted by such measures are those who, first, do not know that the approach is often staged, and, second, are unaware of the nature of the contrived conversion and training methods (the social and psychological manipulation) to which they are subjected. The sects often impose their own norms of thinking, feeling, and behaving. This is in contrast to the Church's approach which implies full-capacity informed consent.
>
> Young and elderly alike who are at loose ends are easy prey to those techniques and methods that are often a combination of affection and deception (e.g., love-bombing, the personality test, or the surrender). These techniques proceed from a positive approach but gradually achieve a type of mind control through the use of abusive behavior modification techniques.
>
> The following elements are to be listed:
>
> - Subtle process of introduction of the convert and his gradual discovery of the real hosts;
> - Overpowering techniques: love-bombing, offering a free meal at an international center for friends, flirting fishing techniques (prostitution as a method of recruitment);
> - Ready-made answers and decisions are being almost forced upon the recruits;
> - Flattery;
> - Distribution of money, medicine;
> - Requirement of unconditional surrender to the initiator, leader;
> - Isolation: control of the rational thinking process, elimination of outside information and influence (family, friends, newspapers, magazines, television, radio, medical treatment, and so forth) which might break the spell of involve-

ment and the process of absorption of feelings and attitudes and patterns of behavior;

- Processing recruits away from their past lives; focusing on past deviant behavior such as drug use, sexual misdeeds; playing upon psychological hang-ups, poor social relationships, and so on;
- Consciousness-altering methods leading to cognitive disturbances (intellectual bombardment); use of thought-stopping cliches; closed system of logic; restriction of reflective thinking;
- Keeping the recruits constantly busy and never alone; continual exhortation and training in order to arrive at an exalted spiritual status, altered consciousness, automatic submission to directives; stifling resistance and negativity; response to fear in a way that greater fear is often aroused;
- Strong focus on the leader; some groups may even downgrade the role of Christ in favor of the founder (in the case of some Christian sects).

Much of the cult controversy relates to the question of whether it is actually possible for groups or authority figures to influence and control the thoughts and behaviors of subject individuals to their detriment.

In the secular world there is general acceptance that such influence and control are very real. Intimidation through force or the threat of it is a powerful controller of behavior, and thoughts tend to follow behaviors through rationalization, self-justification, identification with the aggressor and other mechanisms. Deception is also a well-known method of exploiting people, either through positive misinformation, concealment of important facts, or both. Our statutes, ethical codes, and conventional moralities all recognize and accept the vulnerability of people to intimidation and deception. However, this scenario assumes that the wronged person eventually recognizes and decries his or her victimization. The wronged person presses charges. He or she shows his or her bruises. The wronged person produces evidence that a swindle occurred, that the product was misrepresented, that the lot is under water at high tide. Maybe the wronged person wins the case; maybe not. Perhaps it is deemed the individual's own fault that he or she didn't read the fine print, or that he or she didn't exercise reasonable suspiciousness or prudence. Caveat emptor still obtains despite consumer protection laws. Nevertheless, the reality and effectiveness of intimidation and deception are not at issue per se. Someone has done it to the victim. The victim didn't do it to himself or herself. Cults are able to operate successfully because at any given time most of their members are either not yet aware that they are being exploited, or cannot express such an awareness because of uncertainty, shame, or fear. That there are techniques capable of drawing people into such groups, holding them there, even to their detriment, and influencing their mood, thought and behavior while they remain identified with the group is a hinge of major controversy in this field.

Terms like "brainwashing" are not useful in exploring this question. "Brainwashing" did not prove necessary to account for the unwonted behaviors of prisoners of war (2, 3, 14, 15). "Mind control" is not much better. The realities about techniques of influence do not require neologisms to assert themselves. They may be found in several bodies of literature, to which the reader is here referred through the following list of examples.

1. Laboratory experiments with normal human subjects (16–19).
2. Studies of coercive persuasion or thought reform, outside the cult field (20–29).
3. Studies of accounts by former cult members, surveys and single-group overviews (30–47).
4. Investigative studies of cultlike organizations (48–61).
5. Reports by those who have treated cult victims (62–70).

My own "public health approach" was first proposed at the Bonn conference in 1981 (71). In the six years that have passed since then I have come to believe with even greater certainty that this approach is deserving of consideration because it poses no threat to established religions, new religions, communes, sects (no matter how odd), or even cults if they are of the nontotalist variety. At the same time it tackles the hazards posed by cults, and the harms already suffered by their victims, and strives to protect those who are at risk or may become so.

In public health (including preventive psychiatry) we talk about three types of prevention: primary, secondary, and tertiary. Primary prevention eliminates the causes of illness or unhealthy circumstances. Secondary prevention intervenes early, striving to restore health and prevent recurrence or complications. Tertiary prevention (postvention) comes later, and seeks to diminish the damage and protect the victim from further harm. How can this model apply to cult-related harm?

The definition employed in this chapter is good enough to distinguish cults from genuine churches. Clearly it is essential that, in preventing cults from doing harm, we must not ourselves do harm to organizations that are blameless, and that society needs or desires for its well-being. Returning to the health-related model, one might ask how, for the purposes of treatment, one distinguishes malignant cells from healthy ones in the human body. A good approach, if one is interested in curing cancer, is to find a chemical that kills malignant cells and spares those that are healthy. What would be the effect of approaches which, when applied by society to organizations calling themselves religious, would have no untoward affect upon benign, bona fide religions, but would inhibit the malignant ones, that is, the cults? How could such social medications be prescribed?

Before outlining my suggestions, I wish to say a word about society's responsibility to support research on this problem. We must have a proper evaluation and monitoring of the cult epidemic, and measure the effectiveness of whatever methods we employ. Our society has a large stake in such research, but has not yet come to grips with the necessity to undertake it. If there had been an epidemic of an infectious disease with the morbidity and mortality of this one, research support would abound.

A Public Health Model

I. *Primary Prevention*

With regard to our plague of cults, primary prevention requires strengthening society against them.

A. *Recognition*

The first essential under primary prevention is recognition of the nature and extent of the problem. This must include increasing public awareness and extensive public education. The PTA resolutions and the Wingspread Conference are mere beginnings to this process. Far more must be done.

B. *Religious Outreach Programs*

Many established religious entities have become smug,

self-satisfied, and preoccupied with the material state of the church rather than reaching out vigorously toward the idealism of the young. This cannot—and in my view should not—be accomplished through the schools, or through the dubious electronic propaganda of money-oriented radio and television "ministries." Rather, it should be the responsibility of "mainline" churches to bring to young people the benefits of religion through genuine religious fellowship. There is good reason to believe that such experience will render youngsters less vulnerable to phony but superficially attractive alternatives—cults—masquerading under the guise of religion.

C. *Restoration of Family Values*

While it is not good enough to say that the cult problem or its solution lies in the family, it is true that many families are in trouble. As part of primary prevention, there are many things that could be done to help families. Unfortunately, today there are many social factors, especially in the United States, that seem to militate against family integration. Vulnerability of young people to cults is not the only consequence of this disintegration. Increases in violence, drug abuse, crime, and delinquency all relate to serious problems in families. While it does not appear to me that family problems are significantly more frequent in the backgrounds of cult recruits than in other persons with the same demographic characteristics, it is also true that interventions involving families have often proved helpful in solving cult-related problems.

D. *Risk Factor Review*

How do we review risk factors as part of primary prevention in public health? We inspect. How do we know if it is safe to eat in a restaurant? A trained investigator is legally authorized to examine the food. In fact, inspections of many types of organizations purporting to provide for the physical or mental well-being of the citizenry are legally mandated. This is primary prevention in public health. Even the best hospitals must be inspected regularly. It seems to me that no responsible religious organization should raise objections to comparable inspections with regard to the risk of such harms as are reviewed above. The cults, of course, would be less able to withstand this type of scrutiny.

II. *Secondary Prevention*

The preventive measures discussed below have to do with requirements that I believe society can safely make directly upon the cults. These requirements will act, in the long run, like chemotherapy: to produce a specific effect on that which is harmful or diseased and to preserve the health of that which we desire to preserve.

A. *Revelation*

This means legally requiring any organization that purports to offer services of any kind, including mental or spiritual, to reveal in advance all of the implications of participation or membership. In medicine we call this providing *fully informed consent*. Such a procedure should be made a requirement for any organization that recruits members from the public and in relation to their alleged purposes seeks special status or privilege regarding taxes or anything else. These organizations should be able to show that full disclosure was rendered *before* membership was solicited or accepted. It is not easy to become a Catholic, a Jew, or an Episcopalian. However, it is all too simple to become a Moonie. It usually happens before the recruit even realizes what has been done to bring it about. Most genuine religions, concerned with offering people spiritual fulfillment, strive to ensure in advance that such people know exactly what will be required of them, what their responsibilities will be. Not so the cults.

Many cults—not only the Church of Scientology—couch their claims of benefit in terms of health. We should insist that cult recruiters, like health professionals, if they propose to make you a healthier person, must explain all the risks to your health that the procedure—or membership—may impose, and what its actual limitations are. Under such a set of ground rules, the cheerful, smiling, clean-cut young person (often of the opposite sex) who befriends you and then says, "Would you like to come to a place I know and meet some wonderful people who are interested in the same things you and I are?" would be required to hand you a piece of paper saying "This is an invitation to attend and join the Unification Church. If you do join, the following will be required of you." The list would include, among many other items, surrendering all personal possessions to the church, accepting Sun Myung Moon as the messiah, and living in celibacy until three years after marriage to a partner (who might well be a stranger) chosen by Sun Myung Moon.

B. *Reckoning*

This means accounting for the use of funds. Churches use most of their funds for operational expenses and charitable purposes, that is, for the improvement of the lives and well-being of their members, worthy projects in the community, care for the needy, foreign missions, and so on. There is nothing to fear in accounting for these expenditures. I know many thoughtful people in the clergy who for years have been saying that churches should open their books to appropriate inspection as businesses or hospitals must. Why not? Charitable expenditures should properly be tax exempt. But if the goal of the church's fund-raising is to buy its leader yachts, or jewels, or Rolls-Royce limousines, or firearms, society has a right to know, and there should be a reckoning.

C. *Removal*

This has to do with the vital but delicate subject of removing a member from a cult for a period of objective review. When you look at this proposition as though it were a public health measure, it should not threaten the genuine religions. Simply put, if a reputable person or persons (e.g., a relative or a family) has a basis for being concerned about the health or well-being of a cult member, and a preliminary investigation shows that the concern has merit, that member might be removed from the cult for a short period of time to allow for examination of the situation by an objective agent of society, such as a court. This intervention need not require the type of conservatorship which necessitates proving the member incompetent. The only thing necessary would be to show reasonable grounds for concern about the member's physical or mental health.

Suppose there were a youngster at a Lutheran retreat and his parents thought, "I'm worried about him; his letters seem strange; I want him home." The church would certainly not refuse to tell the parents where their youngster was, or to send him home. If society acknowledges that there are circumstances in which individuals are presently being endangered by certain types of organizations, then society must accept the responsibility to protect those who may be so endangered, by removing them from the suspect situation until safety—and genuine freedom of choice—is assured.

D. *Recovery of Damages*

This is a potent social and legal remedy which derives from the consumer advocacy tradition. If, after leaving an organization to which I previously belonged, I find that I have been harmed as a result of having been in that group, I should be able to sue the organization for the damages that I have experienced. To make a recovery for my losses, I would have to develop proof. The establishment of proof may require investigations, witnesses, and even courtroom procedures.

Suppose someone decided to sue the Roman Catholic church claiming development of bad knees from too much kneeling. Collection of damages would not be likely because the person could have used a pillow, or because the church would not have expelled or punished him for not kneeling. However, suppose someone chooses to sue the Unification Church or the Church of Scientology for having exercised undue influence (a concept that already exists in law) upon his life, resulting in a loss of income, or of position, or of health, or of property, stating further that this undue influence employed deception, lack of initial full disclosure, or failure to give fully informed consent in advance. If proof were forthcoming, then such a lawsuit should lead to a recovery for damages. Ten years ago such suits were almost unheard of. Recently a few have been successful. If lawsuits of this type increasingly lead to recovery of damages from totalist cults, the epidemic of cult-related harms will begin to subside.

III. *Tertiary Prevention*

    A. *Rescue Missions*

Participating in the process of helping refugees from cults has proved to be one way for former victims to be useful and to stay healthy, something like the method used in Alcoholics Anonymous. However, rescuing people from cults can be risky. This brings us back to "removal," but further to the whole question of "deprogramming," which, although it is discussed satisfactorily in the Wingspread report, perhaps deserves a brief comment at this point.

What many parents call "removal" or "rescuing," the cults—and often the police—call kidnapping. I do not advocate kidnapping. But one must ask, what has gone wrong in a society where parents are forced to kidnap their own children through a desperate desire to save them? Many families—normal families by all the usual criteria—have been driven to seizing their own children forcibly to extract them from cults, and then exposing them to the intensive discussions of the cults' practices, including hard facts about the leadership, called "deprogramming."

It has been estimated that two thirds or more of those who have been forcibly "deprogrammed" either never go back to the cults (even though they are free to do so usually in a matter of days or weeks) or return only temporarily. The remainder go back to stay (72). Often when they go back, the cult uses them to intimidate, or even to sue the family. A number of parents in the United States have been charged with kidnapping as a consequence of such failed rescue efforts. However, they are almost never convicted. When the question of criminal intent comes up, the jury rejects the kidnapping charge. Even so, there are the legal costs, the stress of the rescue mission itself, and the terrible subsequent harassment often experienced by the families. Clearly, in order to make such rescue missions and forcible deprogrammings unnecessary, other means should be available to deal with the matter of rescue. (see Removal, above.)

B. *Reentry Counseling*

In the United States, reentry counseling (sometimes called voluntary deprogramming) of people who leave the cults is a relatively effective, legal treatment approach. Most of these patients were not forcibly removed from a cult, but escaped, drifted out, or were ejected from the group, especially if they became ill. The whole question of reentry is something that should be on the conscience of society. What about cult members who do not have families to help them? What about the ones whose families are not sufficiently affluent to pay for reentry counseling services, and where charitable services (like Los Angeles's Cult Clinic) are not available? The problem is there; the seekers for help on reentry are there. Reentry counseling must be considered as a basic element in tertiary prevention. Here we find a neglected social responsibility.

C. *Reconstitution of Relationships*

This means working with the significant others in the life of the individual who is coming back into society. One of the few agencies that is truly providing this service in the United States is the Los Angeles Cult Clinic, which deals with families in a practical way (73). It helps them to keep lines of communication open to their relative in a cult, and productively deals with emotional aspects of the problem, thereby making it possible to reconstitute relationships when the cult member finally returns to the family.

D. *Rehabilitation*

This is an extensive, time-consuming process. The psychopathology of people coming out of cults has been described elsewhere (5). My rough estimate (based on observations not only of cult members but of people returning from prisoner-of-war camps, hostage ordeals, and other types of captivity situations that are similar) is that at least one-third will show some kind of obvious psychopathology. It may take several months before they are ready to work in something resembling ordinary psychotherapy. Prior to that, the method of group therapy employed by Singer (63) seems to be the most effective. Fully to rehabilitate some of these people will take a year or even more, as described by Goldberg and Goldberg (67). Society must be prepared to provide rehabilitation programs for people who are seeking a return to normal, productive lives. If treatment works, the taxes from these refunctioning people will more than pay for it afterwards. Without expert help many of them may become emotionally crippled, public charges, or worse. An honorable and enlightened society cannot fail to provide such care.

Comment

Without apology, as a physician, I look at the cult problem with health and disease in mind. Many people in cults are at risk. Some are already sick. Some are dying. Some are dead. The stress upon their families generates additional casualties. A public health strategy is called for. It is my profound hope that such a strategy—perhaps similar to the one here proposed—will soon be put into effect. Great suffering might be prevented as a result.

Summary

1. The persuasive techniques used by totalist cults to bind and exploit their members, while not magical or infallible, are sufficiently powerful and effective to assure the recruitment of a significant percentage of those approached, and the retention of a significant percentage of those enlisted. (The term "significant" here refers to an amount sufficient for the enrichment of the leadership and their accumulation of power.)
2. Such cults are a genuine menace to society because they cause harm to persons, families, and the community. Whatever good they do could be done as well or better by other organizations (i.e., benign religious groups, legitimate health professions, and so on) that do not pose the same types of risks to individuals and to the public.
3. The extent of cult-related harm during the past 20 years is sufficient to justify describing it as an epidemic, and calling for a public health approach to the problem.

4. The exercise of such an approach should reduce the number and power of cults, and thus reduce the amount of harm they do, without posing any risk to freedom of religion or to nontotalist organizations.

References

1. West LJ: Dissociative reaction, in Comprehensive Textbook of Psychiatry. Edited by Freedman AM, Kaplan HI. Baltimore, Williams & Wilkins, 1967, pp 885–889
2. West LJ: United States Air Force prisoners of the Chinese Communists, in Methods of Forceful Indoctrination: Observations and Interviews. Group for the Advancement of Psychiatry (GAP) Symposium (No. 4), 1957, pp 270–284
3. Farber IE, Harlow HF, West LJ: Brainwashing, conditioning and DDD: debility, dependency, and dread. Sociometry 20:271–285, 1956
4. Allen JR, West LJ: Flight from violence: hippies and the green rebellion. Am J Psychiatry 125:364–370, 1968
5. West LJ, Singer MT: Cults, quacks and nonprofessional psychotherapies, in Comprehensive Textbook of Psychiatry III. Edited by Kaplan HI, Freedman AM, Sadock BC. Baltimore, Williams & Wilkins, 1980
6. Sects or New Religious Movements. Secretariat for Promoting Christian Unity, Rome, May 3, 1986. Washington, DC, United States Catholic Conference, 1986
7. Webster's Third New International Dictionary, Unabridged. Springfield, MA, G. & C. Merriam, 1966, p. 552
8. Lifton RJ: Thought Reform and the Psychology of Totalism. New York, WW Norton, 1963
9. Friedrich CJ (ed): Totalitarianism. Cambridge, MA, Harvard University Press, 1954, pp 156–171
10. Lifton RJ: The Broken Connection. New York, Simon and Schuster, 1979, p 293
11. Zimbardo PG, Hartley C: Who gets recruited during the initial contact phase of cult recruitment? Cultic Studies Journal 2:91–147, 1987
12. Cultism: A Conference for Scholars and Policy Makers. Sponsored by the American Family Foundation; the Neuropsychiatric Institute, University of California at Los Angeles; and the Johnson Foundation. Convened at the Johnson Foundation Wingspread Conference Center, Racine, WI, September 9–11, 1985
13. Delgado R: Religious totalism: gentle and ungentle persuasion under the first amendment. So Cal Law Rev 51:1, 1977
14. Hinkle IE, Wolff HG: Communist interrogation and indoctrination

of enemies of the states. AMA Arch Neurol Psychiatry 76:115–174, 1956
15. Schein E: Coercive Persuasion. New York, WW Norton, 1961
16. Asch SE: Effects of Group Pressure upon the Modification and Distortion of Judgement. New York, Holt, Rinehart, and Winston, 1952
17. Milgram S: Obedience to Authority: An Experimental View. New York, Harper & Row, 1974
18. Zimbardo PG, Ebbesen EB, Maslach C: Influencing Attitudes and Changing Behavior: An Introduction to Method, Theory, and Applications of Social Control and Personal Power. Reading, MA, Addison-Wesley, 1977
19. Orne MT: Demand characteristics and the concepts of quasi-controls, in Artifact in Behavioral Research. Edited by Rosenthal R, Rosnow R. New York, Academic Press, 1969, pp 143–179
20. Meerloo JAM: The crime of mentacide. Am J Psychiatry 107:594–598, 1951
21. Sargant W: The mechanism of conversion. Br Med J 2:311–316, 1951
22. Sargant W: Battle for the Mind: A Physiology of Conversion and Brainwashing. New York, Harper & Row, 1957
23. Sargant W: The Mind Possessed. New York, Penguin Books, 1973
24. Chen TEH: Thought Reform of the Chinese Intellectuals. New York, Oxford University Press, 1960
25. Biderman AD, Zimmer H: The Manipulation of Human Behavior. New York, John Wiley & Sons, 1961
26. Frank JD: Persuasion and Health. New York, McGraw-Hill, 1961
27. Gaylin W: On the borders of persuasion. Psychiatry 37:1–9, 1974
28. Mindzenty J: Memoirs. Glendale, CA, Diane Books, 1974
29. Malcolm A: The Tyranny of the Group. Totowa, NJ, Littlefield, Adams and Co., 1975
30. Warnke M: The Satan Seller. Plainfield, NJ, Logos International, 1972
31. Petersen WJ: Those Curious New Cults. New Canaan, CT, Pivot Edition/Keats Publishing, 1975
32. Patrick T, Dulack J: Let Our Children Go. New York, Dutton, 1976
33. Enroth R: Youth, Brainwashing and the Extremist Cults. Grand Rapids, MI, Zondervan Press, 1977
34. Enroth R: The Lure of the Cults. Chappaqua, NY, Christian Herald Books, 1979
35. Sparks J: The Mindbenders: A Look at Current Cults. New York, Thomas Nelson, Inc., 1977
36. Atkins S, Slosser B: Child of Satan, Child of God. New York, Bantam Books, 1978
37. Conway F, Siegelman J: Snapping: America's Epidemic of Sudden Personality Change. Philadelphia, JB Lippincott, 1978
38. Streiker LD: The Cults Are Coming. Nashville, TN, Abingdon, 1978

39. Edwards C: Crazy for God. Englewood Cliffs, NJ, Prentice-Hall, 1979
40. Mills J: Six Years With God. New York, A&W Publishers, 1979
41. Stoner C, Parke J: All God's Children: The Cult Experience— Salvation or Slavery? Radnor, PA, Chilton Book Co., 1977
42. Underwood D, Underwood B: Hostage to Heaven. New York, Potter, 1979
43. Watkins P: My Life With Charles Manson. New York, Bantam Books, 1979
44. Hunt D: The Cult Explosion. Irvine, CA, Harvest House Publishers, 1980
45. Rudin MR: The cult phenomenon: fad or fact. NY Rev Law Social Change 9:17–32, 1979–1980
46. Zablocki B: Alienation and Charisma. A Study of Contemporary American Communes. New York, Free Press/Macmillan, 1980
47. Wooden K: Children of Jonestown. New York, McGraw-Hill, 1981
48. Brown JAC: Techniques of Persuasion: From Propaganda to Brainwashing. Baltimore, Penguin Books, 1963
49. Yablonsky L: The Tunnel Back: Synanon. New York, Macmillan, 1965
50. Cooper P: The Scandal of Scientology. New York, Tower Publications, 1971
51. Zablocki BD: The Joyful Community. Baltimore, Penguin, 1971
52. Bugliosi V, Gentry C: Helter Skelter. New York, Bantam Books, 1974
53. Verdier PA: Brainwashing and the Cults. North Hollywood, CA, Wilshire Books Co., 1977
54. Wallis R: The Road to Total Freedom, A Sociological Analysis of Scientology. New York, Columbia University Press, 1977
55. Yamamota JI: The Puppet Master: An Inquiry into Sun Myung Moon and the Unification Church. Downers Grove, IL, Intervarsity Press, 1977
56. Bainbridge WS: Satan's Power, a Deviant Psychotherapy Cult. Berkeley, University of California Press, 1978
57. Taylor B: Recollection and membership: converts' talk and the rationalization of commonality. Sociology 12:316–324, 1978
58. Shupe AD Jr, Bromley DG: Moonies in America. Beverly Hills, CA, Sage, 1979
59. Boettcher R: Gifts of Deceit. New York, Holt, Rinehart, and Winston, 1980
60. Klineman G, Butler S, Conn D: The Cult That Died. New York, GP Putnam's Sons, 1980
61. Mitchell D, Mitchell C, Ofshe R: The Light on Synanon. New York, Seaview Books, 1980
62. Singer MT: Therapy with ex-cult members. Journal of the National Association of Private Psychiatric Hospitals 9:13, 1978
63. Singer MT: Coming out of the cults. Psychology Today, January 1979, pp 72–82

64. Etemad B: Extrication from cultism, in Current Psychiatric Therapies, vol 18. Edited by Masserman J. New York, Grune & Stratton, 1979
65. Clark JG: Langone MD, Schecter RE, et al: Destructive Cult Conversion: Theory, Research, and Treatment. Weston, MA, American Family Foundation, 1981
66. Galper M: The cult phenomenon: behavioral science perspectives applied to therapy, in Cults and the Family. Edited by Kaslow F, Sussman M. New York, 1982
67. Goldberg L, Goldberg W: Group work with former cultists. J Nat Assoc Social Workers 27:165–170, 1982
68. Spero M: Psychotherapeutic procedure with religious cult devotees. J Nerv Ment Dis 170:332–344, 1982
69. Langone MD: Treatment of individuals and families troubled by cult involvement. Update 7:27–38, 1983
70. Schwartz LL: Family therapists and families of cult members. International Journal of Family Therapy 5:168–178, 1983
71. West LJ: Die Kulte als problem der offentlichen gesundheit (Cults: A public health approach), in Destructive Kulte. Edited by Karbe KG, Muller-Kuppers M. Gottingen, Federal Republic of Germany, Verlag fur Medzenische Psychologie, 1983, pp 47–64
72. Langone M: Deprogramming: an analysis of parental questionnaires. Cultic Studies Journal 1:63–78, 1984
73. Addis M, Schulman-Miller J, Lightman M: The cult clinic helps families in crises. Social Casework 65:515–522, 1984

Chapter 11

RELIGIOUS CULT MEMBERSHIP: A SOCIOBIOLOGIC MODEL

Brant Wenegrat, M.D.

According to sociobiologists, species-typical social patterns are evolved adaptations. As such, they are due to selective forces akin to those responsible for evolved bodily structures. In itself, this argument is really nothing new. Darwin and other early evolutionists were fully aware of complex subhuman societies. They knew these had to be products of evolution. What is new in sociobiology are recently developed concepts which permit a more detailed calculus of social adaptation than was possible in Darwin's time. Inclusive fitness, kin and reciprocal altruism, parental investment, and evolutionary stability are among these new concepts. For the first time, biologists can calculate the potential adaptive effects of specific social patterns and assess some of the factors that led to their evolution.

The conceptual tools that permit sociobiologists to make more specific statements about social patterns date from the 1960s and 1970s. They have been brought to public attention by several well-known books. *Sociobiology* by E. O. Wilson was the most famous of these books (1). It rekindled a debate, going back to Darwin's time, on the ethical implications of Darwinian theory as applied to human social arrangements (2).

At least some of the current debate is based on a misreading of sociobiologic claims: insofar as sociobiologists treat social patterns as evolved characteristics, they are sometimes mistakenly thought to be saying that environments make no difference. If,

for example, sociobiologists treat male violence as the manifestation of evolved sexual strategies, they are thought to be saying
that males in every society must be necessarily hostile. In fact,
what sociobiologists would say about male violence—and about
other behavioral patterns as well—is that males have evolved
dispositions to be hostile in certain circumstances. Societies that
frequently expose males to those circumstances, and in which
violent behavior is permitted or encouraged as a means of ex-
pressing hostility, will be characterized by male violence. Societies that minimize the deprived and hopeless circumstances
likely to lead to hostility, and with mores prohibiting violent
behavior, will be characterized by public order. A closely related
and equally damaging misconception confuses sociobiologic
claims with behavior genetic statements. Behavior geneticists
measure the extent to which differences between individuals
arise from genetic or environmental sources. Sociobiologic
claims concerning genetic factors are for the most part different:
rather than addressing individual differences, they aim to account for the various common denominators evident in behavior. The differing aims of behavior genetics and sociobiology
result in widely divergent ethical implications.

Wilson's book remains a valuable source for readers wishing
to learn about sociobiology. Books by Clutton-Brock and Harvey
(3), Alexander (4), Reynolds (5), Breuer (6), Trivers (7), and the
King's College Sociobiology Group (8) also provide excellent
overviews. Sociobiologic ideas have important implications for
psychiatric theory and practice. I have discussed these in my
previous work (9).

Mutualism

In the past, talk of species-typical behavior patterns would con-
jure up images of stereotyped motor activities, like the mating
displays of certain fish. These were the "fixed action patterns" of
classical ethology. They were said to be "released" by elementary stimuli, such as a proper sized patch of color, perception of
which was "hard-wired" in the animal nervous system. By
contrast, when sociobiologists talk of species-typical behavior
patterns they are thinking of social strategies. These strategies
may be actualized in highly flexible and even ingenious ways but

remain recognizable by their overall aim. For instance, chimpanzee males compete with each other for dominance, which gives them priority access to reproductively useful resources in chronically short supply. The actual method of competition depends on local circumstance as well as chimp ingenuity. One male chimp was recently observed frightening off his fellows by loudly banging garbage cans obtained from the local research station. This is a long way from the "fixed action pattern."

One important social strategy can be called flexible mutualism. In sociobiologic terms, it is certainly species-typical for human beings. Flexible mutualism is a tendency to form stable groups of individuals who cooperate with each other to their long-term mutual benefit. "Flexible" is an important adjective here: There are species of spiders, for instance, who jointly spin their webs. But this type of mutualism is highly stereotyped. It is more akin to a fixed action pattern than to a genuine strategy. Each spider plays a particular role in the spinning, uninformed by any general social tendency. In flexible mutualism, the social tendency itself is the paramount factor, manifested in specific cooperative ventures.

A flexibly mutualistic social strategy has many adaptive advantages. Stable mutualistic groups can cooperate in defense against predators. Common defense must have been an essential element in allowing previously arboreal primates to adopt terrestrial life. Highly organized common defense is evident in modern baboons, who occupy a terrestrial niche similar to that of the earliest protohominids. Later, when the threat of nonhuman predation had waned, stable protohuman groups must have been better defended against others of their kind. Stable mutualistic groups can also hunt cooperatively. The size of game that can be killed increases disproportionately to the additional caloric needs of a larger hunting party. Additional advantages of life in a stable, flexibly mutualistic group include more rapid technological progress, diminished vulnerability to transient disabling illness, and enhanced accessibility to mating opportunities, among many others.

Of course, natural selection cannot directly produce a flexibly mutualistic species. What it can do is to produce a species with certain communicative, perceptual, cognitive, and affective characteristics. Together these can operate—in the environment to which the species is adapted—to increase the likelihood of mutualistic behaviors. The advantages of mutualism then favor the specific characteristics which have increased its likelihood. The specific characteristics that promote human mutualism are hard to enumerate. As one might expect from the importance of mutualism, the characters that promote it—including communicative skills and emotional preferences—essentially define what it means to be human. Several human characteristics, though, greatly enhance the likelihood of mutualism and deserve special mention.

The first characteristic closely connected with human mutualism is a cognitive bias: individuals everywhere seem to categorize others as being alike or different. Those who are seen as alike, or members of the in-group, however that is defined, are invariably shown more cooperative attitudes than those who are seen as different. Contrariwise, there is invariably a gradient of hostility, which is muted within the in-group and more freely expressed toward outsiders. Second, individuals everywhere seem to feel more comfortable belonging to an in-group of potentially helpful comrades. Perceived alienation from all such groups produces dysphoric feelings, so that persons threatened with alienation will go to great lengths to find some group to belong to. In alienated modern societies, individuals often join subgroups with arbitrary membership signs, including badges, secret handshakes, or salutes, reflecting the strength of their need to belong to some close-knit group, however irrationally constituted. Finally, individuals everywhere tend to accept the worldviews characteristic of their social group. This is more than early enculturation, since numerous studies have shown that people want to conform with those they are close to. In order to conform, they will change their previous views and ignore contradictory evidence. In the small groups of early hominid hunters, cognitive solidarity must have served to reduce strife, diminish leadership conflicts, and prepare the ground for common actions.

Of course, everyone has always known that humans identify with and more or less cooperate with some social group larger than families, that they assume their group's world views, and that their attitude toward outsiders is generally invidious. What is new in the sociobiologic treatment is the concept that these behaviors result from evolved dispositions which had as their selective advantage precisely their tendency to produce what is now a ubiquitous social structure: the mutualistic in-group.

Consider some other possibilities: John Locke believed that human social groups rested on rational contracts: free men and women accepted social constraints in exchange for the benefits of group participation (10). The sociobiologic position is that men and women never decided rationally, but were formed by selective pressures to function in stable groups. Locke's free individual is merely a mythical being. Sigmund Freud believed that the structure of group life resulted from family relationships. The basis of law and the totem, for instance, was a parricidal impulse (11). The sociobiologic position is that group life is itself so advantageous that characteristics producing it have been selected for. There is no rationale for treating group life—and the mutualism it serves—as an epiphenomenon of other adaptive behaviors. Since Emile Durkheim (12), sociologists have generally treated the human group with its culture as having a life of its own. In particular, norms concerning group boundaries—the definition, that is, of in-group and out-group member—and pressures toward conformity have largely been treated as means by which cultural groups perpetuate themselves. Norms and pressures of this sort prevent defections and blunt the effects of competing value systems. The sociobiologic position, by contrast, stresses the individual's view. Groups have boundaries because individuals categorize others as in-group members or outsiders. The pressure to conform reflects a cognitive bias to adopt a consensual worldview. Finally, existential psychologists occasionally treat conformity and the need to belong to a group as means of avoiding fear due to existential isolation [see, for example, Yalom (13)]. By fusing with the group, the individual tries to deny the basic human condition. In the sociobiologic view, however personally important, intrapsychic defensive functions of group life must be epiphenomenal to past selective pressures. These made homo sapiens a primarily social being. Like Locke's rational being, the isolated existential human being may be more abstract than real. Or perhaps the isolated human is a symptom of something gone wrong with modern urban life (see below).

Religion and the Group

Historically, religion and the fate of racial and cultural groups are closely intertwined. Religion has served to sustain racial and cultural groups through severe historic exigencies. The fall of ancient Israel and Judah, in 722 and 586 B.C., followed by exile to distant Mesopotamia, failed to destroy the Jews as a people largely because their religious faith placed their defeat in a cosmological perspective. Because Assyria and Babylon were seen as agents of divine retribution, their victories eventually enhanced faith in the Covenant. Religion has also provided an impetus to racial and cultural groups' grandest historic projects. Before Mohammed, southern Arabian peoples lived in a sort of political-cultural chaos. Families waged blood feuds. Robbers and warlords plundered towns and caravans. Jews, Christians, and Mazdaists killed each other in wars and persecutions. There was little or no sense of wider social cohesion. Mohammed's visions united southern Arabians and gave them a sense of fellowship they had never before experienced. Within several centuries, this previously despised racial and cultural group had mastered much of the civilized world.

In light of its historic connection with the fate of cultural-ethnic groups, it comes as no surprise that classical sociologists have seen in religion mostly its group-dynamic functions. Durkheim saw religion as a form of group-cement, essential to group identity and cohesion (14). Weber and Troeltsch categorized religious bodies according to how they defined their membership (15, 16). This, of course, was a group-dynamic classification, since membership definitions comprise the group boundary norm. Johnson modified the Weber-Troeltsch categories, but retained their emphasis on group-dynamic processes (17). According to Johnson, religious groups could be categorized according to the degree of hostility they manifested toward the surrounding milieu. In a study informed by sociobiologic concepts, Lopreato recently reendorsed the classic sociologic emphasis on religion and group-dynamics (18).

Cult Membership in Sociobiologic Terms

Galanter and Buckley surveyed 119 recent converts to the Divine Light Mission, an Eastern religious cult which once gained notoriety for having a 13-year-old guru, known as Maharaj Ji (19). Converts reported that membership in the Mission had relieved various neurotic symptoms from which they had chronically suffered. The degree of symptom relief correlated strongly with the extent to which converts saw the Divine Light Mission as a cohesive social group. Relief also correlated with the convert's distrust of outsiders. These findings led Galanter to propose that sociobiologic concepts might account for individual motives that lead to cult induction (20).

According to Galanter, disaffiliation from small-scale social groups could produce affective distress, which remits insofar as the cult provides a cohesive in-group experience. This account, of course, rests on the concept of mutualism: affective and cognitive preferences which evolved because they kept individuals in stable mutualistic groups are potentially frustrated by alienated modern life. Bellah and coworkers have noted the extent to which modern life has become atomistic (10). Longings for community are chronically frustrated for Americans in particular. Modern cults may attract and keep their members by counteracting this painful alienation.

The sociobiologic model suggests that the emotional and cognitive biases that make individuals seek in-group experiences are more or less central to human nature. Neither rational self-interest, positive family experience, cultural universalism, nor existential maturity will easily eradicate the desire to join an in-group. Nor will these relieve the distress of being left out of such groups. Insofar as cults meet intransigent needs left unaddressed by the larger culture, they will continue to flourish until the larger culture has changed. From the sociobiologic model proposed by Galanter, cults indirectly measure how well secular culture is constructively meeting some basic human needs.

What is the evidence in favor of this model? First, if the model is correct, persons likely to join a cult should be disaffiliated from other social groups. In their study of conversion to a cult, Lofland and Stark found that converts were globally disaffected from noncult social contacts (21). According to Lofland and Stark, converts were so isolated that they "could, for the most part, simply fall out of relatively conventional society unnoticed." Levine interviewed members of numerous religious cults and observed the same phenomenon (22). Alienation from noncult groups preceded conversion and appeared as an important factor in the conversion process. Levine later studied diaspora Jews who had joined ultraorthodox cults while traveling in Israel (23). Once again, alienation from social groups, compounded by distance from home, seemed to be important to the conversion process. Galanter found prospective evidence for the importance of alienation (24). He studied participants in Unification Church workshops intended to recruit new members. The major predictor of eventual conversion was lack of outside social ties.

Cult recruiters are clearly aware of the importance of social isolation. This is why they direct so much of their effort toward adolescents and young people away from home for the first time. University campuses are particular targets of cult recruiters, especially at the beginning of new academic terms. Adolescents have always been prone to sudden religious conversions. But in modern society there is a notable gap between what Luckmann refers to as primary and secondary socialization (25). Consequently, modern adolescents and college students are particularly likely to be disaffiliated from their families on one hand and from adult groups on the other. The Israeli cults studied by Levine look for potential recruits among young people who look like bewildered travelers.

Most recently, those at the other end of life have also become targets for religious cult recruiters (26). Many elderly persons—especially the bereaved, those living alone, and inmates of nursing homes—are severely socially isolated. They are consequently drawn to cults which offer them companionship.

The sociobiologic model suggests that cult recruitment will proceed by making the subject feel part of the group and not through ideologic persuasion. Etemad pointed out that virtually all cults do recruit members by offering them comradery (27). Potential recruits are invited to a dinner or social meeting at which they are fed and emotionally coddled. Members go out of their way to make them feel special. They become the targets of "love-bombing," as the process has sometimes been called (28). If the potential recruit shows some interest, he or she will be invited to lengthier "retreats." These are most often held at isolated locations. Intensive efforts continue to make the potential recruit feel at home among friends. Practical help may be offered, especially to the elderly (26). Religious dogma is mentioned only after potential recruits are clearly attached to the group. In Lofland and Stark's phrase, adopting the dogma at that point is merely to "accept the opinions of one's friends" (21). In terms of human mutualism, adopting the dogma is doing what comes naturally: accepting the consensual reality of what has become one's perceived social group. The tendency to agree with one's perceived group appears from the outside to override critical faculties. Observers are sometimes astonished by the things recruits will believe to maintain their newfound sense of belonging. The recruit's beliefs are sometimes likened to hypnotic or dissociative phenomena (29). A more apt description, though, stresses what Berger and Luckmann called "the social construction of reality" (30). From his study of cult members, for example, Clark concluded that the mind "is controlled primarily by its identification with the surrounding culture" (31).

A curious historical fact shows how ideologic conversion depends on group dynamics. In the late 1960s, the Unification Church attempted to recruit new members through direct ideologic persuasion in the form of public lectures (32). Few people came to Church lectures and fewer still joined. Unification Church recruiting efforts met with success with American youth only after they turned to love-bombing and put ideology on the back burner.

If cults attract members by offering them an in-group, then maintenance of cult membership should be dependent upon continued feelings of solidarity. Lofland and Stark, on the basis of the study cited above, considered communal residence essential to consolidation of new cult members (21). Galanter and co-workers found that 237 Unification Church members they studied spent 94 percent of their nights in communal living arrangements (33). In the 1960s, Unification Church officials paid less attention to residential arrangements. New converts were frequently given work assignments which led to their isolation from other members. A large proportion quickly reverted to their previous beliefs. Communal living arrangements are currently typical of religious cults in general (34).

Historically, sects that have survived their early years have appeared to benefit from social isolation, whether imposed or voluntary. Mohammed, for instance, was forced from Mecca in 622 A.D. He and a few followers went to strife-torn Medina, whose leaders had invited him in the hopes he could make peace between warring elements. Isolated Medina, which was soon won over to Islam, proved the ideal community in which the new sect could establish itself. Had he remained in Mecca, could Mohammed have kept his followers? There were other inspired prophets who had failed to make a lasting impression on discordant Meccan religious beliefs. American religious history is quite instructive here. Shakers, Amish, Mennonites, and Hutterites, among many other sects, have survived in part by establishing separate settlements. In some cases, the community isolation has been so thorough as to produce genetic differences from outside populations (35). The Mormons, of course, survived by moving to the remotest possible region, where the early converts could live surrounded by fellow believers. Jim Jones and the Bhagwan Shree Rajneesh are the latest cult leaders who have tried to establish isolated communities.

Insofar as the in-group experience motivates cult membership, those who feel that less intensely should be the first to leave. Ungerleider and Wellisch found that subjects who voluntarily left religious cults differed from current cult members, and from "deprogrammed" subjects, in feeling less affiliated while they were active members (36). Significantly, forcible "deprogramming" was less likely to be successful with subjects who had been in a cult for more than one year. Presumably, subjects who had belonged to a cult for more than one year were too thoroughly enculturated to keep them from later returning.

Galanter notes that the emotional distress of separated cult members is treated most effectively in group therapy with other former cult members (34). This type of therapy allows former cult members to discuss the problems they share in common. It might also help to satisfy affiliative needs once met by the cult.

Extrinsic Religion

With the rise of the civil rights movement, attitudinal studies uncovered something surprising: Although churches taught brotherly love, religiously active subjects were more ethnically and racially prejudiced than nonreligious subjects (37–41). This is of obvious relevance to the present point of view. In sociobiologic terms, invidious out-group feeling is the opposite side of the coin to in-group solidarity. Insofar as religious subjects dislike those who are different, they might be using religion to meet their need for an in-group. The affiliative needs met by cults might also fuel mainstream religion!

Allport and coworkers showed that mainstream religious subjects were actually bimodal with respect to degree of prejudice (40, 41). Some religious subjects were less ethnically and racially prejudiced than nonreligious persons. Allport called these subjects, who really believed in brotherly love, the "intrinsically" religious. Other religious subjects, whom Allport called "extrinsics," were far more prejudiced than nonreligious persons. Intrinsics and extrinsics differed on numerous measures other than just prejudice. In large-scale surveys, the effect of "extrinsic" prejudice outweighed "intrinsic" tolerance, making the religious population appear to be generally bigoted. Allport's distinction, which is perhaps the major discovery of modern religious psychology, has been extensively validated (42). Allen and Spilka have defined another dichotomy, committed versus consensual faith, which for all practical purposes is identical to Allport's (43). Committed faith is intrinsic faith; consensual is extrinsic.

As Allen and Spilka imply by using the term "consensual," ethnically and racially prejudiced extrinsically religious persons appear to be after an in-group experience. In sociobiologic terms, extrinsics are mainstream religious persons whose motivations and fears are related to group mutualism. They tend to be conventional and highly attuned to social rules (44). Concerned as they are with social status and categories, they frequently feel controlled by more powerful persons (45). They envy prestige and money (46). Yet, they are unconcerned about justice and tend toward authoritarianism. They are chauvinistic and ethnocentric, and their religion is often exclusionary. Intrinsic religion, by contrast, stresses universalism and the dignity of other faiths.

Extrinsics generally have fewer religious or mystical visions, spontaneous or induced, than their intrinsic counterparts (47–49). Shorn of its group function, religious faith per se may not really interest them as it appears to interest intrinsics.

Some Practical Conclusions

Sociobiologic theories of flexible mutualism suggest that human beings are adapted to stable group life. Numerous affective and cognitive dispositions promote stable group life, but three in particular have been discussed here. The first is a tendency to classify other persons as in-group members or strangers, and to direct hostile behaviors mainly toward the latter. The second is the dysphoria that follows on alienation and resolves with perceived stable affiliation. The third is a tendency to accept the group's consensual views, sometimes by ignoring personal experience. Modern urban society may frustrate these dispositions, which are consequently manifested in religious cult membership. Religious sects and cults may always have served this function. Mainstream denominations probably serve this function for a substantial number of their members, those whom Allport called the extrinsic religious.

This model has certain implications for assessment of practical action with cults and cult members. First, the model draws attention to the motivational import of cults and of other group memberships. Sociobiologic theory indicates that the dispositions subserving flexible mutualism will be powerful and intractable in any environment resembling that of human adaptation. Cultures may channel them toward more or less constructive goals, but the primary dispositions cannot be wished away.

By contrast, other models of group behavior applied to cult phenomena emphasize other factors than the dispositions discussed in this paper. For instance, Locke's model of the human group, which is deeply embedded in modern secular culture (10), implies that group affiliations are readily made and unmade in the service of self-interest. The growth of cults that seem to exploit or mistreat their members and the readiness of devotees to accept seemingly strange ideas seem unintelligible in terms of Locke's model. Since their behavior isn't explicable in purely rational terms, members of cults must be brainwashed or incompetent! Freud's view of group process implies that cult membership will serve personal motives embedded in family and sexual life. Membership in a cult might reduce intrapsychic conflicts or provide objects of transference love. Freud's model ignores the role of alienation. The wish for group membership and tendencies to conform are seen as symptomatic of underlying neurotic needs. The sociologist's model, derived from Durkheim, tells us about the needs of the cult but not of the people who join it. Finally, believing that the wish to belong to an in-group and tendencies to conform are bulwarks against existential fear, the existentialist, like the Freudian, might think they will disappear with adequate analysis.

In terms of the model described in this chapter, cult membership is an indirect measure of a larger social failure: to satisfy in a constructive way group-affiliative needs, particularly of the young. The issue here is not that young people can't make friends, but that our society may be failing to provide them with a sense of real community, which is more than the sum of fragmented dyadic relationships. As noted earlier, this point has been forcefully made by Bellah and colleagues (10). An obvious consequence of this view is that in order to reduce the appeal of cults, efforts should be directed less toward individuals than toward their social circumstances. Some of these efforts may be highly focused on particular institutions. For example, I noted above that large college campuses have become cult recruitment grounds. Greater attention to the constructive social integration of young college students might shut off cult recruiters from some of their likeliest prospects. Freshmen students arriving at large campuses often feel estranged from any real community. Although mainstream religious groups and various campus organizations help students overcome their sense of alienation, communal living arrangements are probably most important in the crucial period when the student has just left home. Fraternities and sororities in particular have the in-group exclusivity, elaborate initiation rites, and group secrets and rituals which prepare them to serve this function. But even the larger dormitories and cooperatives usually have a distinctive culture and provide some sense of membership. However, at the present time many large state-university campuses lack adequate communal residence space to house new students. Freshmen students must compete to obtain the available rooms. For this and other reasons, many students fall through the cracks and remain alienated through their early college years. At least some of these will sooner or later join a cult.

Similar considerations apply in assessing efforts to change those who have already joined a cult. From the present point of view, the success or failure of efforts to "rehabilitate" cult members cannot be judged merely by whether the members stay out of their cults. Instead, success must be judged according to how well ex-cult members sublimate the wish for an in-group which may have led to their joining. Insofar as in-group dispositions are part of the human endowment, success must be judged according to whether these can be harnessed for socially and personally constructive ends. For instance, at least some ex-cult members may become extrinsically religious members of mainstream churches. Although such an outcome might please family members, from the point of view taken here the underlying problems with group-related behaviors have not substantially changed. Similar remarks would apply to ex-cult members who join nonreligious groups with a cultlike social structure or to those who, after the cult, never again find a group to which they feel committed. In terms of the model presented here, the truly "cured" cult member would find in larger society a basis for group identity consistent with personal freedom and dignity and with respect for other peoples. Bellah and coworkers say that that is hard to do in modern American life (10). If so, in the long run the challenge posed by cults is addressed to American culture and not to any single profession or special interest.

References

1. Wilson EO: Sociobiology: The New Synthesis. Cambridge, MA, Harvard University Press, 1975
2. Kaplan AL, ed: The Sociobiology Debate: Readings on Ethical and Scientific Issues. New York, Harper & Row, 1978
3. Clutton-Brock TH, Harvey PH, eds: Readings in Sociobiology. San Francisco, WH Freeman, 1978
4. Alexander RD: Darwinism and Human Affairs. Seattle, University of Washington Press, 1979
5. Reynolds PC: On the Evolution of Human Behavior: the Argument from Animals to Man. Berkeley, University of California Press, 1981
6. Breuer G: Sociobiology and the Human Dimension. Cambridge, England, Cambridge University Press, 1982
7. Trivers R: Social Evolution. Menlo Park, CA, Benjamin/Cummings, 1985
8. King's College Sociobiology Group, eds: Current Problems in Sociobiology. Cambridge, England, Cambridge University Press, 1982
9. Wenegrat B: Sociobiology and Mental Disorder: A New View. Menlo Park, CA, Addison-Wesley, 1984
10. Bellah RN, Madsen R, Sullivan WM, et al: Habits of the Heart. Berkeley, University of California Press, 1985
11. Freud S: Totem and Taboo, in The Standard Edition of the Complete Psychological Works of Sigmund Freud (Vol XIII, pp 1–162). London, Hogarth Press, 1955 (Original work published 1913)

12. Durkheim E: The Rules of Sociological Method. Glencoe, IL, Free Press, 1950
13. Yalom ID: Existential Psychotherapy. New York, Basic Books, 1980
14. Durkheim E: The Elementary Forms of the Religious Life. New York, Collier, 1961
15. Weber M: The Protestant Ethic and the Spirit of Capitalism. New York, Scribner's, 1930
16. Troeltsch E: The Social Teachings of the Christian Churches. New York, Macmillan, 1931
17. Johnson B: On church and sect. Am Sociol Rev 28:539, 1963
18. Lopreato J: Human Nature and Biocultural Evolution. Boston, Allen and Unwin, 1984
19. Galanter M, Buckley P: Evangelical religion and meditation: psychotherapeutic effects. J Nerv Ment Dis 166:685, 1978
20. Galanter M: The "Relief Effect": a sociobiological model for neurotic distress and large-group therapy. Am J Psychiatry 135: 588–591, 1978
21. Lofland J, Stark R: Becoming a world-saver: a theory of conversion to a deviant perspective. American Sociological Review 30:862–875, 1965
22. Levine SV: Role of psychiatry in the phenomenon of cults. Can J Psychiatry 24:593, 1979
23. Levine SV: Alienated Jewish youth and religious seminaries: an alternative to cults? in Psychodynamic Perspectives on Religion Sect and Cult. Edited by Halperin DA. Boston, John Wright, 1983
24. Galanter M: Psychological induction into the large-group: findings from a modern religious sect. Am J Psychiatry 137:1574–1575, 1980
25. Luckmann T: Personal identity as an evolutionary and historical problem, in Human Ethology: Claims and Limits of a New Discipline. Edited by von Cranach M, Foppa K, Lepenies W, et al. Cambridge, England, Cambridge University Press, 1979
26. Brooks A: "Cults" and the aged: a new family issue. New York Times, April 26, 1986
27. Etemad B: Extrication from cultism. Current Psychiatric Therapy 18:217, 1978
28. Halperin DA: Group processes in cult affiliation and recruitment, in Psychodynamic Perspectives on Religion, Sect and Cult. Edited by Halperin DA. Boston, John Wright, 1983
29. Galper MF: The atypical dissociative disorder: some etiological, diagnostic, and treatment issues, in Psychodynamic Perspectives on Religion, Sect and Cult. Edited by Halperin DA. Boston, John Wright, 1983
30. Berger PL, Luckmann T: The Social Construction of Reality: A Treatise in the Sociology of Knowledge. Garden City, NJ, Doubleday, 1966
31. Clark JG: On the further study of destructive cultism, in Psychodynamic Perspectives on Religion, Sect and Cult. Edited by Halperin DA. Boston, John Wright, 1983

32. Long TE, Hadden JK: Religious conversion and the concept of socialization: integrating the brainwashing and drift models. Journal for the Scientific Study of Religion 22:1, 1983
33. Galanter M, Rabkin R, Rabkin J, et al: The "Moonies": a psychological study of conversion and membership in a contemporary religious sect. Am J Psychiatry 136:165–170, 1979
34. Galanter M: Charismatic religious sects and psychiatry: an overview. Am J Psychiatry 139:1539–1548, 1982
35. Reynolds V, Tanner R: The Biology of Religion. New York, Longman, 1983
36. Ungerleider JT, Wellisch DK: Coercive persuasion (brainwashing), religious cults, and deprogramming. Am J Psychiatry 136:279–282, 1979
37. Brown LB: A study of religious belief. Br J Psychol 53:259, 1962
38. Martin C, Nichols RC: Personality and religious belief. Journal of Social Psychology 56:3, 1962
39. Allport GW: The Nature of Prejudice. Cambridge, MA, Addison-Wesley, 1954
40. Allport GW: The religious context of prejudice. Journal for the Scientific Study of Religion 5:447, 1966
41. Allport GW, Ross JM: Personal religious orientation and prejudice. Journal of Personality and Social Psychology 5:432, 1967
42. Spilka B, Hood RW, Gorsuch RL: The Psychology of Religion: An Empirical Approach. Englewood Cliffs, NJ, Prentice-Hall, 1985
43. Allen RO, Spilka B: Committed and consensual religion: a specification of religion-prejudice relationships. Journal for the Scientific Study of Religion 6:191, 1967
44. Hunt RA, King MB: The intrinsic-extrinsic concept: a review and evaluation. Journal for the Scientific Study of Religion 10:339, 1971
45. Pargament KI, Steele RE, Tyler FB: Religious participation, religious motivation, and psychosocial competence. Journal for the Scientific Study of Religion 18:412, 1979
46. Spilka B: Utilitarianism and personal faith. Journal of Psychology and Theology 5:226, 1977
47. Hood RW: Normative and motivational determinants of reported religious experience in two Baptist samples. Review of Religious Research 13:192, 1972
48. Hood RW: Religious orientation and the experience of transcendance. Journal for the Scientific Study of Religion 12:441, 1973
49. Hood RW, Morris R: Sensory isolation and the differential elicitation of religious imagery in intrinsic and extrinsic persons. Journal for the Scientific Study of Religion 20:261, 1981

ENTRY AND DEPARTURE FROM THE SECTS

Chapter 12

THE PSYCHOLOGY OF INDUCTION: A REVIEW AND INTERPRETATION

James T. Richardson, Ph.D., J.D.

In recent years considerable controversy has raged about cults or new religions, representing yet another chapter in the history of conflict over religion in America. The major controversy has centered on induction and resocialization practices of the new religions (1).

Some representatives of a few more traditional religious groups and certain members of relevant disciplines claim that most of the new religions engage in "mind control," "brainwashing," or "thought reform" closely akin to what was assumed to have been practiced by the Chinese communists (2). Some others claim that a new insidious process that goes even beyond brainwashing models is at work (3). Some believe that this type of recruitment tactic demands intervention in order to reunite the member with his or her family and society (4, 5). Other researchers see more normal processes of resocialization taking place and shy away from derivatives of the brainwashing view explanations of the induction process (6–8). Many of these researchers point out that most, if not all, of those who participate in the new religions apparently do so through an exercise of their volition, and that they also usually exercise their volition to leave after a time (9–11). Some of these same researchers do not blame the new religions for disrupting or destroying family relations, and instead may cite both the problems with the family as an institution and the interest of many young people in new religions as symptoms of contemporary problems, rather than variables that are directly, causally related (12).

The level of disagreement between the two camps is not always constant, and not all researchers who study the new religions fit easily into one group or the other. However, the differences of opinion sometimes go beyond the realm of the polite and formal usually exhibited at scholarly conferences. Quite frequently scholars involved in the study of recruitment to new religions find themselves on different sides of heated debates in the media, speaking at conferences and meetings of groups supportive or opposed to new religions, and even opposing one another in significant legal proceedings and legislative hearings.

Such disagreement among those involved in research on the new religions demands attention (13). It is both disquieting and even embarrassing that scholars supposedly studying the same phenomena could have such strong differences of opinion. Discerning why such differences of opinion exist is no simple task, but it is one purpose of this chapter to discuss a few reasons why conclusions about induction into new religions diverge so much. Before that discussion, however, an effort will be made to summarize research results on the induction process itself, using work by scholars from several disciplines. This summary will focus on general features of underlying "deep structure" and ritual behaviors in new religions as they relate to the recruitment or induction process. This section of the chapter is derived in part from an earlier work that focused on similarities between psychotherapies and new religions (13).

Underlying Deep Structure

An underlying "deep structure" is evident in many of the new religious groups. According to Jerome Frank (14), the effectiveness of both psychotherapy and religious conversion generally depends on a common structure by which the therapist or religious group attempts to counteract the person's demoralization. This common structure includes the following: 1) a special supportive, empathic, and confiding relationship between the client and therapist or adherent and religious group; 2) a special setting imbued with powerful symbols of expertise, help, hope, and healing; 3) a special rationale, ideology, or indisputable myth that explains health, illness, and normality and that renders sensible the person's self-preoccupations and inexplicable feelings within a logically tight framework; and 4) a special set of rituals and practices that confirms the person's assumptive world and insures within that context a constellation of new learning experiences and successful outcomes.

These structural elements appear to constitute a necessary condition for successful induction into religious groups, both new and old. The elements are nonspecific in the effects they produce to the degree that they interact independent of a particular form, content, or procedure.

Empirical evidence is accruing that indicates the above structural elements and their nonspecific effects are evident in some new religious and quasireligious group contexts as well (15–27). Galanter and Buckley (17), for example, specifically found that membership in the Divine Light Mission (DLM) was associated with widespread decline in psychological distress and concluded, consistent with Frank's earlier work, "Both techniques provide patients with assistance in dispelling distress by offering them in a supportive manner a series of assumptions about their distress which are consistent with their underlying attitudes" (p. 689). This nonspecific and therapeutic response is evident in some newer religions, self-help groups, consciousness-raising groups, and certain cultic milieus (16). This response has also been demonstrated with individuals from different backgrounds (23), in a variety of different religious groups and movements (22, 26, 28–30), just by attending a series of religious seminars (31), and in one of the more totalistic communal groups (18).

Galanter's 1980 study of the large-group–induction techniques used by the Unification Church can provide us with an example of these common structural elements operative in many new religious conversion settings. [Also see Lofland's (21) discussion of the same group's techniques.] This group, the Unification Church, is somewhat atypical in that they are usually more systematic than most new religious groups in their recruitment efforts. However, the group can serve as a vehicle to examine Frank's ideas.

In his examination of three workshop periods, Galanter found support for 1) a special relationship between the inductees and their hosts—a strong sense of cohesiveness developed during the workshops, especially in the close relationship (i.e., constant supervision, shared reflections, and intense discussions) between the guests and hosts who invited them; 2) a special setting—the workshop center is typically located in a secluded, rustic setting and is symbolically imbued with powerful symbols of hope, healing, and spiritual growth; 3) special rituals—the workshops are structured around a group of activities (e.g., lectures, group discussions, group recreational activities, and reflection periods) which indicate the way a person goes about converting himself or herself; and 4) a special rationale—guests are exposed to and are encouraged to learn the group's creed and religious beliefs which are offered to explain the new recruit's past and present experiences. The presence of these four common elements appear related, in turn, to the improvement in the psychological well-being of members long after joining, and to have contributed to their strong affiliative ties to one another.

Richardson et al. (24) also offer specific detail about the conversion or induction process in the large Jesus Movement group they studied. While they treat the process as a social-psychological one and do not directly apply Frank's ideas of therapeutic structure, it is apparent that the process contains all four elements. The detail available in this study of a communal group clearly shows the special relationship between the member and the group, a special setting imbued with powerful symbols, a specific ideology that is all-encompassing, and special rituals that affirm the world view of the group. Nordquist's (27) careful study of life in an Eastern-oriented group also demonstrates the presence of Frank's underlying structure.

In sum, there is a growing body of empirical research on new religious groups and groups with similar characteristics that is generally supportive of Frank's (14) early comparative analysis of psychotherapy and religious conversion. This common, underlying, deep structure—special setting, relationship, rationale, and rituals—is usually accompanied by a general increase in the adherent's sense of well-being, or a nonspecific "relief effect" (15, 32). Also, corrective experiences and direct feedback are part of most new religious rituals. Beneficial effects from new religious group membership have been subsequently reported for a wide variety of new groups and persons, and they appear to ensue independent of specific cultic beliefs and practices (30).

Induction and Resocialization Rituals

In addition to the underlying structure, religious conversion or induction also serves certain ritual functions. Wallace (33) has contended, for example, that all rituals deal with the problem of transformations of state in human beings or in nature. Two rituals of particular relevance to new religions are those of therapy and salvation. Therapy or healing rituals aim to control human health and tend to embed themselves in past events, whereas salvation rituals aim to renew a damaged identity and to direct themselves toward the future. In new religious groups it is more or less assumed by all parties to the interactions that the adherent is striving to forge a new identity and is in need of some kind of special healing. The combination of healing and salvation rituals as a kind of rite of passage is probably what makes religious conversion or induction, functionally speaking, such a powerful socializer of human behavior. Renunciation, expiation, and cleansing manifest themselves in such contexts. Individuals successfully inducted into most of the new religions emerge in a metaphorically transformed sense as individuals resocialized into a new psychological or social world.

The "rite of passage" nature of such healing and salvation rituals in new religions typically involves three stages: separation (whether physical or psychological); transition (learning the new role and worldview); and incorporation (adopting the standards of the system and living by it). Moreover, they effectively impress on the initiate: 1) how a change in one's self is sequentially managed within a particular structure with the assistance or guidance of a particular person or group; and 2) how the outcomes can be ultimately attributed to one's own efforts.

Richardson and Kilbourne (34) have recently applied the above reasoning in a comparison of the use of the brainwashing-thought-reform models of the 1950s with their contemporary application to new religions. They believe that the four major models of "brainwashing"—the neo-Freudian (35), the physiologic (36), the Pavlovian and psychoanalytic (37), and the cognitive and social-psychological (38)—can be similarly conceptualized in terms of a three-stage "rite of passage" ritual to explicate the resocialization process [also see Somit (39)]. These three stages consist of an individual's initial socioemotional breakdown, followed by a period of developing commitment to and identification with the captors (in the Korean War situation), and the person's resulting immersion into a new group and legitimated normative structure. Each stage is associated with a particular kind of control over the person (i.e., stimulus control, response control, and normative control, respectively) and seems highly ritualized, as are many religious settings (40, 41).

Applications of so-called brainwashing or thought reform models to the new religions have major difficulties. Richardson and colleagues (42) point out that the Lifton thought reform model does not fit the Jesus Movement in several ways, including the all-important absence of any physical coercion. Taylor's (43) careful study of recruitment processes in the Unification Church also notes significant differences between Lifton's research and his own. He concludes that "the recruitment process . . . resembles evangelistic exhortation more than coercion" (p. 89). However, it is plain there are some similarities, if only because both the brainwashing-thought-reform setting and participation in a new religion involve resocialization. But a key difference between the Korean War prisoner situation and participation in a new religion is that of volition (43). Nevertheless, even this distinction needs to be qualified, since the initial context of some of the key brainwashing research contained evidence of considerable volitional change. For instance, Lifton's (35) classic study of thought reform closes with a chapter discussing reeducation and "open" (i.e., voluntary) personal change in the context of the communist revolution in China. This more volitional aspect, which is seldom cited in contemporary application of Lifton's work, also contains the three-stage ritual process of healing and salvation seen in so many resocialization settings.

Ofshe et al. (44) have suggested a similar three-stage "rite of passage" healing and salvation ritual in relation to their studies of Synanon, and have contended that the key to self-change and commitment resides in the group or group leader, causing the target person and others to produce behaviors signifying to the target person and others that self-change and commitment exist. By making small demands on the individual within a context of voluntarism or illusory voluntarism, the individual comes to view himself or herself as autonomous, and eventually conforms to the new role requirements. Ofshe (45) further points out the importance of creating some kind of intense emotional or high arousal experience in a ritualistic fashion in order to provide the individual with a credible account (46, 47) by which to justify a major life decision or life change. We can see, then, how the rituals of healing and salvation and their "rite of passage" nature ultimately function as legitimating interactional episodes (48), both to move the person in the direction of desired change and to confirm the new worldview and sense of self.

Controversy over Induction Process

The foregoing has been a straightforward discussion of research findings about the process of affiliation with newer religions or so-called cults. Data have been presented from a number of reputable scholars in several disciplines, all of whom seem to share a general agreement that what happens in new religious groups' recruitment and induction efforts is fairly easy to understand, and follows normal rules of behavior as propounded by sociologists, social psychologists, psychiatrists, and psychologists. However, as is well known, there is considerable controversy over the meaning of the process. Other scholars claim vastly different results from research on new religious recruitment, and there is a significantly different interpretation offered in the popular media as well (49). This difference of opinion cannot be fully examined in this context. However, it demands some attention, and to this I now turn.

First I will offer a view of the differences between scholars that attends to variations in general perspective toward the subject matter. I will then present a discussion of differences in background and social location of researchers that contributes to differences in ideological orientation. Then I will deal with the fact that researchers are often studying different things in actuality and that they have tendencies to overgeneralize findings. Lastly there will be some comments on the implication of different methodologies of research employed by scholars in this area of study.

Differences in Perspective

This broad consideration, which will be covered in some depth, covers a "multitude of sins." An earlier report on changing paradigms in conversion research (50) discusses the way that many scholar's views of the recruitment or induction process have changed in recent years. This change has occurred mainly because of research on induction into newer religions, but also as a result of related research on participation in political movements of the past few decades in America.

The major thesis of this report was that something akin to a new alternative paradigm in the Kuhnian sense is development in research and conversion and induction, especially research in sociology and social psychology. The old paradigm, with its assumptions about the passivity of human beings, and its overemphasis on the individual, is giving way, at least partially, to another view. This new view stresses humans as volitional entities who assign meaning to their action and to the actions of others within a social context. This paradigm shift may well be a part of related developing concerns within the disciplines of psychology, sociology, and social psychology. However, research in the area of recruitment to new religions is contributing its own independent impact.

The Old Paradigm of Conversion or Induction

The traditional conceptualization of the induction process derives from the culture of which it is a part. The prototype is the common interpretation of the conversion of Paul on the road to Damascus. The "Pauline experience" has been a major basis for understanding religious induction experiences for people of Western European culture, especially since the time of the Reformation. The revivalist tradition in America continued and even augmented the focus on Pauline-like conversion experience because of the emphasis on recruitment that was brought on by the "free market" in religion resulting from the lack of an official state church. This prototype has gained new impetus of late via some of the new religious movements of Christian origin, such as the Charismatic Renewal and the Jesus Movement (51). Even some of the Eastern-oriented religions, such as Hare Krishna, have adopted a view of recruitment to new religions that seems similar in important ways to the Pauline experience (52).

A characterization of common perceptions of the Pauline experience on the road to Damascus yields some interesting insights into how most people in Western culture have typically viewed the act of joining a religious group. First, the experience had been perceived to be sudden, dramatic, and emotional; it had a definite irrational quality to it. It was inexplicable in any terms except those that included an active agent not under the person's control. A powerful external agent over which Paul held no sway caused Paul to be converted. Traditional views of this event attribute agency to an omnipotent god; more recent "sophisticated" views attribute agency to unconscious psychological influence or similar concepts. Whatever the characterization of the active agent, that agent is definitely not the person. In Paul's case an ostensibly powerful man was totally incapacitated by the actions of the external causal agent focusing on him as an individual.

The Pauline experience also is viewed as a single event thoroughly changing one's life. Thus the event was viewed in individualized and psychologized ways. A single individual was changed via a total break with the past in a relatively permanent way. One static personal situation was dramatically modified into another static situation. The conversion involved an apparent total negation of the old self and the implantation of a new self, at least as it was experienced by Paul and represented by many since.

The Pauline experience is also often interpreted in cognitive terms. It was thought that what happened to Paul caused him to change his beliefs immediately, and that behaviors congruent with the new beliefs then were developed. Behaviors follow beliefs, then, in the traditional paradigm.

In sum, the traditional view of this experience is psychological, deterministic, and assumes a passive subject. It is usually viewed as predestinational (using a theologically connoted term) or predispositional (to use a more psychological term). More sociological terms that might be fitted into this deterministic model include such notions as situationally determined.

The Old Paradigm and Brainwashing Models

Brainwashing is a popularized term that has been applied to a supposedly mysterious process whereby Chinese and Russian communists extracted confessions from prisoners and seemed to change, at least temporarily, the beliefs, and even the values, of these individuals. A number of classic studies and interpretations of this phenomenon have been offered by scholars, including especially the four mentioned (35–38). Nearly all such studies, with the partial exception of Schein et al.'s work (38), treat brainwashing in a way that exemplifies the traditional conversion and induction paradigm.

Most interpretations of brainwashing assume a relatively passive subject under the control of all-powerful external agents who use omnipotent and evil techniques. The change associated with brainwashing involves a total negation of the old self and the substitution of a new one in its place. The change is viewed as relatively sudden, dramatic, and emotional. Physical and mental coercion are assumed to be crucial in bringing about significant cognitive changes.

As pointed out in Richardson and Kilbourne's (34) discussion of brainwashing models, Biderman (53) offered some 20 years ago an analysis of why the term brainwashing came to prominence in the 1950s and 1960s in the West. He noted that most of the researchers were caught up in the anticommunist rhetoric of the cold war, which permeated their analysis. Biderman said that there seemed to be an assumption that communist beliefs were "fundamentally alien to human nature and social reality. The acceptance of communist beliefs is consequently regarded as ipso facto evidence of insanity or a warped, evil personality, or both" (p. 560). This anticommunist sentiment was also antitotalitarian and anticollectivistic in orientation, with even an element of racism included. Such an ideologically based view contributed to a misunderstanding of so-called brainwashing phenomena in the 1950s that still persists, as evidenced by the casual use of such approaches being offered today by some scholars and laypeople in discussions of new religions' induction processes. Sociologist Tom Robbins has referred to applications of such views to induction into new religions as the "invasion of the body snatchers" or "Little Red Riding Hood" view, terms that seem apropos in light of the historical development of the concept (34).

Emergence of a New "Activist" Perspective

Within the social and behavioral sciences there have always been those who opted for a more humanistic perspective that allowed for an acting and conscious human agent. Within the psycho-analytic tradition Jung broke dramatically with Freud and claimed that religion can often help people integrate their lives. The very title of Jung's best-known book, *Modern Man in Search of a Soul* (54) illustrates his more "active agency" view. The work of Gordon Allport (55) in the area of psychology of religion also tends toward this different view, as does the work of Viktor Frankl, whose *Man's Search for Meaning* (56) involves a rejection of Freudian-dominated perspectives. William James's work, partic-ularly his discussion of "volitional conversion" as contrasted to "the conversion of self-surrender," is also germane (57).

Within sociology we have seen newer, more humanistically oriented, interpretations being offered—views that take a some-what "softer" line toward such matters as religion, religious experiences, and other activities, which were previously viewed as frivolous, that might be viewed as fulfilling for individuals (58). Within social psychology a rejection of the mechanistic view of the human being has attempted to turn that discipline on its head and encourage it to overcome the domination of the labora-tory as the only acceptable research site (59–62).

It is within this broad, more humanistic tradition in sociology and social psychology, but also somewhat independent of it, that a new paradigm has begun to develop. Recent work on new religious movements by some sociologists, social psychologists, and a few psychologists and psychiatrists has helped produce an alternative view of conversion and induction into the new reli-gions consonant with this paradigm.

Although there are a number of different developments within sociology and social psychology that relate to the rise of an alternative paradigm, one of the most important occurred with the publication of the oft-cited article by John Lofland and Rodney Stark (63). They presented a model of "conversion to a deviant perspective" that incorporated both predispositional and situational elements. This model was developed out of re-search on the beginnings of the Unification Church in America (64, 65), which makes it very germane to the subject of induction into new religions. Their work can be viewed as the beginning of sociological and social psychological studies of participation in new religious movements. At the time of their work no one guessed that either the specific group studied or the larger movement itself would gain the attention that it has, and no one could have anticipated the major impact of their conversion model.

The Lofland and Stark model was an important step in the process of developing an alternative paradigm because it served as a bridge between old and new approaches. The model contained a logically complete and up-to-date statement of the traditional psychological predisposition perspective (often referred to as the "motivational" model in the literature) that focused on the forces that might "push" a person into conversion. This view is derivative of the "Pauline paradigm" described herein. But the model also spoke of the future of research on conversion by focusing on the process of conversion which, of course, was a recognition that conversion has a definite organizational aspect and is a social event. One other key aspect of the model was the incorporation of subjects who would sometimes self-define themselves as religious seekers and take action to change by deciding to interact with selected people and allowing affective ties to develop with them. Thus the Lofland and Stark model contained an implicit focus on a volitional subject, along with more traditional deterministic elements.

Lofland has moved more overtly in the direction of the activist perspective, as evidenced by his book *Doing Social Life* (66) and his more recent major updating of the earlier model (65). He says of this shift:

> I have since come to appreciate that the world-saver model embodies a thoroughly "passive" actor—a conception of humans as a 'neutral medium which social forces operate'. . . . It is with such a realization that I have of late encouraged students of conversion to turn the process on its head and to scrutinize how people go about converting themselves. Assume, that is, that the person is active rather than merely passive. (p. 22)

Straus, a Lofland student who has done research on Scientology and other new religious groups, in a report published as part of Lofland's book *Doing Social Life* (67), develops a model of "seeking" or "creative transformation" that relies on a view of human beings as active and meaning-seeking entities. He decries earlier work in the area of "identity change" that employs a "passive image of humans," and instead opts for a perspective that assumes "the individual human acting creatively within a natural life setting in order to construct a satisfying life" (p. 252). His model of creative transformation is apparently the first explicit treatment in the literature on conversion and induction to adopting such an explicitly activist view of human beings. Included in this provocative work are discussions of initial "creative bumbling," and "strategies for creative exploitation" (by individuals seeking to join a new group, in contrast to usual interpretations of the conversion situation). In a later work (8) Straus discusses in more depth the activist paradigm that he was positing in the earlier work. He says:

> Sociologists have conventionally approached religious conversion as something that happens to a person who is destabilized by external and internal forces and then brought to commit self to a conversionistic group by social forces applied by that 'trip' . . . and its agents. This stands in contrast to an alternative paradigm of the individual seeker striving and strategizing to achieve quantum changes in his or her life experience, and which treats the groups and others involved in this process as salesmen, shills, coaches, guides and helpers—themselves typically converts further along in their own personal quests. (p. 158)

Also of note is the work of Balch and Taylor, who studied a much publicized UFO group (68, 69). In their 1978 report they include a section on "The Role of the Seeker," in which they delineate the active searching behavior of most of their respondents. This seeking approach to life is of such importance that some people become members, in spite of the absence of some usually expected pressures such as the development of interaction and affective ties between members and prospects. In a later work, Balch (70) deliberately contrasts the two perspectives, referring to one as "structural-functional" (by which he means our "passive model") and the other (using Straus's term) as "activist." He says:

> The most conspicuous failure of the structural model is its inability to account for decisions to join the UFO cult. Much has been written about the devious ways that cults lure unsuspecting recruits into their psychological traps. The prevailing view is that recruitment techniques systematically exploit powerful social and psychological forces that weaken the prospective members' critical judgment. . . . This argument is not

a very useful explanation of recruitment and conversion to the
UFO cult. . . . Recruitment was structured to reduce contacts
between members and would-be recruits. . . . Interaction was
severely circumscribed. . . . [The leaders offered] their message on a take-it-or-leave-it basis . . . the UFO cult did not
systematically manipulate social pressures to get people to
join. (pp. 8–9)

Balch states that the critical similarity among those who joined
was (70) (p. 9): "All of them defined themselves as seekers before
joining." He also noted how the prospects then decided to
cooperate with efforts to convert themselves and willingly
played the role of new converts, which involved many changes
of behavior and belief. Balch pursues this role-playing idea in
another work (71) in which he explicitly rejects brainwashing
interpretations of joining a new religion in favor of a more
mundane role theory interpretation. He says: "their overt behavior was misleading. They looked tuned in, appeared committed,
but were simply playing a role that concealed their true feelings"
(p. 4). Balch stresses then the volitional aspects of role-playing
and urges: "Don't be deceived by appearances" (p. 42) into
inferring total commitment from behavior.

Bromley and Shupe (72), who have studied the Unification
Church and other groups, have also applied a role theory perspective to conversion to new religious movements. Bromley
and Shupe conclude that the old motivational model focusing on
predispositions is inadequate. Instead they note that the rapid
conversion syndrome which has gained so much attention is
more easily explicable in terms of "socially structured events
arising out of the role relationship" (p. 161). They discuss the
pattern of people deciding to play roles and getting involved in a
group, with a more thoroughgoing acceptance of beliefs occurring later in the recruitment process. As such, their model is at
least implicitly more activist in orientation because of its stress on
the decision to become involved in the role.

Kilbourne and Richardson (73) have related sociological role
theory to Robert Lifton's protean-human concept, albeit with a
more positive interpretation than is usually given the concept.
They define a new "social experimenter role" in society as one
"played" for at least a time by many people in our society who
try out different therapies, life-styles, or religions in an experi-

mentally oriented way, seeking to have self-growth experiences and change their identities. [See Kilbourne and Richardson (13) for a discussion of the competition among various alternative therapies and the new religions.]

Downton (28), in his study of joining the Divine Light Mission, posited an active subject seeking out new ways to live and new interpretations of life. While he did integrate some of the notions of external pressures that usually accompany more deterministic sociological work, he was in the main activist in orientation and put the major responsibility for conversion on the seeking subject. His book explained in great detail the way in which DLM converts managed their own induction into the DLM.

Travisano (74), building on Berger's notion of "alternation" (58), has presented an interpretation of conversion in the symbolic interactionist tradition. Travisano's seminal report implies an active subject more or less in control of his or her own destiny, seeking out changes in identity. This work has been used by Gordon (75) in a study of a Jesus Movement group, but the active agent perspective is somewhat subdued. Richardson (6) critiques and builds on the work of Travisano and Gordon in developing a more explicit application of symbolic interaction theory to recruitment in new religions. In doing so, he applies an activist orientation in explaining the "conversion careers" of individuals participating in the new movements. He states that one of the factors crucial in explaining what happens is "the explicit plans, desires, or motives of people involved in conversion careers" (p. 50). Pilarzyk (52) also applies Berger's phenomenological perspective in a very insightful comparison of recruitment and induction processes used by the DLM and the Hare Krishna group. He concludes that there are vast differences between the two group's approaches, which he labels "sectarian conversion" in the Hare Krishna group and "cultic alternation" in the DLM. However, both types of induction imply an active, meaning-seeking subject.

More recently, in the study of new religions an explicit focus on leaving new religions has developed. This area of study has developed as researchers recognized that only a small minority of those who join such groups actually stay for lengthy periods of time (9, 11, 76). The act of leaving (or disaffection, deconversion, or disaffiliation) has, by its very nature, led to greater recognition of the volitional nature of such actions. Thus this area of study contributed its own impetus to the emergence of an alternative paradigm in conversion and recruitment research as more and more research focused on the high turnover rates in newer religions (10, 16, 26, 32, 47, 77–81).

Thus it appears that a steady evolution of a new view of conversion and induction into the study of new religions can be traced in the work of a number of researchers over the past 15 or 20 years. That work has taken several theoretical paths, but an overall trend seems unmistakable. These several scholars have, explicitly or implicitly, recognized a more active subject, "working out," or at least actively contributing to, his or her own induction. They have noted that induction into new religions often means a series of affiliative and disaffiliative acts that constitute a conversion career, and that individuals are often only deciding to behave, at least for a time, as a convert, playing the convert role, as they experiment with ways to affirm their personhood. These researchers have found that induction is a social phenomenon, with affection and emotional ties playing key roles in the affirmative decision to negotiate with a group about possible participation and commitment. This new emerging paradigm competes against modern versions of the traditional "Pauline paradigm" that has been dominant for decades. The most notable version of the traditional paradigm relevant to this chapter is, of course, the "brainwashing" view already briefly described.

Why the Difference in Perspective?

As suggested, a major shift of perspective may be occurring in the area of recruitment/induction to new religions. If so, it is important to know why this is happening. Even if there is no paradigm shift taking place, it is important to attend to the general views taken by scholars studying induction into new religions, and to make an effort to explain differences that exist. The following is based in part on an earlier effort (82), offered to add to the dialogue about the meaning of the new religions in our society. A number of ideas will be presented which, taken as a whole, may shed some light on the controversy about induction into new religions.

Ideological Orientation

First, at the risk of offending some, it should be noted that many members of the social and behavioral science disciplines are at least implicitly antireligion in their approach to life and scholarship. And some who are not antireligion "in general" may be personally opposed to specific versions of religion. Others may be somewhat proreligion, or at least sympathetic to specific versions of religion. Thus some of the willingness to adopt one perspective or another on cults may derive from something of an ideological bias, either for or against religious or quasireligious solutions to problems.

Certain theoretical perspectives seem to be in competition with religious worldviews, and perhaps this influences the work of some scholars in significant ways. For instance, what little writing there has been about new religions by scholars of a more Marxian perspective (83) seems as negative toward them as that of at least one sociologist who is an avowed evangelical (84). Sociologists within the deviancy tradition may make certain assumptions about those they study, especially if such researchers operate within what is sometimes referred to as the "nuts and sluts" tradition, which seems to study "weirdos" partially for the entertainment value of such work. It is also not surprising to find some more psychoanalytically oriented therapists espousing negative views about religion, new or old (2). Indeed, some variants of this broad perspective, in ways analogous to the view of religion by Marxists, treat religions as at least a symptom, if not a direct cause of bad personal states (13). One prominent therapist (4) whose work is often associated with the anticult movement, has demonstrated this position by stating in a professional paper that the urgent question motivating his work is, "What kind of nutty people get into these crazy groups?" Moving from such mental constraints to examine the phenomenon of new religions from an objective view may be very difficult for those heavily committed to alternative perspectives.

The social location of the researcher is related to the perspec-

tive issue, but is a more straightforward sociological notion. By
this term is meant the more simple considerations such as age,
social class, occupation, and so on. It seems a reasonable conclusion to draw that people are influenced by the social situations of
which they are a part. Thus it is very understandable that some
individuals involved with family therapy would tend to blame
new religions for heaping more trouble on an obviously already
overburdened institution of the family (85–87). And it is just as
easy to understand why some who view themselves as young
rebels against society's dominant institutions and values would
respond favorably toward groups that also seem opposed to
these things, even if the groups' ways of showing rebellion
seems a bit odd. Conversely, some people whose profession
inclines them toward accepting the dominant values of society
and helping people adjust to those values, may be less apprecia-
tive of groups and individuals who want to do things differently.
But for someone not so enamored with society's values and
norms, identification with "underdog" groups (which certainly
includes most new religions) may come easy.

It seems reasonable to assume that most involved in this area
of research take the view they do based on sound motives and
sincerely held beliefs. This is a normal state of affairs. However,
we should recognize that the "place from whence we come"
influences our scholarly perspective. A corollary of that position
is that there may not be just one brand of truth available in this
area of study, and no one person or group has a monopoly on
"The Truth." This comment leads directly to the next point.

Studying Different Things

Another major reason why researchers draw different conclusions from their work is the rather simple fact that they are often
studying different phenomena. One is reminded of the fable of
the blind men trying to describe an elephant by feeling just one
part of the huge animal. Some people are studying life in the
groups making up the broader new religious movement (18, 21,
23, 24, 27). Such scholars often use a combination of methods,
including both formal and informal interviews, applying standardized assessment instruments of various kinds, and participant observation, which means that the researcher stays with
the group for at least a reasonable time, observing what they do.

Quite often the focus of study in such research is on questions of how and why people join, and what effects this has on them. Some researchers, on the other hand, are studying people who have left such groups (4, 5, 88), for whatever reason and through whatever method, and who also have some perceived difficulty with readjustment such that they or someone close to them has referred them for therapy. Thus the therapy situation becomes a research data-gathering setting, a situation not without some epistomological problems.

But that comment is not meant to suggest that the first research situation described is not without its own perils. Researchers living with groups are not by definition brainwashed by them, but are plainly studying a group of people relatively content with remaining in the group, even if temporarily. This fact should be recognized so that the participant-observer researcher is not fooled by a description of what are normal social processes of self-justification and the building of definitions or reality that the group shares. It may in fact be the case that the people who are still in the group think it perfect and ideal, and it may in fact be just that for those who are present. But those doing such research must recognize that the "knife" of high attrition rates for new religious groups cuts both ways. Those doing therapy on an extremely small sample of members who leave the groups are probably being misled about life in the new religion (11, 79). However, those studying a larger but still small proportion of members who experience new religions and who are present in the group at the time of the research also must be somewhat limited in what they can conclude from such research.

The latter line of research is studying life inside the group(s) as depicted by and through the group of people there at the time, most of whom are there for a relatively short time. What this kind of research most often misses, however, is any data on those who have already left the group. Granted that most of those interviewed may later leave, nevertheless this is seldom recognized as any "before" stage of a classic "before and after" research design. Yet, the data are often reported as if the group were a stable organization with permanent members. Thus conclusions that do not fit all, or even a majority, of the participants in a given group may be propounded by the researcher, if there is a failure to recognize limitations of the data.

This problem is mirrored and demonstrated in the extreme by some who do research on the very narrow sample of those who have left and experienced serious enough problems to be referred to a therapist (4). Studying this select group and accepting them for what they are is no problem, because there are plainly some people who experience problems as a result of their experiences in new religions, a not-too-surprising fact. All groups and social institutions have participants who experience difficulties in adjustment (which is not to say that all groups and social institutions are alike), and we need to know about such situations in order to ameliorate any difficulties of readjustment. Thus we have marriage counselors, family counselors, occupational counselors, school counselors, therapists, and social workers of various kinds who attempt to help people adjust to their difficult life situations. Such activities are a part of American life, and we are used to the notion that many people during their lives will need some sort of therapy.

But, what is surprising is the fact that some professionals engaged in work with those who have problems upon leaving the new religions use this as a data base to generalize back to life in the group, often in a very condemnatory fashion. As described earlier, the writings of some who do research on groups by living with them may reflect a certain naiveté by overlooking the fact that many have not found life in new religions so ideal, and have moved on to other commitments. But this pales when compared with the work of those who would feel free to describe life inside the groups for all participants based almost completely on data gathered in therapy situations with an extremely small subset of those who have been involved in the new religions. Some of these same researchers refuse to enter the groups at all, and appear to be practicing "cerebral hygiene" similar to August Comte, one of the founders of sociology, who refused to read any more books after a certain time in his life so as not to contaminate his mind.

What is taking place in most therapy situations is that someone is trying to help someone else restructure his or her life and interpret past experiences in a way that will allow that person to adjust and function within society. Thus the therapist is often furnishing a specific interpretation, if not a broader worldview, to the client (14). To treat this situation as a valid data gathering situation is somewhat analogous to doing research on something by interviewing oneself over and over. The comments may be brilliant and insightful, but the data base is plainly a bit limited.

Even if we did not find this problem of the therapist furnishing an interpretation to the client and then treating this as data, there would still be the problem of treating the information gathered in the therapeutic setting as indicative of what life is like in the new religious groups for most participants. Not many of us would write a definitive statement about the meaning and value of higher education in America by interviewing a select sample of college dropouts who had enough difficulty dropping out to be perceived by themselves or someone else as requiring therapy to readjust to society. But some mental health practitioners apparently think they can make definitive statements about new religions on the basis of information gathered from a select sample of people who have had readjustment difficulties after being associated with a new religion, and some assume that the problems the person has were caused directly and only by the religious group.

This difficulty is exacerbated by the fact that many of those dropouts being studied have been deprogrammed in one way or another. One prominent therapist (5) who writes on the new religions admits that 75 percent of the clients she interviewed have been the subject of legal conservatorships, and another well-known team of writers (88), in a recent article that claimed to explain effects of life in the groups, admitted that 71 percent had been deprogrammed. Such work is plainly not research on life within new religions, and the limitations of such work should be recognized (29, 89). This is especially true in light of Solomon's (79) work and Wright's (10, 80) research, which indicates that one major effect of deprogramming is to convince ex-members that they were originally brainwashed by the new religion. Those who study deprogrammed ex-members of new religions should clearly label their research as such, just as those who only study those who are still in new religions should admit that there are limitations to their own work.

Overgeneralizing

There is a natural tendency in all of us to overgeneralize our findings and to make broader claims than our data will support.

Thus some of us who have done research on recruitment into several different religions may be prone to conclude that conversion processes and resocialization are similar in other groups, that the processes used vary only in degree of sophistication, and that those participating in such processes are doing so willingly and often for their own purposes (9). But we must be wary of extending our conclusions too far. There could be something new just around the corner, although careful ethnographic work on more and more groups, coupled with the high attrition rates which are a part of virtually all newer religions (10, 12, 90) suggests that the likelihood of such an outcome is low.

But, having said this, it nonetheless seems that some people associated with the anti-cult position have turned overgeneralization into an art form. It is distressing to hear all induction processes into new religions discussed as if they were exactly like alleged practices of one segment of one notorious new religion which may well have engaged in deceptive induction practices during a time in its history. Otherwise knowledgeable scholars talk as if that group is always and forever the same, and that they cannot change. If this group used deception in their recruitment, this means that one relatively small newer religion did something that many in our society (including this writer) would consider unethical. Why for some this automatically means that virtually all new religions are deceptive and require rigorous regulation, control, and even termination, is puzzling. The plain fact is that we have very little information on most new religious groups. Most of the research has focused on only a handful of the hundreds of groups that dot the contemporary religious landscape. Much more research is needed, but this must be preceded by a recognition of all involved that the phenomenon of new religions is multifaceted and well differentiated, and any type of generalization is fraught with difficulty.

Research Methodologies

What has already been said involves the recognition that research methodologies differ considerably in studies of recruitment to new religions. This should not be surprising, however, since the types of questions being asked also differ. It is unrealistic to expect the researcher interested in comparing theological developments within certain groups to use the same methods as someone wanting information on resocialization processes.

Those studying organizational change in new religions would not use the same methods as someone interested in personality assessment. Yet difficulties arise when the same question is being addressed using different methodologies. This is especially true when global judgments are being made about whether or not new religions are good or bad, and whether they help or hinder members in personal growth or in becoming functioning members of society. This, of course, relates to the earlier made points about differences in perspective, in subject matter of study, and tendencies to overgeneralize. The situation of some researchers who may have initially positive feelings toward new religions going into a group, talking with and testing relatively contented members, and then drawing wide-ranging conclusions about the positive value of new religions in our society, is mirrored by the situation of someone with somewhat negative feelings toward religion doing research while also engaged in therapy on a select sample, and then using these data to draw over-reaching conclusions of a more negative nature. And there are those who do no empirical research at all on the process, but speak anyway, perhaps basing their ideas on one or two idiosyncratic encounters with the cults.

I am not saying that all who do research on new religions fall into one or the other of these categories. Indeed, few are actually prototypical cases. But all of us must guard against such tendencies and the possible interaction of methodological approach with perspective. There can be a compounding or additivity of effects which detracts greatly from the value of a person's work. We simply must recognize that one's research methods may impact on the type of information gathered and the conclusions drawn from it, and that one's perspective and discipline influence, if not dictate, the methods used to gather information. Being cognizant of these potential problems will lead to better research as well as more tolerance and understanding among researchers, not to mention more information on why people join new religions.

References

1. Bromley D, Richardson JT, eds: The Brainwashing/Deprogramming Controversy. Lewiston, NY, Edwin Mellen Press, 1983

2. Verdier P: Brainwashing and the Cults. Redondo Beach, CA, Institute of Behavioral Conditioning, 1977
3. Conway F, Siegelman J: Snapping. New York, Delta Books, 1979
4. Clark J: Problems in referral of cult members. Journal of the National Association of Private Psychiatric Hospitals 9:19–21, 1978
5. Singer M: Coming out of the cults. Psychology Today, January 1979, pp 72–82
6. Richardson JT: Conversion careers. Society 17:47–50, 1980
7. Robbins T, Anthony D: The limits of coercive persuasion as an explanation for conversion to authoritative sects. Political Psychology 2:27–37, 1980
8. Straus R: Religious conversion as a personal and collective accomplishment. Sociological Analysis 40:158–165, 1979
9. Bird F, Reimer B: Participation rates in the new religious movements. Journal for the Scientific Study of Religion 21:1–14, 1982
10. Wright S: Defection from new religious movements, in The Brainwashing/Deprogramming Controversy. Edited by Bromley D, Richardson JT. Lewiston, NY, Edwin Mellen Press, 1983 pp 106–121
11. Richardson JT, Van der Lans J, Derks F: Leaving and labelling: voluntary and coerced disaffiliation from religious social movements, in Research in Social Movements, vol 9. Edited by Lang K. Greenwich, CT, JAI Press, 1986
12. Kilbourne B, Richardson JT: Cults versus families: a case of misattribution of cause. Marriage and Family Review 4:81–100, 1982
13. Kilbourne B, Richardson JT: Psychotherapy and new religions in a pluralistic society. American Psychol 39:237–251, 1984
14. Frank J: Persuasion and Healing: A Comparative Study of Psychotherapy. New York, Schocken, 1974
15. Galanter M: The "relief effect": a sociobiological model for neurotic distress and large-group therapy. Am J Psychiatry 135:588–591, 1978
16. Galanter M: Psychological induction into the larger group: findings from a modern religious sect. Am J Psychiatry 137:1574–1579, 1980
17. Galanter M, Buckley P: Evangelical religion and meditation: psychotherapeutic effects. J Nerv Ment Dis 166:685–691, 1978
18. Galanter M, Rabkin R, Rabkin F, et al: The "Moonies": a psychological study of conversion and membership in a contemporary religious sect. Am J Psychiatry 136:165–169, 1979
19. Lieberman MA, Gardner JR: Institutional alternatives to psychotherapy: a study of growth center users. Arch Gen Psychiatry 33:157–162, 1976
20. Lieberman MA, Solow N, Bond GR: The psychotherapeutic impact of women's consciousness-raising groups. Arch Gen Psychiatry 36:161–168, 1979
21. Lofland J: Becoming a "world-saver" revisited, in Conversion Careers: In and Out of the New Religions. Edited by Richardson JT. Beverly Hills, CA, Sage, 1978, pp 10–23

22. McGuire MD: Pentecostal Catholics. Philadelphia, Temple University Press, 1982
23. Nicholi AM: A new dimension of the youth culture. Am J Psychiatry 131:396–401, 1974
24. Richardson JT, Steward MW, Simmonds RB: Organized Miracles. New Brunswick, NJ, Transaction Books, 1979
25. Simon J: Observations on 67 patients who took Erhard seminars training. Am J Psychiatry 135:686–691, 1978
26. Underleider JT, Wellisch D: Coercive persuasion (brainwashing), religious cults and deprogramming. Am J Psychiatry 136:279–282, 1979
27. Nordquist T: Ananda Cooperative Village. Uppsala, Sweden, Religionhistoriska Institunionen, 1978
28. Downton JV Jr: Sacred Journeys. New York, Columbia University Press, 1979
29. Kilbourne B: The Conway and Siegelman claims against religious cults: an assessment of their data. Journal for the Scientific Study of Religion 22:380–385, 1983
30. Richardson JT: Psychological and psychiatric studies of new religions, in New Perspectives in the Psychology of Religion. Edited by Brown LB. New York, Pergamon, 1985
31. Lovekin A, Maloney HN: Religious glossolalia: a longitudinal study of personality changes. Journal for the Scientific Study of Religion 16:383–393, 1977
32. Galanter M: Engaged members of the Unification Church. Arch Gen Psychiatry 40:1197–1202, 1983
33. Wallace A: Religion: An Anthropological View. New York, Random House, 1966
34. Richardson JT, Kilbourne B: Classical and contemporary applications of brainwashing models: a comparison and critique, in The Brainwashing/Deprogramming Controversy. Edited by Bromley D, Richardson JT. Lewiston, NY, Edwin Mellen Press, 1983, pp 29–45
35. Lifton R: Thought Reform and the Psychology of Totalism. New York, WW Norton, 1963
36. Sargant W: Battle for the Mind. Garden City, NY, Doubleday, 1957
37. Meerloo J: The Rape of the Mind. New York, Grosset & Dunlap, 1956
38. Schein E, Schneier I, Barker CH: Coercive Persuasion. New York, WW Norton, 1961
39. Somit A: Brainwashing. International Encyclopedia of the Social Sciences. New York, Macmillan and Free Press, 1968
40. Bird F: The nature and function of ritual forms. Studies in Religion 9:387–402, 1980
41. Holloman R: Ritual opening and individual transformation: rites of passage at Esalen. American Anthropologist 26:265–289, 1974
42. Richardson JT, Simmonds RB, Harder M: Thought reform and the Jesus movement. Youth and Society 4:185–200, 1972

43. Taylor D: Thought reform and the Unification Church, in The Brainwashing/Deprogramming Controversy. Edited by Bromley D, Richardson JT. Lewiston, NY, Edwin Mellen Press, 1983, pp 73–90
44. Ofshe R, Berg NE, Coughlin R, et al: Social structure and social control in Synanon. Journal of Voluntary Action Research 3:67–77, 1974
45. Ofshe R: The social development of the Synanon cult: the managerial strategy of organization transformation. Sociological Analysis 41:109–127, 1980
46. Beckford JA: Accounting for conversion. Br J Sociol 29:249–262, 1978
47. Beckford JA: Through the looking-glass and out the other side: withdrawal from Rev. Moon's Unification Church. Archive de Science Sociales des Religious 45:95–116, 1978
48. Berger P: The Sacred Canopy. New York, Doubleday, 1967
49. Van Driel B, Richardson JT: Print media and new religious movements. Paper presented at Western Social Science Association annual meeting, Reno, NV, 1986
50. Richardson JT: The active vs. passive convert: paradigm conflict in conversion/recruitment research. Journal for the Scientific Study of Religion 24:163–179, 1985
51. Richardson JT, Reidy MTV: Form and fluidity in two glossalalic movements. Annual Review of the Social Sciences of Religion 4:183–220, 1980
52. Pilarzyk T: Conversion and alternation processes in the youth culture: a comparative analysis of religious transformations, in The Brainwashing/Deprogramming Controversy. Edited by Bromley D, Richardson JT. Lewiston, NY, Edwin Mellen Press, 1978, pp 51–72
53. Biderman A: The image of "brainwashing." Public Opinion Quarterly 26:547–563, 1962
54. Jung CG: Modern Man in Search of a Soul. New York, Harcourt, Brace & Co, 1933
55. Allport G: The Individual and His Religion. New York, Macmillan, 1950
56. Frankl V: Man's Search for Meaning. Boston, Beacon, 1962
57. James W: The Varieties of Religious Experience. New York, New American Library, 1958
58. Berger P: Invitation to Sociology. New York, Doubleday, 1963
59. Sampson EE: Scientific paradigms and social values: wanted—a scientific revolution. J Pers Soc Psychol 38:1332–1343, 1978
60. Gergen KJ, Morawski J: Emergence of an alternative metatheory of social psychology, in The Review of Personality and Social Psychology. Edited by Wheeler L. Beverly Hills, CA, Sage, 1980
61. Ginsburg G: Emerging Strategies in Social Psychological Research. New York, John Wiley & Sons, 1979

62. Backman C: Epilogue: a new paradigm? in Emerging Strategies in Social Psychological Research. Edited by Ginsburg GP. New York, John Wiley & Sons, 1979
63. Lofland J, Stark R: Becoming a world saver: a theory of conversion to a deviant perspective. American Sociological Review 30:863–874, 1965
64. Lofland J: Doomsday Cult. Englewood Cliffs, NJ, Prentice-Hall, 1966
65. Lofland J: Becoming a "world-saver" revisited, in Conversion Careers: In and Out of the New Religions. Edited by Richardson JT. Beverly Hills, CA, Sage, 1978, pp 10–23
66. Lofland J: Doing Social Life. New York, John Wiley & Sons, 1976
67. Straus R: Changing oneself: seekers and the creative transformation of life experience, in Doing Social Life. Edited by Lofland J. New York, John Wiley & Sons, 1976
68. Balch RW, Taylor D: Salvation in a UFO cult. Psychology Today 19:58–66, 106, 1976
69. Balch RW, Taylor D: Seekers and saucers: the role of the cultic milieu in joining a UFO cult, in Conversion Careers: In and Out of the New Religions. Edited by Richardson JT. Beverly Hills, CA, Sage, 1978
70. Balch RW: Two models of conversion and commitment in a UFO cult. Paper presented at annual meeting of the Pacific Sociological Association, Anaheim, CA, 1979
71. Balch RW: Looking behind the scenes in a religious cult: implications for the study of conversion. Sociological Analysis 41:137–143, 1980
72. Bromley D, Shupe A Jr: Just a few years seem like a lifetime: a role theory approach to participation in religious movements, in Research in Social Movements, Conflict, and Change. Edited by Krisberg L. Greenwich, CT, JAI Press, 1979, pp 159–186
73. Kilbourne B, Richardson JT: Social experimentation: self process or social role. Int J Soc Psychiatry 31:13–22, 1985
74. Travisano RV: Alternation and conversion as qualitatively different transformations, in Social Psychology Through Symbolic Interaction. Edited by Stone GP, Garverman M. Waltham, MA, Ginn-Blaisdell, 1970
75. Gordon D: The Jesus People: an identity synthesis. Urban Life Culture 3:159–178, 1974
76. Levine S: Radical departures. Psychology Today 18:20–27, 1984
77. Derks F, Van der Lans J: The post-cult syndrome: Fact or fiction? Paper presented at Conference of Psychologists of Religion, Catholic University, Nijmegen, The Netherlands, 1981
78. Skonovd N: Leaving the cultic religious milieu, in The Brainwashing/Deprogramming Controversy. Edited by Bromley D, Richardson JT. Lewiston, NY, Edwin Mellen Press, 1983, pp 91–105
79. Solomon T: Integrating the "Moonie" experience: a survey of ex-

members of the Unification Church, in In Gods We Trust. Edited by Robbins T, Anthony D. New Brunswick, NJ, Transaction Books, 1981, pp 275–294

80. Wright S: Post-involvement attitudes of voluntary defectors from controversial new religious movements. Journal for the Scientific Study of Religion 23:172–182, 1984

81. Jacobs J: The economy of love in religious commitment: the deconversion of women from non-traditional religious movements. Journal for the Scientific Study of Religion 23:155–171, 1984

82. Richardson JT: Methodological considerations in the study of new religions, in Scientific Research and New Religions: Divergent Perspectives. Edited by Kilbourne B. San Francisco, CA, AAAS, Pacific Division, 1985

83. Foss D, Larkin R: Worshipping the absurd. Sociological Analysis 39:157–164, 1978

84. Enroth R: Youth, Brainwashing, and the Extremist Cults. Grand Rapids, MI, Zondervan, 1977

85. Zerin MF: The pied piper phenomenon: family systems and vulnerability to cults, in Scientific Research and New Religions: Divergent Perspectives. Edited by Kilbourne B. San Francisco, American Association for the Advancement of Science, Pacific Division, 1985

86. Markowitz A: The role of family therapy in the treatment of symptoms associated with cult affiliation, in Psychodynamic Perspectives on Religion, Sect, and Cult. Edited by Halperin DA. Littleton, MA, John Wright-PSG, 1983

87. Halperin DA: Self-help groups for parents of cult members, in Psychodynamic Perspectives on Religion, Sect, and Cult. Edited by Halperin DA. Littleton, MA, John Wright-PSG, 1983

88. Conway F, Siegelman J: Information disease: have cults created a new mental illness? Science Digest 90:86–92, 1982

89. Kilbourne B: A reply to Maher and Langone's statistical critique of Kilbourne. Journal for the Scientific Study of Religion 25:116–123, 1986

90. Barker E: The ones who got away: people who attend Unification Church workshops and do not become members, in of Gods and Men. Edited by Barker E. Macon, GA, Mercer Press, 1983

Chapter 13

Deprogramming (Involuntary Departure), Coercion, and Cults

J. Thomas Ungerleider, M.D.
David K. Wellisch, Ph.D.

There has been continuing concern in this country during the past decade about the phenomenon of cults (or sects), most specifically over the circumstances of young adults joining and remaining in them. Issues of so-called brainwashing (coercive persuasion or thought reform) have been raised and much parental and societal anxiety has been generated. This concern is due to many factors, including members' rejection of traditional values, alienation from their families, and concern that the energies of members will be utilized in the furthering of the cults' economic and social goals. One remedy has been called deprogramming or involuntary departure, a procedure applied by laypersons. We will consider various aspects of the deprogramming issue.

Deprogramming (Involuntary Departure)

Involuntary departure from a cult can be subdivided into two stages. The first is "obtaining" the person (preparatory phase) and the second is the procedure he or she is then subjected to in

The authors thank Jan C. Costello, J.D., Professor at Loyola Law School, for help with the legal sections of this chapter.

order to change his or her thinking about the cult (deprogramming technique).

Preparatory Phase

A common method to gain physical control of the convert involves waiting for him or her to appear alone on a street or other public place. The convert can then be physically forced into a car and taken to the site chosen by the deprogrammer. Another technique is to devise a fictitious story, possibly involving family illness or death, which will draw the convert away from the cult residence (1).

The father of deprogramming is generally regarded as Ted Patrick, a controversial, charismatic, and oft-jailed layperson who has described his deprogramming technique in his own writing (2). A vivid description from Patrick:

> Suddenly Lockwood grabbed the boy without warning and hurled him head first onto the seat. . . . Wes came bowling out into the street next to the car shrieking and waving his arms, yelling at the top of his voice 'Help! Help! they're kidnapping me! Call the police! Help me!'. . . . I reached down between Wes's legs, grabbed him by the crotch and squeezed—hard. He let out a howl and doubled up, grabbing for his groin with both hands. Then I hit, shoving him head first into the back seat of the car and piling in on top of him. (2)

Deprogramming Techniques

Once the convert is obtained the techniques applied by the deprogrammers may vary considerably. Because deprogramming is a lay procedure, described anecdotally by those to whom it has been applied, there are few first-hand accounts in the scientific literature. Psychotherapeutic intervention or evaluation in a psychiatric hospital, outpatient visits to a therapist, or counseling by a member of the clergy in a church or temple office are not strictly classified as deprogramming procedures, as the patient is a voluntary one, free to leave or terminate at any time. Lay deprogramming is often done in a hotel room or isolated site which can be secured against anticipated escape attempts (i.e., one may be on the second floor with windows nailed shut, all doors locked, and telephone removed). Former cult members may assist the deprogrammer.

Anecdotal stories of these techniques abound, including the use of sexual partners (for celibate cult members) and drugs (alcohol) to lessen their resistance (3). There have also been alleged use of guard dogs and shotgun-at-the-chin techniques designed to more directly instill fear.

Then a period of confrontation, "dialogue," and exhortation ensues, with alleged control of the member's physical environment (food, sleep, and so on) until the member realizes the error of his or her ways. This may take hours, days, or even weeks. It may also terminate if the deprogrammee directly escapes or (falsely) convinces the deprogrammers that he or she has recanted, only to leave and rejoin the cult after eventual release. In the book *Snapping* the authors have described the physical details of deprogramming and have obtained accounts from ex-cult members of their own deprogramming experiences (4). This presents a vivid picture of the phenomenology of this procedure and experience. The ex-members generally describe a process whereby they initially tried to ignore or suppress the intrusions of the deprogrammers' thoughts into their own cult-based doctrine-laden thinking. This became impossible (for some, not all) and they began to once again utilize the discriminative part of their egos and self-evaluative capacities.

Lifton, in his book *Thought Reform and the Psychology of Totalism* describes a process of surrender of the ego to the group as a prerequisite toward membership in a totalistic milieu such as a cult (5). The dynamic thrust of the deprogramming process, therefore, seeks to reverse this surrender to the cult and reinvest evaluative capacity in the individual. One important variable to consider in predicting "success" of the deprogramming process is how long the individual had been in the cult and thereby surrendered his or her evaluative capacity in exchange for the doctrine of the group. In our study of those who returned to cults after deprogramming (versus those who were deprogrammed and did not return) those unsuccessfully deprogrammed had been in the groups longer than those successfully deprogrammed. It appeared that cult membership of one year was a sharp dividing line in terms of return versus nonreturn to the cults postdeprogramming (6).

Patrick has his own description of deprogramming and its aftermath. He states:

> Deprogramming is like taking a car out of the garage that has not been driven for a year. The battery has gone down, and in order to start it up, you've got to put jumper cables on it. It will start up then but if you turn the key off right away, it will go dead again. So you keep the motor running until it builds up its own power. This is what rehabilitation is. Once we get the mind working, we keep it working long enough so that the person gets in the habit of thinking and making decisions again. (4, p. 69)

The ex-members who describe their deprogramming go beyond the simple renunciation of the cult's doctrine in exchange for that of conventional society. They describe the switch from "a cult state of mind" to another mode of thought process, that of individualized, evaluative thought. Many ex-members, at least temporarily, become deprogrammers themselves or join other deprogrammers. Since the cultlike qualities of these deprogramming teams has been noted by a number of observers, it is uncertain just how much evaluative thought has returned after deprogramming.

Some deprogrammers have intimate knowledge of the particular cult and challenge their ideologies (i.e., "heavenly deception" in the Unification Church, "fair game" in Scientology, and so forth). Some of their deprogramming techniques are designed to counteract either what the particular deprogrammer has experienced when he or she, or his or her aides, were themselves in cults or what he or she fantasizes has been done or told to the member. Reports exist of deprogrammers joining cults to extricate someone and then becoming converted themselves to the cult and having to be rescued and "deprogrammed" by others. Apparently the group process in relation to surrender of one's own ego and self-evaluative capacity is so strong that even Ted Patrick, the master deprogrammer, felt its effects. Commenting on his experiences when he infiltrated the "Children of God," he stated:

> You can feel it coming on. You start to doubt yourself. You start to question everything you believe in. Then you find yourself saying and doing the same things they are. You feel like you're sinking in sand, drowning—sometimes you get dizzy. (4, p. 65)

The issue has been raised whether the techniques are not reprogramming the person back to his or her previous belief system, rather than freeing the individual to make a rational choice. If the member never does renounce the cult then he or she is regarded by deprogrammers as an unsuccessful attempt or failed deprogramming, not as one who now has free will and has still chosen to remain with the cult. A key theme indicated by successfully deprogrammed ex-members is the highly accurate knowledge of their cults utilized by the deprogrammer. This constantly reoccurs in their descriptions of what finally "got to them" in the experience.

The Mental Health Professional, the Law, and Deprogramming

Mental health professionals have become involved in this lay procedure of deprogramming in a variety of ways along a spectrum of participation from direct to very indirect. Although no studies of such involvement have been done, it seems clear that direct involvement by mental health professionals is the exception rather than the rule. Sometimes they have advised parents about the need for deprogramming. Sometimes they have "observed" (or been consultants to) the deprogramming after the cult member has been removed to the site of the deprogramming. Far more often, they have advised parents or the courts about the (psychological/psychiatric) need for legal intervention. Sometimes mental health professionals have testified in subsequent court cases about the prior mental capacity of those cult members who had previously been deprogrammed (7). Moreover, mental health professionals who have advised the courts in these matters sometimes have done so without examining the patient-cult member. For example, in 1977, a psychologist submitted a statement about a young person who had joined a cult to a United States court. The psychologist admittedly had never examined the patient nor seen anyone from that cult but he described the effects of extremist religious cults on persons who become members. In his affidavit to the judge he stated (in part): "lack of emotional commitment to established social institutions . . . delay of personal integration into the mainstream of community life . . . impaired sense of meaning in basic life direction . . . stultifying effect on inner forces of psychological growth and maturation . . . impairment in the development of a clearly defined sense of identity" (8). The most surprising part of this was not its submission by the psychologist, nor its acceptance by the judge but that this procedure of advising the judge has not been deemed unethical by the psychiatric professional societies (Robert Moore, M.D., personal communication). In another instance a psychiatrist testified in a controversial proceeding after observing the cult member—at a distance—speaking with her parents but never actually examining her or attempting to interact with her. Ethical behavior on the part of the psychiatrists vis-à-vis cults and their members has been only addressed, in a question and answer format, in the *Opinions of the Ethics Committee* of the American Psychiatric Association where it is stated that it is not "ethical" for a colleague to make a diagnosis of mental illness, solely because the individual has joined a "new religion" or cult (9).

All of this controversy has occurred in a milieu where U.S. psychiatrists and the American Psychiatric Association have been critical of our Soviet counterparts, even adopting a resolution (at the Sixth World Congress of Psychiatry in Honolulu, Hawaii, in August 1978) condemning the alleged unethical use of psychiatry to curtail political and religious dissent in the Soviet Union (The Declaration of Hawaii) (8).

Mental health professionals have also counseled or evaluated ex-cult members who have been deprogrammed elsewhere and seek help in subsequent adjustment to life outside the cult (10). This last involvement is a more traditional psychotherapeutic one since the ex-cult member seeks treatment voluntarily: in that sense, he or she is no different from any other psychiatric patient. This is not a topic for discussion here.

Much controversy concerning deprogrammings has come to light via legal proceedings. To avoid being open to charges of kidnapping, parents (along with deprogrammers) have requested temporary conservatorships[1] so they can turn the cult member over—not for psychiatric evaluation, hospitalization, or treatment—but for deprogramming. To "qualify" for a conservatorship (in California) the person must be suicidal, homicidal, or gravely disabled (unable, as a result of mental disorder, to provide for his basic personal needs for food, clothing, or shelter). Being psychotic or under the influence of "mind control" does not, in and of itself, fulfill these qualifications.[2]

In California, as in other states, a temporary conservatorship may be sought and imposed ex parte; that is, based solely upon the allegations of the moving party, and without giving the proposed conservatee a chance to appear and present a defense.[3] Use of ex parte proceedings is sometimes recommended by deprogrammers, on the theory that it will provide at least a short period of time within which to attempt the deprogramming. Even if the temporary conservatorship is vacated at a subsequent full due process hearing, or overturned on appeal, the cult member may by then have changed his or her mind about cult membership, that is, may have been successfully deprogrammed.

Legal Barriers to Deprogramming and the Liability of Mental Health Professionals

The California case of *Katz v. Superior Court* has been widely cited as establishing the illegality of using conservatorships to facilitate deprogramming (11). In that case five adults who were the subject of conservatorship proceedings brought by their parents appealed the trial court's temporary conservatorship orders. The trial court had acted based in part upon the parent's allegations that the children had become involved with a religious organization that placed psychological pressures on them, causing impairment of their physical and mental health and loss of their free will. The temporary conservatorships were appointed under a provision of the California probate code which permitted protection of the property of a conservatee who "is likely to be deceived by artful and designing persons."

On appeal, the conservatorships were found to be unjustified even if the evidence before the trial court was given its most favorable interpretation, and vacated.

The Court of Appeals declared that the only criterion that justified imposing conservatorship over an adult's person (and permitting the conservator to subject him to involuntary treatment) was "grave disability." At the conservatorship hearing there was no showing that the proposed wards were physically unhealthy or deprived of or unable to secure food, clothing, and shelter. Although the parents' expert mental health witnesses (a psychiatrist and a psychologist) testified concering the negative emotional effects of "coercive persuasion," the Court of Appeals noted that they could not assign the proposed conservatees a psychosis diagnosis, or any other category under the American Psychiatric Association's *Diagnostic and Statistical Manual* (11, pp. 976–980).

Since the *Katz* conservatees were not shown to be either mentally ill or thereby incapable of caring for their basic needs, they could not lawfully be placed under conservatorship. Moreover, the Court of Appeals stressed, if they had been mentally ill, it would still have been inappropriate for the trial court simply to place the adult children in their parents' custody (presumably for deprogramming purposes); under California law the conservatees were instead entitled to a mental health evaluation and treatment. "To do less is to license kidnapping for the purpose of thought control" (11, p. 983).

The *Katz* decision identified an additional, serious difficulty with applying conservatorship procedures to cult members. The parents in this case essentially asked the trial court to investigate the validity of their children's religious beliefs in order to determine that the proposed wards were "deceived"; the conservatees, in their own defense, introduced mental health professionals' testimony that their experiences and behavior were "no more than usually accompany devotion to a religious belief." Such an action by a court would violate the "wall of separation" between church and state mandated by the First Amendment. Consistent with this concern, the *Katz* court struck down the probate code language referring to deception by "artful and designing persons" as unconstitutionally vague when applied "to the world of ideas. . . . In the field of beliefs, and particularly religious tenets, it is difficult, if not impossible, to establish a universal truth against which deceit and imposition can be measured" (11, p. 970).

Nine years after *Katz*, a California Court of Appeals again relied upon the First Amendment in finding that former cult members could not proceed with tort suits against the religious organizations, in *Molko and Leal v. Holy Spirit Association for the Unification of World Christianity* (7). The trial court correctly declined to consider the psychiatrist's and psychologist's testimony introduced by plaintiffs to show that cult members were so "persuasively coerced that they could not engage in the free exercise of their own will and intellect." The First Amendment barred any judicial attempt to distinguish whether plaintiffs' motivation for joining the church were as a result of "brain-washing" or religious faith.

> The idea that religious doctrine can be (or as some would have it, invariably is) manipulatively employed to subvert reason . . . which it may be noted, is an idea that has been used to condemn *all* religions as deceptively exploitive of certain universal human needs (see, e.g., Freud, *The Future of Illusion* (1927) . . . is one we may entertain as individuals but which the First Amendment forbids us to consider as judges." (7, p. 19)

The court noted that "both doctors seem to have reasoned backwards from their disapproval of those methods (Unification Church methods) to the conclusion that the plaintiffs were not thinking freely because they were persuaded by them" (11, p. 16, no. 9). Legal arguments to reinterpret the First Amendment in order to legitimize deprogramming have been made but are beyond the scope of this chapter (12).

The *Molko* decision, in addition to underscoring the First Amendment issues, cautioned against the danger of relying upon value judgments disguised as expert psychiatric opinion (7, p. 19).

Finally, *Molko* is significant because the Court of Appeals, while affirming the trial court's dismissal of the ex-cult members' claims against the religious organizations, found that the trial court had wrongly dismissed the defendants' counterclaims. Thus, the Unification Church may file an amended complaint against the plaintiffs for, among other things, conspiracy to prevent (by deprogramming), members of the Church from freely exercising their religious beliefs.

Both cult members who are unsuccessfully subjected to deprogramming, and religious organizations themselves, can and have brought civil suits seeking both damages and injunctions against the deprogrammers. In *Taylor v. Gilmarten*, an adult plaintiff whose parents had unsuccessfully attempted to deprogram him into leaving the Monastery of the Holy Protection of the Blessed Virgin Mary, sued employees of the Freedom of

Thought Foundation, which carried out the deprogramming attempt after plaintiff's father obtained a temporary guardianship over him (13). Finding that the federal trial court erred in dismissing the plaintiff's claims, the United States Court of Appeals held that plaintiff could pursue his claims of false imprisonment, intentional infliction of emotional distress, and conspiracy by private persons to cause the state to deprive him of his constitutional rights.

The *Taylor* court found that the guardianship order was invalid, because it was not based upon a finding that the proposed ward was mentally ill, violent, might hurt himself or others—or was unable to care for his basic needs. The Court of Appeals stressed that "the judge fashioned this order to suit something that was not even provided for in any statute" and that the order was therefore void. Although a valid conservatorship or guardianship order would be a defense to the false imprisonment claim, "[a]n unauthorized judicial command furnishes no protection to those who act under it" (13, pp. 1352, 1353). The Tenth Circuit roundly condemned

> the appellees' attempted use of these insanity statutes in an effort to develop an immunity defense in which evidence of insanity is subjected to excessive conduct. This is a misuse of the . . . statutes having a clear purpose to get some kind of court protection of deprogramming. This should not be allowed. (13, p. 1361)

The language of *Taylor v. Gilmarten* strongly suggests that tort liability will attach to a mental health professional who forms part of a private conspiracy to use a conservatorship or guardianship procedure to make deprogramming possible. A mental health professional who is directly involved in confining a cult member or subjecting him or her to deprogramming similarly could be sued for false imprisonment or intentional infliction of emotional distress. The mere fact that a guardianship order was obtained from a judge is not adequate to protect the mental health professional, where the order itself was void. Currently the imposition of a guardianship or conservatorship to make deprogramming possible (as opposed to permitting involuntary treatment of a mentally ill person who meets the statutory criteria) is nowhere provided for in state or federal law.

Diagnostic Criteria

The *Diagnostic and Statistical Manual of Mental Disorders*, 3rd ed. (DSM-III) addresses cult membership under atypical dissociative disorders (DSM-III, 300.15). This description is for "prolonged dissociative states that may occur in persons who have been subjected to periods of prolonged and intense coercive persuasion (brainwashing, thought reform, and indoctrination) while the captive of terrorists or cultists." But unlike most conditions listed in DSM-III *no* signs, symptoms, or other criteria for diagnosis are listed! No psychological tests exist that diagnose the syndrome of coercive persuasion and we have found no indication of overt mental illness in our cult population study (6).

Summary

The dimensions of deprogramming of members of cults are unclear. No figures are available to evaluate the frequency of deprogramming or the effectiveness of this intervention, much less the variety of procedures classified under this rubric. However, the evolution of legal and ethical issues cited in this brief report clearly indicate a thoughtful and reasoned posture for the mental health professional in regard to deprogramming.

First, the criteria, in many states, for an ex-parte conservatorship for purposes of obtaining the cult member for deprogramming will require a finding of mental illness and resulting inability to care for one's basic needs. In addition, good clinical practice requires a face-to-face evaluation of any person thought to be gravely disabled and thus must be done by conventional procedures including clinical interviewing and possibly psychological testing. The person being examined should be told what is happening and be made aware that he or she is not in a casual conversation or social situation. If the cult member is found to meet the conservatorship criteria, the psychiatric unit or hospital, and not a locked hotel room or isolated house, is the proper milieu for treatment. To do less or otherwise is an unacceptable and unethical practice, not to mention illegal, in light of the reasoning of *Katz*.

We believe that the mental health professional testifying in court (or advising the court) in support of a conservatorship who claims expertise and special knowledge of cults but who has never actually evaluated the member in question, is unprofessional in behavior. Similarly a mental health professional who cooperates in an attempt to obtain a conservatorship over an individual who does not meet the statutory criteria for incompetency, and where the intent is to subject the individual to deprogramming—versus mental health treatment—places himself or herself in legal jeopardy.

There is another role for the mental health professional, however; some cult clinics have developed models that dynamically facilitate constructive parental involvement with their cult member children. Not only does this keep the lines of communication open with the children but helps the parents cope emotionally with this situation, and educates parents in the complexity of the psychology of the cults and cultic thinking. It also reduces disabling parental guilt and will facilitate postcult recovery when the child leaves the cult. This ongoing dialogue with their cult member children helps arm parents with proper information, mount sensible arguments, and emphasizes retention of critical evaluative skills for the children vis-à-vis their cults. This places a modicum of power back into the hands of the parents. In all of this the mental health professional can play a vitally important role.

Conclusion

Coercive involuntary departure from cults, called deprogramming, has been considered here. A variety of issues pertaining to the role of the mental health professional, both ethical and legal, have been raised. Pertinent legal decisions have been described.

We have discussed topics that question the propriety of the mental health professional as exemplified by him or her as

1. a cult or anticult advocate.
2. an advisor to the court or a judge in a conservatorship procedure:
   - with special knowledge of cults but without examining the cult member at all, or

- without a traditional examination but rather by "eye-balling" the cult member at a distance.
3. alleged sole possessor of the special knowledge to diagnose brainwashing (coercive persuasion), by previous experience with related situations [e.g., examination of prisoners of war (POWs) in Korea].
4. diagnosis of all members of cults as ipso facto suffering from mental illness (i.e., atypical dissociative reaction), without examining these members.

We have also raised social policy and philosophical issues: How active can the mental health professional be within and without the courts in promulgating the concept that it is better (healthier) for all to remain with their parents, and with traditional ways of believing and to stay in the establishment than to break with all of the above and join a cult? Does one have a legal "right to be weird" (not gravely disabled) in this world? and lastly, What is the difference between these issues for our nation's mental health professionals and these issues in the Soviet Union, where religious and political dissidents are diagnosed as "sluggish schizophrenics with reformist delusions" and incarcerated in mental institutions?

References

1. Siegel TI: Deprogramming religious cultists. Loyola of Los Angeles Law Review 11:807–828, 1978
2. Patrick T: Let Our Children Go. New York, E. P. Dutton, 1976
3. Ungerleider JT, Wellish DK: Psychiatrists' involvement in cultism, thought control, and deprogramming. Psychiatric Opinion 16:10–15, 1979
4. Conway F, Seigelman J: Snapping. New York, Dell Publishing, 1978
5. Lifton RJ: Thought Reform and the Psychology of Totalism. New York, WW Norton, 1956
6. Ungerleider JT, Wellisch DK: Coercive persuasion (brainwashing), religious cults, and deprogramming. Am J Psychiatry 136:279–282, 1979
7. *Molko and Leal v. Holy Spirit Association for the Unification of World Christianity*, No. A925338, Slip Opinion, Cal Ct Ap, 1st Dist, March 31, 1986

8. Ungerleider JT: Casting the first stone. Medical Tribune 19:23, 1978
9. American Psychiatric Association: Section 13, in Opinions of the Ethics Committee on the Principles of Medical Ethics. Washington, DC, American Psychiatric Association, 1985, p 13
10. Singer MT: Coming out of the cults. Psychology Today Jan 1979, pp 72–82
11. *Katz v. Superior Court of the City and County of San Francisco,* 73 Cal App 3d 952, 141 Cal Rptr 234, 1977
12. Delgado R: Religious totalism: gentle and ungentle persuasion under the First Amendment. Southern California Law Review 51:1–98, 1977
13. *Taylor v. Gilmarten,* 686 F 2d 1346, 10th Cir, 1983

Notes

1. All states have civil court procedures which permit a person found "incompetent" by reason of mental illness or disability to be placed under the care and custody of a guardian or conservator. State laws vary widely as to both the criteria for "incompetency" and the powers given to the conservator or guardian. In general, however, to justify the imposition of a conservator or guardian over an adult individual, that individual must be found to "lack sufficient understanding or capacity to make or communicate responsible decisions concerning his person." *See* National Conference of Commissioners on Uniform State Law, Uniform Probate No. 5 at 203 (4th ed., 1975). Moreover, that lack of understanding must be attributable to the mental or physical disability specified in the guardianship or conservatorship statute, for example, mental illness, mental retardation, alcoholism. Many states use a separate procedure for civil commitment of mentally disabled persons to psychiatric hospitals; some, however, use a conservatorship or guardianship proceeding for this purpose. For a general discussion of conservatorship, guardianship, and civil commitment law in the different states, see Parry J: Incompetency, guardianship, and restoration, in *The Mentally Disabled and the Law.* Edited by Brakel S, Parry J, Weiner B. American Bar Foundation, 1985, pp. 269–434.
2. Cal. Welf. and Inst. Code No. 5350 *et seq.* set out procedures for conservatorship and involuntary treatment of gravely disabled persons. Cal. Probate Code No. 1731 *et seq.* permits appointment of a conservator of the person or property of an adult person who is unable properly to provide for his or her personal needs for physical health, food, clothing, or shelter. A conservatorship over an adult's *property* can be appointed where the adult is substantially unable to manage his or her own financial resources, or resist fraud or undue influence. It is noteworthy that the latter conservatorship does not permit involuntary treatment of the adult subject to "undue influ-

ence"; to authorize involuntary *treatment*, an individual must be found gravely disabled under Cal. Welf. and Inst. Code No. 5350.

3. The constitutional right of due process applies to any individual proposed for conservatorship or guardianship, because of the loss of liberty at stake. State laws vary as to the degrees of procedural protection allowed, but in order to justify a *permanent* (long-term) conservatorship or guardianship, due process requires notice, opportunity to be heard, and the assistance of legal counsel or other advocate. See Parry J: Incompetency, guardianship and restoration, pp. 379–382. For this reason, *ex parte* proceedings can authorize only a short-term conservatorship, usually subject, as in California, to subsequent judicial review. Cal. Welf. and Inst. Code Nos. 5350, 5353.

LEGAL AND SOCIAL IMPLICATIONS

Chapter 14

THE CIVIL LIBERTIES OF RELIGIOUS MINORITIES

Ted Bohn, M.S.W., J.D.
Jeremiah S. Gutman, LL.B.

The emergence over the last two decades of new religions and
religions new to the United States (e.g., The Unification Church,
the Hare Krishnas, etc.) has been occasioned by much controversy and debate related principally to the legitimacy of the
religions themselves. Far from being ignored by the American
populace and law enforcement officials, however, these newly
emergent religions soon spawned a countermovement referred
to by its practitioners as "deprogramming." Amid allegations
that the subject religions recruited new members through the
use of coercive techniques, and convinced that their children
were being held against their wills, parents of church members
typically arranged with professional deprogrammers to have
their children abducted and subjected to prolonged sessions in
which the abducted individual was "persuaded" to renounce
his or her religious beliefs and rejoin the family unit in pursuit of
more commonly accepted goals. Thus, an indispensable premise of the deprogramming industry is that the religious beliefs
espoused by members of newly emergent religions are so unpopular as to cast doubt that adherence to them could be accomplished by other than coercive means. That is to say that deprogrammers labor under the asserted belief that adherents of

The authors thank Paul G. Stack, P.L.S, for his technical assistance in the
preparation of this chapter.

newly emergent religions have been "brainwashed." Not surprisingly, then, the natural consequence of this posture involves
restoring a member to what parents and deprogrammers view as
a legitimate belief system through the "deprogramming" process. In *Colombrito v. Kelly* (1), the Court accepted Le Moult's
(1978) definition of the deprogramming process:

> Deprogrammers are people who, at the request of a parent or
> other close relative, will have a member of a religious sect
> seized, then hold him against his will and subject him to
> mental, emotional, and even physical pressures until he re-
> nounces his religious beliefs. Deprogrammers usually work for
> a fee, which may easily run as high as $25,000.
>
> The deprogramming process begins with abduction. Often
> strong men muscle the subject into a car and take him to a place
> where he is cut off from everyone but his captors. He may be
> held against his will for upward of three weeks. Frequently,
> however, the initial deprogramming only lasts a few days. The
> subject's sleep is limited, and he is told that he will not be
> released until his beliefs meet his captors' approval. Members
> of the deprogramming group, as well as members of the fam-
> ily, come into the room where the victim is being held and
> barrage him with questions and denunciations until he recants
> his newly found religious beliefs. (2)

Although few if any empirical data are available on the scope
of the deprogramming phenomenon in the United States, a
complaint prepared for submission to the United Nations Committee on the Protection of Minorities recites 500 known instances of deprogramming in the United States in the last decade
(3). The practice of deprogramming is not unique to the United
States, however, having its counterparts in Great Britain and
France, for example (4).

We turn now to an examination of the legal implications to
which the practice of deprogramming gives rise.

Freedom of Religion in the United States

There are two sources of protection of religious freedom in the
United States, the latter, decisional caselaw, being dependent
upon the former, the First Amendment to the Constitution of the
United States, for support.

As it pertains to religion, the First Amendment (5) is divided into two distinct clauses: the Establishment Clause and the Free Exercise Clause. The Establishment Clause provides: "Congress shall make no law respecting an establishment of religion," while the Free Exercise Clause adds to the language above the words: "or prohibiting the free exercise thereof." The Establishment Clause prohibits the federal or state governments from recognizing or indicating a preference for one religion over another, while the Free Exercise Clause prohibits government from interfering with the *absolute* freedom to adhere to religious beliefs of the individual's choice.

For the sake of clarity, it should be noted that although the Amendment would seem to prohibit Congress alone from abridging religious freedom, the prohibitions of the First Amendment were made applicable to the States through the Due Process Clause of the Fourteenth Amendment in *Everson v. Board of Education* (6) (Establishment Clause applies to States through Due Process Clause of Fourteenth Amendment) and *Cantwell v. Connecticut* (7) (Free Exercise Clause made applicable to States through Due Process Clause of Fourteenth Amendment). Thus, no governmental entity, whether federal or state, or any subordinate operatives thereof (e.g., municipal legislatures, mayors, school boards, or police officers) may enact legislation or take official action inconsistent with either the Establishment Clause or the Free Exercise Clause.

The Amendment does not apply to private conduct, being silent on the subject entirely. Thus, private actors who fail to respect either of the clauses do not violate the Constitution, although certain private behavior that seeks to violate the clauses may well fall with the purview of other laws, as the discussion which follows reveals.

Caselaw

Of the two clauses, newly emergent religions clearly derive the greater protection from the Free Exercise Clause, since it is this clause that seeks to prohibit the government from interfering with religious beliefs. A threshold question that the Supreme Court early confronted was, "What do the words 'Free Exercise' mean?" In *Reynolds v. United States* (8), the Court drew a critical distinction between religious beliefs and conduct arising out of religious tenets. In *Reynolds*, a member of the Mormon Church challenged the government's right to criminalize polygamy, a practice which he asserted was mandated by his religion. In sustaining both the criminal statute and the state's power to enact it, the Court held there were certain types of conduct that so threatened the social fabric that they could not be said to fall within the protections afforded by the First Amendment, and the Court noted that polygamy was one such variety of conduct. (There is now some doubt among constitutional lawyers and scholars as to whether *Reynolds* was correctly decided and whether it would have been decided differently had the issue arisen later.) The early distinction between beliefs and conduct survives in the constitutional arena; and while conduct having its origins in religious teachings enjoys limited protection from governmental incursions, religious beliefs are entitled to absolute protection (i.e., the government may never interfere with an individual's right to adhere to any religious belief of his or her choice).

In a multitude of Free Exercise cases in the intervening years, the Court has never had reason to alter its original deference to pure religious beliefs and has only occasionally, for that matter, limited the protection afforded religious conduct as well.

In *United States v. Ballard* (9), a criminal prosecution brought against defendants who had secured donations of money from the public by claiming that they had supernatural powers and divine authority, the Court refused to permit the jury to consider the truth or falsity of the defendants' religious beliefs. In an oft-quoted opinion, Justice Douglas wrote, quoting the first two sentences from *Cantwell*, above:

> "[T]he Amendment embraces two concepts—freedom to believe and freedom to act. The first is absolute but, in the nature of things, the second cannot be." Freedom of thought, which includes freedom of religious belief, is basic in a society of free men. It embraces the right to maintain theories of life and of death and of the hereafter which are rank heresy to the followers of the orthodox faiths. Heresy trials are foreign to our Constitution. Men may believe what they cannot prove. They may not be put to the proof of their religious doctrines or beliefs. Religious experiences which are as real as life to some may be incomprehensible to others.
> Yet the fact that they may be beyond the ken of mortals does not mean that they can be made suspect before the law. Many take their gospel from the New Testament. But it would hardly

be supposed that they could be tried before a jury charged with the duty of determining whether those teachings contained false representations. The miracles of the New Testament, the Divinity of Christ, life after death, the power of prayer are deep in the religious convictions of many. If one could be sent to jail because a jury in a hostile environment found those teachings false, little indeed would be left of religious freedom. The Fathers of the Constitution were not unaware of the varied and extreme views of religious sects, of the violence of disagreement among them, and of the lack of any one religious creed on which all men would agree. They fashioned a charter of government which envisaged the widest possible toleration of conflicting views. Man's relation to his God was made no concern of the state. He was granted the right to worship as he pleased and to answer to no man for the verity of his religious views . . . if those doctrines are subject to trial before a jury charged with finding their truth or falsity, then the same can be done with the religious beliefs of any sect. When the triers of fact (i.e., the jury) undertake that task, they enter a forbidden domain. (Citations omitted.) (10)

Thus the substance of the particular religious beliefs being asserted in a Free Exercise claim are not to be submitted to the court or jury for judgment. As the Court has subsequently held in several opinions, all that is needed to prevail on a Free Exercise claim is that those asserting the claim maintain a sincere and genuine belief in the religion asserted and that those beliefs occupy a position of central importance in the teachings of the religion. Nothing else is required of the plaintiffs in a Free Exercise claim.

Illustrative of the deference accorded religious beliefs by the Court is *Sherbert v. Verner* (11). In *Sherbert*, the Court was faced with a challenge by a Seventh Day Adventist to South Carolina's disallowance of her claim for unemployment benefits. The claimant had been discharged from her job because she was unwilling to work on Saturdays, the Adventist Sabbath. When she subsequently made application for unemployment benefits, the State sought to disallow her claim, asserting that, because of her unwillingness to work on Saturdays, she was not "available for employment" as the statute required. The Court refused to examine the legitimacy of the Adventist's religious beliefs and simply held that in disallowing her claim the state had violated the Free Exercise Clause. Absent a "compelling state interest," the Court noted, the state put the claimant to an impermissible choice, namely, choosing between her religion and a job. (It should be noted that the claimant was otherwise available for work that did not require Saturday labor.)

In *United States v. Seeger* (12), the Court was faced with the difficult task of evaluating the conscientious objector status of a petitioner seeking, on the basis of his religious beliefs, to avoid conscription. Section 6 (j) of the Universal Military Training and Service Act (13) at the time exempted from service in the armed forces "those persons who by reason of their religious training and belief are conscientiously opposed to participation in war in any form." The Act defined "religious training and belief" as "an individual's belief in a relation to a Supreme Being involving duties superior to those arising from any human relation, but not including essentially political, sociological, or philosophical views or a merely personal moral code." The Court, unable to ascertain the boundaries of "religion," framed the issue for determining the legitimacy of a conscientious objector's claim as "whether a given belief that is sincere and meaningful occupies a place in the life of its possessor parallel to that filled by the orthodox belief in God of one who clearly qualifies for the exemption" (14). Further on in the opinion, the Court stated:

> [T]he claim of the registrant that his belief is an *essential* part of a religious faith must be given great weight. . . . The validity of what he believes cannot be questioned. Some theologians, and indeed some examiners, might be tempted to question the existence of the registrant's "Supreme Being" or the truth of his concepts. But these are inquiries foreclosed to Government. . . . Local boards and courts in this sense are not free to reject beliefs because they consider them "incomprehensible." Their task is to decide whether the beliefs professed by a registrant are *sincerely held* and whether they are, in his own scheme of things, religious. . . . But we hasten to emphasize that while the "truth" of a belief is not open to question, there remains the significant question of whether it is "truly held." This is the threshold question of sincerity which must be resolved in every case. [Emphasis added.] (15)

Thus, the Court refused to examine the substance or verity of Respondent's asserted religious beliefs and concluded only that the claimant must have a sincerely held belief that occupies an essential part of his or her faith and that this belief occupies a position of importance in the scheme of his religion, parallel to that which God occupies in the more traditional religions.

Similarly, in *Welsh v. United States* (16), the Court reversed a conviction for avoiding conscription. The petitioner had there refused to state "I am, by reason of my religious training and belief, conscientiously opposed to participation in war in any form," as the application for exemption required. Instead, he crossed out the words "religious training and," thus intimating that his objections to war in any form issued principally from his *beliefs*, which, it could be inferred, were not "religious" in nature. Since Congress specifically excluded from the conscientious objector category those whose objections were primarily political, sociological, or philosophical, or even the result of a "merely personal moral code," the Court was here put to the test. The Court noted that "When a registrant states that his objections to war are 'religious,' that information is highly relevant to the question of the function his beliefs have in his life. But . . . a registrant's statement that his beliefs are nonreligious is a highly unreliable guide for those charged with administering the exemption" (17). The Court also noted, in determining that the petitioner's objections were "religious" after all, that the Act would not be construed so as to afford differential treatment to "theistic and nontheistic" religions, a result that would raise issues with respect, not only to due process of law, but to whether theism was being "established."

In *Gillette v. United States* (18), the Court refused to permit conscientious objector status because there the petitioners asserted a particularized objection only to the Vietnam War as an "unjust" war and were unwillingly to state that their objection to war had its origins in religious beliefs that found all war objectionable. The Court decided the case on the basis of the statute, which required an objection to all war. The Court noted, "The specified objection must have a grounding in 'religious training and belief,' but no particular sectarian affiliation or theological position is required" (19); and "The relevant individual belief is simply objection to all war, not adherence to any extraneous theological viewpoint. And while the objection must have roots in conscience and personality that are 'religious' in nature, this requirement has never been construed to elevate conventional piety or religiosity of any kind above the imperatives of a personal faith" (20).

The Court rejected the petitioners' claim that in requiring objection to all war, Congress implicitly violated the Establishment Clause because it favored religions that opposed all war over religions that opposed only "unjust" ones. The Court noted that Congress's reasons for requiring objection to all war were purely secular in nature and not motivated by a desire to favor one set of religious beliefs over another.

In *Wisconsin v. Yoder* (21), the Court reversed convictions of Amish parents for violating the compulsory school attendance law. The parents refused to send their children to public or private school after the eighth grade, in contravention of legislation which required school attendance until the age of 16. Despite the interests of the state in guaranteeing an educated citizenry and protecting children from ignorance, the Amish provided the Court with copious evidence that "the traditional way of life of the Amish is not merely a matter of personal preference, but one of deep religious conviction, shared by an organized group, and intimately related to daily living" (22). The Court noted: "That the Old Order Amish daily life and religious practice stems from their faith is shown by the fact that it is in response to their literal interpretation of the Biblical injunction from the Epistle of Paul to the Romans, 'Be not conformed to this world. . . . ' " This command, the Court noted, "is fundamental to the Amish faith" (23). Moreover, the Court found that the statute placed an impossible burden on the Free Exercise rights of the Amish.

In a recent case of first impression, the California Superior Court had occasion to consider whether a religious entity could ever be sued for recruiting new members. In *Molko v. Holy Spirit Association* (24), apostate members of the Unification Church sued the Church alleging that their membership had been induced and continued, until their respective abductions and deprogrammings, by fraud and deceit; that they had been unlawfully "imprisoned" by brainwashing and mind control; that one of them had been induced by the same means to make a large donation that he wanted returned. Plaintiffs relied upon expert opinions from both a psychiatrist and a psychologist. The Court dismissed the complaints before trial, refusing to permit the state, by its court, even to consider the physically noncoercive indoctrination techniques or the truth or falsity of religious "misrepresentations." Since even to consider the propriety of "psychological techniques" of recruitment and retention of members is impossible "without questioning the authenticity and the force of the Unification Church's religious teachings," such judicial inquiry "is constitutionally forbidden." The Court continued:

> The idea that religious doctrine can be (or, as some would have it, invariably is) manipulatively employed to subvert reason— which, it may be noted, is an idea that has been used to condemn *all* religions as deceptively exploitative of certain universal human needs (see, e.g., Freud, *The Future of an Illusion* [1927])—is one we may entertain as individuals but which the First Amendment forbids us to consider as judges. Embodied in this constitutional prohibition is not simply a recognition of the value of the religious sensibility in its inevitably diverse and often conflicting forms, but as well an acknowledgment of the powerlessness of reason, and therefore the powerlessness of the law, to compass the mystery of religious faith.

With respect to the inadmissibility of the testimony and opinions of the psychiatrist and the psychologist, the Court stated, "Thus, from the point of view of the law, the opinions of plaintiffs' experts are neither true nor false. As the trial court observed, these opinions are simply 'veiled value judgments concerning the entire outlook of the Unification Church.' " It seems apparent, then, that courts will not sit in judgment of the authenticity of religious beliefs in *any* context.

Free Exercise and the Newly Emergent Religions

Despite the repeated emphasis that the Supreme Court has given the deference to religious belief principle in its numerous opinions, a number of suits involving newly emergent religions have nonetheless led some courts into the philosophical quagmire of determining not merely the bona fides with which the belief is held, but the verity of the particular religious tenets involved. The Supreme Court has made it clear that plaintiffs asserting a Free Exercise claim need show only a "genuine and sincere belief" in the principles of the subject religion, and that the principles themselves are absolutely immune from judicial scrutiny. Whether the suit presses the right of a religion to be free from state harassment, or the harassment of individuals in league with state or federal officials, therefore, its members need only demonstrate that they adhere to a genuine and sincere belief in the principles of that religion and that those principles are central to the religion itself, not that the principles in which they vest that belief are in any sense theologically defensible, true, authentic, or acceptable.

Despite the proscription that the Court has fashioned insulating the substantive principles of religions from judicial inquiry, several fora have held that, where a *statute* grants special status or privileges to religious entities or their members, judicial inquiry into the substantive tenets of the asserted religion is permissible.

Thus, in *Unification Church v. Immigration and Naturalization Service* (25), where the Unification Church invoked that section of the Immigration and Naturalization Act (26) permitting aliens to be admitted to the United States upon a blanket labor certification if they have "a religious commitment . . . to work for a nonprofit religious organization," the court held that the Unification Church qualified as a "religion" within the meaning of the Immigration and Naturalization Act, but only after inquiry into the principles of the religion itself.

Similarly, in *Holy Spirit Association for the Unification of World Christianity v. Tax Commission of the City of New York* (27), where the Unification Church sought tax exemption as a religious entity, New York's highest court again found it appropriate to inquire into the nature and theological justification of the religion, even though it ultimately held that the Unification Church qualified for the benefits sought.

Thus, while judicial inquiry into the substantive teachings of an asserted religion is at the very best a highly questionable practice, even where such intrusions have occurred, the religions in question are normally determined to be bona fide.

In the context of deprogramming litigation, however, inquiry into the substantive tenets of the adherent's religion is undeniably improper, for a requirement that the adherent first prove the authenticity of his chosen religion before prevailing on damage claims essentially obviates the protections of the First Amendment entirely. As noted earlier, the Free Exercise Clause exists precisely in order to protect even the most unpopular religions. Requiring the deprogramming victim plaintiff to demonstrate the "legitimacy" of that religion flies in the face of First Amendment law.

Moreover, given that the objective of deprogramming is to coerce the adherent to renounce his or her religious *beliefs*, deprogramming would seem at once violative of the Free Exercise Clause. However, the problem is that, in many cases, purely private parties are involved, and, as noted earlier, the Amendments to the Constitution are generally applicable only to government actors. Nonetheless, fearing the consequences of illegally seizing a religious sect member for the purpose of deprogramming, the professional deprogrammers began to devise stratagems of camouflage.

While private parties such as deprogrammers might hope to escape liability for claims brought directly under the Constitution, they could not hope to fare so well under standard tort law and criminal statutes which forbid kidnaping. Fearing the consequences (both criminal and civil) of seizing a religious sect member for the purpose of deprogramming, the professional deprogrammers devised a scheme that they hoped would insulate them from liability for their deprogramming activities. This strategy involves using the state civil conservatorship and guardianship statutes, those normally employed for the purposes of civil commitment, to "legitimate" the deprogramming effort by lending color of judicial approval to the procedure. Thus, the early deprogramming cases saw the deprogrammers or the parents applying to courts for conservatorship orders in typically ex parte (i.e., one-sided, without notice) proceedings, wherein it was merely alleged that an adult son or daughter was being held against his or her will or was somehow unable to resist the influence of the religious sect. In the vast majority of cases, there was absolutely no testimony by witnesses other than parents, much less experts who had personally evaluated the religious adherent, to substantiate the assertion that any form of mental illness made the intended conservatee unable to resist the coercive techniques that the parents alleged.

We now turn to a consideration of the use of conservatorship statutes to initiate the deprogramming procedure and to lend judicial gloss to it.

Seizure Pursuant to a Judicial Order
of Conservatorship

An individual may be deprived of his or her liberty only pursuant to a criminal conviction or by one of several forms of civil jurisdiction that may be asserted by private parties, such as guardianships or conservatorships. In several cases involving members of newly emergent religions, parents and deprogrammers have sought temporary conservatorships over adherents in an attempt to legitimate the deprogramming effort. It was hoped that the award of temporary conservatorship over a son or daughter would comport legally with due process and therefore immunize the parents and deprogrammers from liability for constitutional deprivations of liberty and the right to freedom of travel and religious freedom, as well as liability under various other laws of the United States and state tort law.

Thus, a fundamental legal distinction was thought to exist between seizure of the person pursuant to a valid conservatorship order and seizure of the person without any conservatorship order at all (28).

Unless the individual has not yet reached the age of majority, any seizure made without a conservatorship order at once implicates a variety of statutes, including, at the very least, state kidnap statutes (29). If, in the course of the abduction, the parents or deprogrammers bring the seized individual across state lines, federal statutes are also implicated (30).

But the distinction between seizure pursuant to a conservatorship order and seizure without benefit of such an order is finally an illusory one following the decision in *Katz v. Superior Court of California* (31), which held that California's conservatorship laws (32) could not be used to obtain control over a person for the purpose of subjecting him or her to religious deprogramming. The distinction between seizure pursuant to a conservatorship order and seizure without such an order may therefore now be an irrelevant one for purposes of the seizure's legality. The *Katz* (33) opinion would seem to intimate that, absent a showing of mental incompetence, a person can never be legally seized for the purpose of subjecting him or her to deprogramming.

In *In re Katz* (34) and *Katz v. Superior Court* (35), the parents of five members of the Unification Church sought temporary conservatorships over the persons of their sons and daughters for the expressed purpose of having them "deprogrammed." The Court there looked to two separate grounds on which to base its decision that parents (or other parties in interest) could not avail themselves of the conservatorship statutes for the purpose of subjecting a daughter or son to religious deprogramming. The Court first examined the statute under which the parents sought the conservatorship order. The California statute provided:

> Upon petition as provided in this chapter, the superior court, if satisfied by sufficient evidence of the need therefor, shall appoint a conservator of the person and property or person or property of any adult person who, in the case of a conservatorship of the person is unable properly to provide for his personal needs for physical health, food, clothing or shelter, and, in the case of a conservatorship of the property, is substantially unable to manage his own financial resources, or resist fraud or undue influence. . . . (36)

The Court first noted that there was no expert testimony that the intended conservatees were in any respect unable to care for themselves or their property. The Court stated:

> It is a fundamental principle, based upon the plainest dictates of justice that before a person can be deprived of his liberty and his property on account of his mental incompetency, he must be brought clearly within the terms of the statute, and the evidence must show that his mind is so far gone and so weak and feeble that he does not realize and comprehend the value and prudent management of his property, and is not sufficiently normal to care for it in the usual acceptation of that term. (37)

The Court then added: "In the field of beliefs, and particularly religious tenets, it is difficult, if not impossible, to establish a universal truth against which deceit and imposition can be measured" (38). Conservatorship for purposes of deprogramming, the Court said, was a misuse of the statute.

> If there is coercive persuasion or brainwashing which requires treatment, the existence of such a mental disability and the necessity of legal control over the mentally disabled person for the purpose of treatment should be ascertained after compliance with the protection of civil liberties. . . . To do less is to license kidnaping for the purpose of thought control. (39)

Next, the Court examined the constitutional infirmities involved in seeking to obtain control over church members for the purpose of "deprogramming." The Court analyzed the assertions of the parents, who claimed that the Unification Church was not a "true" religion and that therefore the First Amendment's Free Exercise Clause ought not protect the conservatees in this instance. The Court recalled the *Ballard* (40) and *Cantwell* (41) standards, that those asserting Free Exercise claims ought not to be subjected to proving the truth or substantive authenticity of their religion in order to invoke the protection of the First Amendment, and held those standards applicable so long as the adherents maintained a genuine and sincere belief in the religion asserted. Inquiry beyond this initial level of sincerity determination is forbidden domain, the Court noted. But the Court also held that, even if the Church members were to concede that the Unification Church offered nothing in the way of religion, the First Amendment nonetheless protected freedom of association, and the parties seeking conservatorship were therefore faced with a virtually insurmountable barrier to conservatorship, for the parents would have to demonstrate a *compelling state interest* in order to overcome the protections afforded the intended conservatees by the First Amendment. The Court concluded by stating:

> [I]n the absence of such actions as render the adult believer himself gravely disabled as defined in the law of this state, the process of this state cannot be used to deprive the believer of his freedom of action and to subject him to involuntary treatment. (42)

Thus, the *Katz* (43) case casts serious doubt upon the ability of parents ever to obtain control over sons or daughters for the purpose of "deprogramming," absent a showing of serious mental incapacity, presumably involving the testimony of several experts, pursuant to the state conservatorship statute. This being the case, any seizure of the person in California and jurisdictions in accord therewith would ipso facto constitute kidnaping.

Similarly, in *Taylor v. Gilmartin* (44), the Court of Appeals for the Tenth Circuit held that temporary guardianship orders procured for the purpose of subjecting members of religious groups to deprogramming were illegal and a misuse of the statute. The

Court noted that Oklahoma's guardianship statute was to be used for the purpose of protecting the mentally ill or individuals dangerous to themselves or others. The federal Court in *Taylor* (45) found the reasoning of the state court in *Katz* (46) persuasive, and continued to consider the tort liabilities to which the deprogrammers subjected themselves by misusing the guardianship statute in this way. The Court noted that obtaining the conservatorship order did not have the intended effect of immunizing the deprogrammers from the civil rights statutes and tort laws of the state.

Thus, since deprogrammers are now "on notice" that guardianship and conservatorship statutes may not be used for the purpose of lending judicial legitimacy to the deprogramming process, family members and deprogrammers alike who continue to avail themselves of such statutes in the future could also be called to answer in damages for "abuse of process." Moreover, because the complaints filed by parents and deprogrammers with whom they are in league typically lack any but conclusory and unsupported allegations of mental illness, it is conceivable that the petitioners in a conservatorship or guardianship proceeding initiated for the purpose of lending judicial gloss to a deprogramming process could be assessed attorneys' fees for the intended conservatee, since any such proceeding is clearly frivolous and without merit. In order to constitute a meritorious cause under such statutes, the complainants must establish at least some factual basis for mental incapacity on the part of the intended ward. Because conservatorships for deprogramming are routinely ex parte (or one-sided), such a remedy may be rare, but subsequent fee awards in abuse of process, other tort, and civil rights cases are likely consequences.

In any case, the importance of the *Katz* (47) and *Taylor* (48) opinions is that they make all conservatorship orders procured for the purpose of religious deprogramming illegal both as a matter of statutory interpretation and constitutional law, thus abolishing the distinction between seizures made with, and those made without, a conservatorship order (49).

Of interest to the mental health profession is the curious fact that, in a surprisingly large number of deprogramming cases, professionals, including psychiatrists, have supported applications for conservatorships based upon purported conclusions of the mental ill health of a proposed conservatee who had never been examined, and in many cases never even seen. In one case, a diagnosis and recommendation were made upon the basis of observing the proposed conservatee in a courtroom. In another case, the physician, not a psychiatrist, expressed his opinion of the need for conservatorship of a man he had never set eyes upon based upon the physician's personal family experience when a relative joined a different religious group he denominated a "cult." Mental health professionals who engage in vicarious diagnoses and recommend deprivations of freedom and personal integrity upon anything other than personal evaluation not only do damage to the credibility of the mental health professions and expose themselves to personal liability for malpractice, but risk professional censure and discipline.

Criminal Remedies

The only known criminal prosecutions of abductions in deprogramming cases have been undertaken by state prosecutors pursuant to state criminal statutes. The state criminal statutes under which deprogrammers may be liable include kidnap (50), unlawful imprisonment (51), assault (52), battery (53), and conspiracy to commit any of these substantive offenses (54). In *People v. Patrick* (55), for example, the court sustained the conviction of a deprogrammer under California's kidnap and false imprisonment statutes and rejected his contention that the abduction was defensible as a result of "necessity." The "necessity" defense has been variously defined as involving an action, otherwise unlawful, which the actor nonetheless undertakes in order to prevent an immediate, greater harm (56). The defendant asserted that he abducted the victim of the deprogramming because the danger posed by not deprogramming her was greater than that posed by the kidnap. The court found the defense to be without merit.

Since the standard of proof required to convict in a criminal proceeding is far more stringent than that needed to prevail in a civil context (57), the deprogrammer who is convicted of any of the criminal offenses set forth above can expect to be called to answer civilly for the offense, since an award of damages after a criminal conviction is very much more likely.

The federal law also recognizes criminal kidnaping (58), although the offense must involve crossing state lines in order to fall within the purview of federal criminal jurisdiction. With respect to federal prosecutions, however, the United States Department of Justice has failed to prosecute any of the more than 500 cases of deprogramming known to have occurred in the United States in the last decade, claiming, inter alia, that the kidnap never crossed state lines (a matter of *factual* determination), or, that if it did, it was essentially a matter of intrafamily concern into which the Justice Department has no desire to venture (59). The state prosecutions, however, call the wisdom and good faith of the policy of the federal government into question, revealing that state courts and juries are not convinced of the "innocent" "intrafamily" nature of the act of deprogramming. Recalling LeMoult's definition of deprogramming (60), cited, in *Colombrito v. Kelly* (61), it becomes apparent that deprogrammings often involve a great deal of physical force, including even the occasional use of firearms, in order to secure the "cooperation" of the adherent. Moreover, no known cases exist in which the state has sought to prosecute parents, but only the professional deprogrammers who are, more often than not, only too well aware of the fact that they are violating criminal laws (having in some cases been previously convicted of the same offenses), but seek to profit handsomely from that criminal behavior.

But the federal kidnap statutes are not the only criminal sanctions available to federal prosecutors in deprogramming cases. Two statutes, the KKK law, now 18 U.S.C. §§ 241 (62) and 242 (63), can be invoked to prosecute deprogrammers whose intent is to coerce adherents of newly emergent religions into renouncing their religious beliefs, and, thus to deprive them of the constitutional right to freedom of religion.

Section 241 provides:

> If two or more persons conspire to injure, oppress, threaten, or intimidate any citizen in the free exercise or enjoyment of any right or privilege secured to him by the Constitution or laws of the United States, or because of his having so exercised the same; or
>
> If two or more persons go in disguise on the highway, or on the premises of another, with intent to prevent or hinder his free exercise or enjoyment of any right or privilege so secured—

They shall be fined not more than $10,000 or imprisoned not more than ten years, or both; and if death results, they shall be subject to imprisonment for any term of years or for life.

Because the rights involved in deprogramming cases are secured by the First Amendment, and are applicable to the states through the Due Process Clause of the Fourteenth Amendment (which applies only to the actions of the state and not to the actions of private parties), securing a conviction under § 241 would be impossible without a showing that the abduction involved participation by state officials (e.g., the police who refuse to intervene despite knowledge of the illegality of the abduction, or possibly issuance by a state judge of a conservatorship order, despite his or her awareness of its invalidity, for the purposes of deprogramming). Several cases have recognized that private actors who carry out the criminal deprivation of a constitutional right in concert with state officials are criminally liable under § 242, which provides:

Whoever, under color of any law, statute, ordinance, regulation, or custom, willfully subjects any inhabitant of any State, Territory, or District to the deprivation of any rights, privileges, or immunities secured or protected by the Constitution or laws of the United States, or to different punishments, pains, or penalties, on account of such inhabitant being an alien, or by reason of his color, or race, than are prescribed for the punishment of citizens, shall be fined not more than $1,000 or imprisoned not more than one year, or both; and if death results shall be subject to imprisonment for any term of years or for life.

Section 242 clearly applies only to state officials (e.g., police) or to those private citizens found to have acted in concert with such state officials (64). There is thus no question that a federal prosecutor could reach, if so inclined, the conduct of police officers who, knowing of the illegal abduction of a religious sect adherent, refused to intervene. If it could be shown that there existed any sort of conspiratorial relationship between the deprogrammers and the police in this regard, the prosecutor could also reach the conduct of the deprogrammers, otherwise purely private parties, under § 242 because the private parties are said to be shrouded with state authority by virtue of the involvement of state officials, whether those state officials acted within or without the scope of their authority (65).

However, we are deposited once again at the threshold problem confronted in § 241 if absolutely no state involvement can be shown, that is, if the deprogrammers, purely private parties, have undertaken the abduction without aid or benefit of judicial order or police indifference. Because the right to religious freedom arises under the First Amendment and finds its way to the states through the Due Process Clause of the Fourteenth Amendment, the 1870 statute is held not to have been intended by Congress to impose criminal responsibility. As to rights derived from the pre–Civil War Constitution, however, protection is afforded. In *United States v. Guest* (66) and *United States v. Johnson* (67), involving purely private conspiracies to deprive citizens of constitutional rights, the Court noted that the federal prosecutor could reach purely private conduct provided that the rights violated were secured to the individual aggrieved independent of the Due Process Clause of the Fourteenth Amendment. In *Guest* (68), for example, the Court noted that § 241 could be invoked to prosecute private interference with the right to travel interstate, which right has as its source Article III § 2 of the Constitution and is not dependent for its genesis on any of the Amendments which apply to the states through the Fourteenth Amendment.

The identical debate over the "state action" requirement has arisen in the civil context (see below). At least one court has held, however, that, since a kidnap or illegal abduction at once deprives the victim of his or her constitutional right to freedom of travel, private parties will be held to answer civilly for violations of that right in the deprogramming context (69). Thus, in addition to prosecution under the federal kidnap statute, it appears that federal prosecutors could reach deprogrammers under 18 U.S.C. § 241 and, in many cases, 18 U.S.C. § 242 as well.

Not surprisingly, however, since the Justice Department has refused to exercise its prosecutorial discretion in the decision not to prosecute under federal kidnap statutes, it can hardly be within the realm of reasonable expectation to think that it will prosecute under the civil rights statutes.

Perhaps somewhat paradoxically, the civil rights statutes were enacted by Congress in order to reach the criminal behavior of state actors who notoriously violated the constitutional rights of citizens. The Congress saw the statute as a method of prosecuting state officials and private parties who acted to deprive citizens of their constitutional rights as well (e.g., the Ku Klux Klan), for riding roughshod over the rights of individuals. More often than not, state courts, juries, and prosecutors failed to secure convictions of those involved, being infamously of the same prejudices and attitudes as those on trial. Thus, the Congress saw no alternative but to secure the Constitutional rights of citizens by making available the federal laws, courts, and prosecutorial power for the purpose of guaranteeing federal constitutional rights. Ironically, however, in the context of First Amendment rights and the violations thereof inhering in the practice of deprogramming, the state courts, prosecutors, and statutes have been far more active in bringing criminal prosecutions than the federal prosecutors and courts (70).

An interesting question is whether, by virtue of its deliberate failure to safeguard the rights of religious minorities, the federal government has violated the Establishment Clause by favoring some religions over others. For purposes of this argument, however, the problem is that the failure of the Justice Department to prosecute these violations of Constitutional rights is properly described as a "practice," that is, it cannot be said to be the result of *legislation*. The First Amendment is silent where mere practices of state officials are concerned—its prohibitions speak only to legislation that violates the Establishment of Religion or the Free Exercise thereof. Thus, while the policy of the federal government may be one of willfully failing to enforce the First Amendment rights of religious sect members, technically, it may be argued, the Constitution has not been offended because this practice is not legislative in its origins. While the result is thus a de facto preferential enjoyment of religious freedom by adherents of mainstream religions, and a corresponding lack of those same freedoms by members of newly emergent religions, because the result is not legislatively mandated, the Establishment Clause can be said not to have been violated. The better and dominant view of this point, that the First and Fourteenth Amendments reach inaction and action by executives and judges as well by legislators, is for another forum.

Moreover, since the decision to prosecute is wholly within the discretion of the prosecutor, there is no way to compel prosecution in deprogramming cases. No doubt, federal prosecutions would have the desired effect of deterring deprogrammings that by now, it should be evident, are illegal on both statutory and constitutional grounds.

Finally, federal prosecutors could seek indictments under 18 U.S.C. § 245, which provides in relevant part:

> (b) Whoever, whether or not acting under color of law, by force or threat of force willfully injures, intimidates or interferes with, or attempts to injure, intimidate or interfere with—
>
> * * *
>
> (2) any person because of his race, color, religion or national origin and because he is or has been—
>
> * * *
>
> (E) traveling in or using any facility of interstate commerce, or using any vehicle, terminal or
>
> * * *
>
> facility of any common carrier by motor, rail, water, or air;
>
> * * *
>
> (4) any person because he is or has been, or in order to intimidate such person or any other person or any class of persons from—
>
>> (A) participating, without discrimination on account of race, color, religion or national origin, in any of the benefits or activities described . . . or
>> (B) affording another person or class of persons opportunity or protection so to participate; or
>
> (5) any citizen because he is or has been, or in order to intimidate such citizen or any other citizen from lawfully aiding or encouraging other persons to participate, without discrimination on account of race, color, religion or national origin, in any of the benefits or activities . . . or participating lawfully in speech or peaceful assembly opposing any denial of the opportunity so to participate—
>
> shall be fined not more than $1,000 or imprisoned not more than one year, or both; and if bodily injury results shall be fined not more than $10,000, or imprisoned not more than ten years, or both; and if death results shall be subject to imprisonment for any term of years or for life. . . .

Thus, it seems clear that § 245 (b) (2) (E) provides a basis for criminal prosecution, wholly independent of state action, and able to reach private action that interferes with the rights to peaceful assembly and travel interstate, as all abductions in furtherance of deprogramming necessarily do.

However, as with federal kidnap statutes, and §§ 241 and 242, no prosecutions have yet been brought by the federal government in deprogramming cases.

Federal Civil Remedies

42 U.S.C. §§ 1983 and 1985(3)

In the context of criminal remedies, we examined §§ 241 and 242 and looked briefly at § 245 of the Civil Rights Act. Not surprisingly, Congress also enacted civil analogues to §§ 241 and 242; 42 U.S.C. 1983 and 1985(3) provide civil relief for violations of constitutional rights or federal statutes, and again the distinction between state action and private action is critical. By far the most frequently asserted (and successfully litigated) federal civil remedy is 42 U.S.C. § 1985(3), which provides:

> If two or more persons in any State or Territory conspire or go in disguise on the highway or on the premises of another, for the purpose of depriving, either directly or indirectly, any person or class of persons of the equal protection of the laws, or of equal privileges and immunities under the laws and in any case of conspiracy set forth in this section, if one or more persons engaged therein do, or cause to be done, any act in furtherance of the object of such conspiracy, whereby another is injured in his person or property, or deprived of having and exercising any right or privilege of a citizen of the United States, the party so injured or deprived may have an action for the recovery of damages, occasioned by such injury or deprivation, against any one or more of the conspirators.

Section 1985(3) is the civil analogue of 18 U.S.C. § 241 and is intended to reach *purely private conspiracies* which seek to deprive the victim of any constitutional or federal statutory right. Again, however, the question arises whether Congress has the authority to reach purely private conspiracies to deprive individuals of constitutional rights, since the First Amendment is made applicable to the states only through the Due Process Clause of the Fourteenth Amendment, which requires "state action" to be enforceable. In *Griffin v. Breckenridge* (71), the Court held that, where the right alleged to have been violated by the private conspiracy has its source in the Constitution proper, rather than in one of the amendments thereto, the power of Congress to reach conspiracies in derogation thereof is plenary. Thus, the Court sustained the right of the plaintiffs to maintain an action under § 1985(3) against private conspirators who deprived them of the right to interstate travel, having its source in Article IV § 2 of the Constitution proper.

Several state (72) and federal courts (73) have relied upon the *Breckenridge* opinion to give rise to a cause of action under § 1985(3) against purely private action by deprogrammers.

Only one opinion which denied a § 1985(3) claim in the religious deprogramming context could be found (74), and this case was clearly an aberration.

In *Cooper v. Molko* (75), for example, parents arranged to have their son, a member of the Unification Church, abducted and deprogrammed. The son was held forcibly and subjected to five days of coercion. He thereafter escaped. Plaintiff filed under §§ 1983 and 1985(3), alleging that the police knew of the abduction and failed to take any corrective action.

Section 1983 provides:

> Every person who, under color of any statute, ordinance, regulation, custom, or usage, of any State or Territory, subjects or causes to be subjected, any citizen of the United States or other person within the jurisdiction thereof to the deprivation of any rights, privileges, or immunities secured by the Constitution and laws, shall be liable to the party injured in an action at law, suit in equity, or other proper proceeding for redress.

Thus, plaintiff claimed, the police had entered into a conspiracy with the deprogrammers. The involvement of state officials (the police) was not only sufficient to state a cause of action under § 1983, but the court held that the private defendants could also be sued under § 1983 because state officials conspired with private parties. Under the logic of *United States v. Price* (76), private parties who act in conspiracy with state officials may be sued under both §§ 1983 and 1985(3). Similarly, under § 1985(3), the involvement of the police confers the state action necessary to reach a First Amendment claim [*Adickes v. S. H. Kress & Co.* (77)]. Perhaps most significant in the *Cooper* (78) opinion is the holding that police *inaction* was sufficient to state a claim under §§ 1983 and 1985(3). The court noted that "It is clear that § 1983 was intended to apply to acts by police officers of omission as well as commission" (79).

As to the claim under § 1985(3), the *Cooper* (80) court noted that plaintiff had to show 1) the existence of a conspiracy 2) for the purpose of depriving him or her, either directly or indirectly, of the equal protection of the laws or of any privileges and immunities secured to citizens under the laws 3) that the conspirators did, or caused to be done, any act in furtherance of the object of the conspiracy 4) such that plaintiff was injured in person or property or deprived of having and exercising any right or privilege of a citizen of the United States; 5) plaintiff must show violation of a protected right 6) and an invidiously discriminatory, class-based animus that motivated the violation.

The Court held that, while in *Griffin v. Breckenridge* (81), the Supreme Court left open the question of what classes besides race could be protected by § 1985(3), an invidiously discriminatory motive to deprive plaintiff of his First Amendment right to freedom of religion, motivated by animus toward his or her religion, was sufficient to state a claim under § 1985(3). Citing to *Marlowe v. Fisher Body* (82) and *Baer v. Baer* (83), the Court held that religious groups such as the Unification Church are protected by § 1985(3).

The deprogrammers in *Cooper* (84) attempted to defend against the animosity requirement by noting that they were motivated, not by animus toward plaintiff's religion, but instead by parental concern. The Court stated:

> We note, moreover, that whatever good ultimate purpose the defendants may have had in mind, that good motive would not necessarily negate their alleged animus against plaintiff's religious group. (85)

Moreover, in *Colombrito v. Kelly* (86), the court noted:

> [P]arental concern and a class-based animus may coexist or indeed sometimes merge. It could reasonably be inferred from the present record that although the parents acted out of

concern for their son's well being, they simultaneously were motivated by an intense animosity toward the Unification Church, to which he had been converted and toward its beliefs and practices. (87)

Other Courts have also sustained the §§ 1983 and 1985(3) claims against deprogrammers [e.g., *Katz* (88)], which held that even purely private conspiracies could be reached under § 1985(3) where they involved a fundamental right not having its genesis in the Bill of Rights, but arising independently from the Constitution proper, such as the right to interstate travel.

Courts have also been quick to recognize that plaintiffs who prevail on either § 1983 or § 1985(3) claims would qualify for attorneys fees under 42 U.S.C. § 1988, which provides:

In any action or proceeding to enforce a provision of sections 1981, 1982, 1983, 1985, and 1986 of this title, Title IX of Public Law 92-318, or Title VI of the Civil Rights Act of 1964, the court, in its discretion, may allow the prevailing party, other than the United States, a reasonable attorney's fee as part of the costs.

Constitutional Claims

A plaintiff can also establish a claim directly under the United States Constitution against any federal agents or officers if he or she can prove their involvement in the deprogramming, either directly or by omission. In *Bivens v. Six Unknown Named Agents of the Bureau of Narcotics* (89), the Court noted that § 1983 applied to the actions of *state* officers and not to those of federal officers or officials. It seemed hardly possible that a plaintiff could have a cause of action against state operatives who deprived him or her of a constitutional right but have no claim for relief against the federal government for identical behavior. Thus, the Court in *Bivens* (90) held that a plaintiff who could make out constitutional violations directly under the Constitution or its Amendments could have his remedy in damages, injunctive relief, or both. *Bivens* (91) arose in the context of a Fourth Amendment (search) violation, and the Court did not provide an exhaustive list of which constitutional rights would give rise directly to actions under the Constitution itself. However, lower courts (92) have read *Bivens* (93) broadly to include a cause of action for First Amendment violations.

Injunctive Relief

Injunctive relief against deprogrammers is available against state actors or private conspirators in any manner linked with state action under §§ 1983 and 1985(3) and directly under the Constitution under *Bivens* (94) as well as under Fed. R. Civ. P. 65.

Federal Tort Law

A plaintiff whose rights have been violated by a federal agent (e.g., an FBI agent who has knowledge of the abduction but fails to intervene) may also state a claim under the Federal Tort Claims Act (95). Plaintiff must show both that he or she has exhausted any administrative remedy and "demonstrate that the act complained of would constitute a tort in the state where it was committed" (96). There is no reason in theory that a plaintiff could not assert both a *Bivens* claim for violations of constitutional rights as well as a tort action if the facts will support it; however, the 1974 amendments to the Tort Claims Act state that it shall be the exclusive remedy for certain police torts (97).

Federal Habeas Corpus

Finally, if an adherent has been abducted, the religious group of which he or she is a member may file a writ of habeas corpus demanding the release of the member. If the group members know where the adherent is being held, the writ, once issued by a court, will be enforced by the federal marshals.

State Civil Remedies

Tort Law

The adherent who has been abducted can state a claim in tort for kidnaping, false imprisonment, assault, battery, intentional infliction of emotional distress, and, if he or she has been abducted pursuant to a conservatorship without any sound belief or proof that she or he is mentally incompetent, possibly abuse of process as well. Moreover, if the plaintiff is able to show, perhaps through the existence of prior decisional law combined with testimony, that the defendants knew that the use of the conservatorship statute was a misuse of the statute for deprogramming purposes, punitive damages as well as attorneys' fees may be recovered.

State Constitutions

A member of a newly emergent religion who has been abducted may also state a claim for violations of rights secured to her or him by the *state* constitution, and the right so to file will arise directly under the state's own constitution. In some cases, the state's constitution may confer even greater substantive rights than does the federal constitution.

Injunctive Relief

The religious group or the aggrieved member may file for injunctive relief pursuant to the constitution of the state involved if a right alleged to have been violated thereunder can be found.

State Habeas Corpus

All states also have habeas corpus (98) constitutional guarantees and statutes that enable a state court to secure the release of the person from illegal custody.

Federal and State Defenses and Immunities

As to tort claims, both the state and federal governments may enjoy immunity from suit on the theory of sovereign immunity. However, with the advent of the Federal Tort Claims Act (99) and similar state statutes, it is unlikely that the state or federal governments would prevail in a tort action commenced because of tortious conduct on the part of their agents. Indeed, plaintiff need assert only the relationship of agency in order to stand on a theory of respondeat superior (i.e., that the employer is liable for the acts of the employee in the scope of the employment).

Immunities to suit under the civil rights statutes are another matter entirely, however. First, should a court find that a judge has erroneously issued a conservatorship order and thereby violated the plaintiff's First Amendment right to freedom of religion, the judge will nonetheless enjoy absolute immunity from suit (100). Thus, a § 1983 or 1985(3) action will never prevail against a judge who had jurisdiction to issue the order.

Police officers do not enjoy absolute immunity from suit under the civil rights statutes, but enjoy only a qualified, good faith immunity. In *Monell v. New York City Department of Social Services* (101) and *Owen v. City of Independence* (102), the Court held that municipalities and their officials qualify as "persons" within the meaning of § 1983. Municipal officials such as council members, clerks, and police officers enjoy only a qualified, good faith immunity, which is an evidentiary issue.

An important point also decided by *Owen* (103) was that a plaintiff in a § 1983 or § 1985(3) claim can*not* reach the municipality simply by virtue of the *respondeat superior* theory; that is, plaintiff cannot prevail on a suit against the municipality simply by virtue of the fact that the municipality is the untoward police officer's employer. While such a theory will normally prevail in a tort action, the same is not necessarily true of civil rights claims brought against police officers. The municipality may elect to indemnify the officer, meaning that the municipality believes the officer acted within the scope of his or her authority, and the municipality will then be held responsible for the deprivations of civil rights committed by him or her. On the other hand, if the municipality believes that the officer did not act within the scope of his or her authority, it may assert a good faith immunity under *Owen* (104), and only the officer will answer for the deprivations individually. For this reason, *respondeat superior* is not available in civil rights actions; otherwise, the municipality would automatically be called, by virtue of the employer-employee relationship, to indemnify the officer who acted outside the scope of his or her authority.

Conclusion

The modern dilemma posed by the failure of the federal government to enforce the First Amendment right to freedom of religion on behalf of members of newly emergent religions is unprecedented in American history. While the federal and state governments both have certainly been lax in the area of civil rights in the past, never has the religious freedom issue occupied such a central place in the civil rights arena. The First Amendment's protections were designed to extend to the most unpopular beliefs, and instead we find its protections being offered only to the established mainstream religions. Unfortunately, this makes a mockery of the First Amendment, which is now applied to protect only those religions that require its protections least. It is the thesis of this chapter that adherence to the tenets of a religious or other group, no matter how bizarre or inconsistent with societal norms, can never justify conservatorship and that religious deprogramming itself, whether with or without color of conservatorship, is never justified legally, psychiatrically, or ethically; that absent a showing that an individual is in fact mentally incompetent, a conservatorship is improper; that it is a sound conclusion that has been reached by one commentator (105) and several courts (106) holding the use of conservatorship to gain control of the initiate for the purpose of subjecting him or her to deprogramming is prima facie a misuse of the statute and a First Amendment violation. It is also the conclusion that, because the expressed purpose of deprogrammers is to cause the adherent to renounce her or his religious beliefs, this dirty business, which flourishes with the tacit approval of the Justice Department, can be deterred only by vigorous enforcement of state criminal statutes and by similarly vigorous suits for civil remedies against all the individuals involved. While the Constitution and its Amendments may not reach purely private violative behavior, nonetheless, the government and courts should not and will not permit anyone to profit from violations of the rights of others. In addition to civil redress, it is the obligation of both state and federal officials to press prosecutions to safeguard the constitutional freedoms and civil liberties of those affected and threatened by deprogramming behavior.

Notes

1. 764 F.2d 122, 125 (2nd Cir. 1985).
2. LeMoult, Deprogramming Members of Religious Sects, 46 Fordham L. Rev. 599, 604, 605 (1978), cited in Colombrito v. Kelly, supra (see note 1 and text).

3. Draft complaint against the United States in files of Jeremiah S. Gutman.
4. Complaint filed with United Nations Subcommission on the Protection of Minorities against the United Kingdom and France.
5. U.S. Constitution, Amendment I (1791).
6. 330 U.S. 1 (1947).
7. 310 U.S. 296 (1940).
8. 98 U.S. 145 (1878).
9. 322 U.S. 78 (1944).
10. 322 U.S. at 86–88.
11. 374 U.S. 398 (1963).
12. 380 U.S. 163 (1965).
13. 50 U.S.C. App. § 456(j).
14. 380 U.S. at 166.
15. 380 U.S. at 184, 185.
16. 398 U.S. 333 (1970).
17. 398 U.S. at 341.
18. 401 U.S. 437 (1971).
19. 401 U.S. at 450, 451.
20. 401 U.S. at 454.
21. 406 U.S. 205 (1972).
22. 406 U.S. at 216.
23. *Idem.*
24. District Court of Appeal Division Two, Nos. A025338 and A020935 (March 31, 1986).
25. 547 F. Supp. 623 (D.D.C. 1982).
26. 8 U.S.C. §§ 1182(a) (14) and 1153(a) (6) in conjunction with 20 C.F.R. 656.10(c) (2) (1982).
27. 55 N.Y.2d 512 (1982).
28. There exists some debate over the validity of seizures made pursuant to an invalid conservatorship order, though the majority view is that seizure made pursuant to an invalid conservatorship order is unlawful, and therefore actionable in damages [(e.g., Taylor v. Gilmartin, 686 F.2d 1346 (10th Cir. 1982), *cert. den.*, 459 U.S. 1147 (1983)].
29. For example, New York defines "abduct" [Penal Law § 135.00 (2)]:

"Abduct means to restrain a person with intent to prevent his or her liberation by either (a) secreting or holding the person in a place where he or she is not likely to be found, or (b) using or threatening to use deadly physical force.

and punishes abduction as its highest grade of crime [Penal Law § 135.25]:

A person is guilty of kidnapping in the first degree when he or she abducts another person and when:

     1. His or her intent is to compel a third person to pay or deliver money or other property as ransom, or to engage in other particular conduct, or to refrain from engaging in particular conduct; or . . . .

30. 18 U.S.C. § 1201 (1948), which reads in relevant part:

    (a) Whoever unlawfully seizes, confines, inveigles, decoys, kidnaps, abducts, or carries away and holds for ransom or reward or otherwise any person, except in the case of a minor by a parent thereof, when:
    (1) the person is willfully transported in interstate or foreign commerce . . . shall be punished by imprisonment for any term of years or for life.

31. 141 Cal. Rptr. 234 (Ct. App. 1977).
32. Cal. Prob. Code § 1754.1 (West Cum. Supp. 1977).
33. 141 Cal. Rptr. 234.
34. No. 216828 (San Francisco County Super. Ct. Mar. 24, 1977), *rev'd sub nom.* Katz v. Superior Court, 73 Cal. App. 3d 952, 141 Cal. Rptr. 234 (1977).
35. 141 Cal. Rptr. 234.
36. Cal. Prob. Code, § 1754.1 (West Cum. Supp. 1977).
37. *Citing* to In Re Coburn, 11 Cal. App. 604, 606, 105 P. 924, 925 (1909); 141 Cal. Rptr. at 242.
38. 141 Cal. Rptr. at 244.
39. 141 Cal. Rptr. at 253.
40. 322 U.S. 78 (1944).
41. 310 U.S. 296 (1940).
42. 141 Cal. Rptr. at 256.
43. 141 Cal. Rptr. 234.
44. 686 F.2d 1346 (10th Cir. 1982), *cert. den.,* 459 U.S. 1147 (1983).
45. *Idem.*
46. 141 Cal. Rptr. 234.
47. *Idem.*
48. 686 F.2d 1346 (10th Cir. 1982), *cert. den.,* 459 U.S. 1147 (1983).
49. That conservatorship orders obtained for the purpose of deprogramming *should* be barred by the First Amendment is the conclusion of an unusually articulate commentary found at Note, *Conservatorships and Religious Cults, Divining a Theory of Free Exercise,* 53 N.Y.U.L. Rev. 1247 (1978).
50. For example, see New York Penal Law, §§ 135.20 and 135.25.
51. See, for example, New York Penal Law, §§ 135.10 and 135.15.
52. See, for example, New York Penal Law, §§ 120.20 and 120.25.
53. See, for example, New York Penal Law, §§ 120.00, 120.05, and 120.10.
54. See, for example, New York Penal Law, Article 105.

55. 179 Cal. Rptr. 276 (App. 1982), *hearing den.* (1982).
56. See LaFave and Scott, *Criminal Law* (1972).
57. *Idem.*
58. 18 U.S.C. § 1201.
59. Private correspondence to Jeremiah S. Gutman from U.S. Department of Justice.
60. See note 2, above.
61. 764 F.2d 122 (2nd Cir. 1985).
62. Enacted in original form in 1870.
63. Enacted in original form in 1870.
64. See, for example, Cooper v. Molko, 512 F. Supp. 563 (N.D. Cal. 1981).
65. For example, United States v. Guest, 383 U.S. 745 (1966).
66. 383 U.S. 745 (1966).
67. 390 U.S. 563 (1968).
68. 383 U.S. 745.
69. See, Cooper v. Molko, 512 F. Supp. 563 (N.D. Cal. 1981).
70. See, for example, People v. Patrick, 179 Cal. Rptr. 276 (App. 1981), *hearing den.* (1982).
71. 400 U.S. 88 (1971).
72. For example, Katz v. Superior Court, 141 Cal. Rptr. 234 (Ct. App. 1977).
73. For example, Eilers v. Coy, 582 F. Supp. 1093 (D. Minn. 1984); Taylor v. Gilmartin, 686 F.2d 1346 (10th Cir. 1982), *cert. den.*, 459 U.S. 1147, and 103 S. Ct. 3570 (1983); Ward v. Conner, 657 F.2d 45 (4th Cir. 1981); Cooper v. Molko, 512 F. Supp. 563 (N.D. Cal. 1981); Mandelkorn v. Patrick, 350 F. Supp. 692 (D.D.C. 1973).
74. Weiss v. Patrick, 453 F. Supp. 717 (D.R.I. 1978).
75. 512 F. Supp. 563.
76. 383 U.S. 787 (1966).
77. 398 U.S. 144 (1970).
78. 512 F. Supp. 563.
79. 512 F. Supp. at 567.
80. 512 F. Supp. 563.
81. 403 U.S. 88 (1971).
82. 489 F.2d 1057 (6th Cir. 1973).
83. 450 F. Supp. 481, 490, 491 (N.D. Cal. 1978).
84. 512 F. Supp. 563.
85. 512 F. Supp. at 570.
86. 764 F.2d 122 (2nd Cir. 1985).
87. 764 F.2d at 131.
88. 141 Cal. Rptr. 234.
89. 403 U.S. 388 (1971).
90. *Idem.*
91. *Idem.*
92. Stanley v. United States, 54 U.S.L.W. 2573 (11th Cir. No. 84-5273 Apr. 21, 1986); Dellums v. Powell, 566 F.2d 167, 194 (D.C. Cir. 1977), *cert. den.*, 438 U.S. 916 (1978); Yiamouyiannis v. Chemical

Abstracts Service, 521 F.2d 1392 (6th Cir. 1975), *cert. den.*, 439 U.S. 983 (1978); Skehan v. Trustees of Bloomsburg State College, 501 F.2d 31 (3rd Cir. 1974); Green v. Laird 357 F. Supp. 227 (N.D. Ill. 1973); Rodriguez v. Barcelo, 358 F. Supp. 43 (D.P.R. 1973); Revis v. Laird, 391 F. Supp. 1133 (E.D. Cal. 1975); Gardels v. Murphy, 377 F. Supp. 1389 (N.D. Ill 1974); Peacock v. Board of Regents, 380 F. Supp. 1081 (D. Ariz. 1974); Butler v. United States, 365 F. Supp. 1035 (D. Hawaii 1973).

93. 403 U.S. 388 (1971).
94. *Idem.*
95. 28 U.S.C. §§ 2671–2680 (as amended, 1974).
96. Dorsen, Bender, Neuborne, and Law, *Political and Civil Rights in the United States*, Vol. 2, 1979, at 485.
97. *Idem.*
98. New York, for example, Constitution, Art. I § 4, and Civil Practice Law and Rules, Article 70.
99. 28 U.S.C. §§ 2671–2680 (as amended, 1974).
100. Pierson v. Ray, 386 U.S. 547 (1967).
101. 436 U.S. 658 (1978).
102. 48 U.S.L.W. 4389 (1980).
103. *Idem.*
104. *Idem.*
105. See note 49, above.
106. For example, Katz v. Superior Court, 141 Cal Rptr. 234 (Ct. App. 1977); Taylor v. Gilmartin, 686 F.2d 1346 (10th Cir. 1982), *cert. den.*, 459 U.S. 1147, and 103 S. Ct. 3570 (1983).

Chapter 15

OPTIONS FOR LEGAL INTERVENTION

Richard Delgado

The Options

Options for intervening in connection with the activities of cult groups are as varied as the legal imagination. This section lists a number of the options, subdivided into two broad categories. Succeeding sections discuss the need for such interventions, as well as their status under prevailing moral and legal norms.

Preinduction Remedies

To avert, or minimize, the various harms that are found sometimes to be associated with living in a cult group, a number of preinduction remedies are available. These remedies, as a group, aim at avoiding the harm, rather than undoing it or compensating for it once it has occurred.

One such preventive remedy is a simple requirement of identification—a legal requirement that cult proselytizers identify themselves to potential recruits and disclose specified information about the name of the group, its leader, location, and demands placed on members. Failure to provide the required information would be punished by fines or a prison sentence. A number of young people who have left cults have complained that the recruiters and leaders misled them into thinking the group was nonreligious—a discussion group or Peace Corps type organization, for example. Many cults use pseudonyms or front names. Eventually, of course, the recruit learns the truth about the organization, but often too late—he or she has been so "softened up" by chanting, sleep deprivation, "love bombing," and peer pressure that he or she is unable to make an independent evaluation of his or her growing commitment to the group. A requirement of identification could help avert these problems, and could be compared to consumer and truth-in-lending laws currently in effect. Recently, the United States Supreme Court has struck down disclosure rules that disproportionately burdened small, unpopular religious groups in fund-raising. But the greater stake in connection with recruitment—one's person, rather than one's money—should adequately distinguish the two types of statutes.

A further preventive remedy is public education. School- or college-age youth could be given classes or seminars on the methods and consequences of cult induction and taught to be skeptical of nebulous "pitches" and extravagant claims. Such training could be likened to courses in sex and drug education; the intent would be to make students careful, alert consumers in the area of high-demand groups. A number of school districts have such courses in place, and the national Parent-Teacher Association (PTA) has encouraged this trend.

Another group of devices would aim at incorporating opportunities for reflection, or communication with the outside world, at some specified point in the indoctrination process. These devices could be compared to currently existing "cooling off" legislation in the consumer protection area—measures that enable a purchaser to return a product and rescind a sale undertaken in the heat of the moment (purchase of an expensive set of books by a welfare family, for example). Examples of such devices in the cult context might include a legal requirement that cults—and perhaps all religious groups—permit reasonable, nondisruptive communication with persons outside the group. Alternatively, groups could be required to give their members "sabbaticals," periods when the member would leave the training area for reflection and contemplation. Even a brief respite from the intense conditioning required by some cult groups could enable members to assess their growing commitment to the group and decide whether they wished to return for more.

A final preinduction remedy would be provision for giving effect to a document, similar to the "living will" or durable power of attorney, that calls for rescue should the signor come under the influence of specified cults or cultlike groups. Such a document would constitute evidence of a person's desires at a time when he or she was free of unusual pressures and focusing autonomously on his or her desires and life plan. Of course, it would be necessary to recognize the possibility of a person's rescinding such a document, but the existence of opposing statements by the same individual would at least call a court's attention to the environmental and social factors responsible for the disparate statements. Moreover, the filing of the first statement might ease the burden of parents and mental health professionals attempting to cope with the dilemmas of particular cult inductions; it would put them on notice that membership might be against the convert's considered judgment.

Postinduction Remedies

One set of postinduction remedies includes civil or criminal actions against cult leaders for various torts or crimes committed as part of the induction process. There have been a few convictions of cult leaders under federal antipeonage legislation (laws that forbid slavery), and some have proposed the application of the federal kidnapping ("Lindbergh") statute to cult cases. Far more frequent, however, are civil suits for such torts as fraud, unlawful imprisonment, or intentional infliction of emotional distress. Mental health professionals are frequently called upon to testify as expert witnesses in such trials. A number of such suits have resulted in large recoveries (while others have yielded only modest relief or none at all). Successful lawsuits seem to have been responsible for some cults' changing their recruitment practices and, as such, have had some discernible deterrent effect.

A related postinduction feature is not an independent remedy but rather operates as a defense to legal action directed against would-be rescuers of cult victims. Sometimes parents, relatives, or religious leaders who were associated with a cultist in his or her former life become concerned over his or her mental-physical condition. Believing other avenues of relief to be fruitless, they may forcibly abduct the member from the commune or other living area and attempt to "deprogram" or otherwise bring the member to his or her senses. When the attempt is successful, legal action rarely ensues because there is no one to bring charges. If it fails, however, the cult member and his or her leaders may persuade the local district attorney to bring charges. Frequently, the parents or other would-be rescuers admit the actions but argue that they were justified by the defense of necessity—the so-called "choice of evils" defense. The defense, recognized by the Model Penal Code and about one half of American jurisdictions, excuses conduct that would otherwise be criminal if the perpetrator shows that he or she acted under a belief that intervention was necessary to avert an even greater evil than that sought to be prevented by the criminal statute violated. In some of these cases, mental health professionals have sometimes been called to the stand to testify to conditions within the cult that allegedly justified the parents' actions. The defense of necessity seems to have been successful in roughly one-half of the cases in which it was used.

At other times, deprogramming or "exit counseling" (the current euphemism) is carried out voluntarily—the parents and counselor manage to gain access to the cult member and attempt to persuade him that his thought processes have been blunted and that he should disengage himself from the group before it is too late. Voluntary extrication of members presents no legal problem; indeed, a recent court decision holds that the First Amendment rights of parents and counselors would be violated by limiting their freedom to talk with, remonstrate with, and attempt to persuade cult members to leave the group.

Sometimes exit counseling is carried out under the authority of a court order of conservatorship or guardianship. When carried out in this fashion, legal liability for counselors and parents is much reduced, of course, but not all states permit orders to be issued for such purposes. A California intermediate-level appellate court decision [*Katz v. Superior Court*, 73 Cal. App.3d 952, 141 Cal. Rptr. (1977)], held conservatorships for religious deprogramming unconstitutional. Although the California decision is not binding on other states, it has had some influence beyond that state's borders. Although courts in some states have continued to issue conservatorships for the purpose of helping extricate a cult member, the number of such orders has declined in recent years.

Evaluating the Options: Moral and Legal Analysis

Each option—indeed, each case—presents a different constellation of moral and legal interests. Yet, it is possible to make a number of generalizations, at least at the level of indicating what elements should play a part in assessing the various options.

Intervention of any kind inevitably will encroach to a greater or lesser extent on religious liberty, in our society a highly protected value. Thus, any practice aimed at curtailing a cultic practice must be supported by a strong reason. (In the language of the law, there must be a "compelling state interest.") In general, that reason for intervention will take the form of some alleged harm, or group of harms, found to be caused by the cult. Such harms could be individual or societal. The case for intervention is also affected by the extent to which intervention interferes with religious belief or practice: the greater the interference, the higher the justification must be. Also, the requirement of justification increases if intervention is aimed at a central, or vital, tenet or practice of the group. Finally, the case for intervention weakens if the harm at which intervention is aimed is voluntarily incurred by competent adults. The remainder of this chapter takes up these matters, in turn.

First Amendment case law indicates that certain harms rise to the level of compelling state interest—precipitation of serious physical or emotional injury; severe harm to autonomy; installation of disabling guilt; maturational arrest. Religion cases also indicate that harm to broad social interests or institutions (such as harm to the family) may also constitute compelling state interests.

Whether the practices of particular cult groups cause such harms, and if so, to what extent, is an empirical question. The literature that I have reviewed—primarily legislature hearing reports, legal depositions and judicial opinions, and the writings of journalists and social scientists who have studied cults—indicates that each of the harms described in the preceding paragraph is associated with some, or many, cult groups. The degree varies, and apparently not all who associate with the groups emerge harmed. Not all cults cause each of the harms, and those that do cause a particular harm may change their practices from time to time, becoming more or less harmful. The practices of certain large or geographically dispersed cult groups, like the Unification Church, may vary from place to place. Some investigators, for example, have reported significant differences in the methods of operation of the Unification Church on the west and east coasts.

Moreover, the interpretation to be placed on empirical findings of harm seems to vary remarkably from observer to observer. When the harm consists of an intangible effect (such as loss of autonomy or the capacity to make independent decisions) this is understandable, but different observers appear to place different values on incidence of tangible, physical harms (such as severe malnutrition, mass suicide, or use of dangerous drugs, such as toluene). Some are satisfied that these effects occur and are serious enough to call for measures aimed at averting them; others seem prepared to dismiss them as infrequent or atypical. Objective, accurate empirical studies would certainly aid analysis.

In addition to the requirement that intervention be justified by a strong state interest, intervention must not encroach any more than necessary on protected religious liberty. Constitutional analysis also pays attention to the role the interdicted practice plays in the religion's scheme of belief and practice. Interventions that impinge on central, essential elements are scrutinized more carefully than ones that interfere with inessential practices or minor elements of worship or organization.

Thus, a court might find that a requirement of self-identification by proselytizers (exemplified, for example, by a requirement that they wear an identifying badge) constituted a minor, permissible interference with religious liberty. At the same time, the arrest and incarceration of the group's spiritual leader (as occurred recently with the Unification Church), or a law that permitted forcible abduction and deprogramming on the basis of an ex parte hearing would receive much closer scrutiny.

Two further factors affect the balancing of cult versus state interest. One is the extent to which the harms associated with cult membership are consensual, that is, voluntarily incurred. If it should appear that the harms—or, at any rate the individual ones, such as physical sickness, emotional disease, lost opportunities for maturation and advancement, suppressed autonomy, and so on—are voluntarily incurred, then the case for intervention obviously weakens. The same would be true if the individual undergoing them did not perceive them as harms (even though others might). The other factor is the ability to draw lines—to indicate in what respects the practices of cult groups differ in their effects, either in kind or degree, from those associated with groups we are prepared to tolerate—Jesuit seminaries, the Boy Scouts, boot camp, Outward Bound, and the like.

Consensuality

The antipaternalistic bias that informs our political and legal system predisposes us to reject governmental action aimed at protecting us from ourselves. Thus, if it were to appear that the harms suffered by cult members were voluntarily incurred, or if the members did not see them as harms at all, but, rather as mild prices to be paid for enlightenment or bliss, then the case for state intervention would weaken. Consent, then, becomes an important ingredient in the way in which we look at cults. But before analyzing issues of consent and voluntariness, it might be urged that such values play no part, or play a reduced part, in the analysis of religious joining. Religious devotion and affiliation, it might be asserted, are areas in which faith and discipleship, not consent and choice, operate.

I believe this objection to be misguided. Self-determination is deeply rooted in our treatment of and notions of religion. Although some religious groups, it is true, emphasize passive acquiescence and obedience, the legal system has always required that religions treat individuals as though commitment to religion is an affirmative act they alone are free to make. The drafters of the Constitution saw religion in these terms. For example, in drafting the preamble to Virginia's religious-freedom statute, Jefferson wrote: "God made man's mind free, and deliberately chose that religion should be propagated by reason and not by coercion." Locke, whose writings strongly influenced the American framers of the Constitution, wrote that religion is "the inward persuasion of the mind," and spoke of a church as a "voluntary society of men, joining themselves together of their own accord." Modern decisions also emphasize the voluntary aspect of religious affiliation, by upholding laws against religious fraud, for example, or requiring that religious beliefs, to be entitled to exemption (from military service, for example), be sincere. A few cases [e.g., *Campbell v. Cauthron*, 623

F.2d 503 (8th Cir. 1980)] uphold a right against imposed religiosity directly. Others uphold the principle indirectly. [See, e.g., *Wooley v. Maynard*, 430 U.S. 705 (1977) (striking down, under free-speech portion of the First Amendment, state statute under which every automobile license plate was inscribed with motto, "Live Free or Die"); *Torcaso v. Watkins*, 367 U.S. 488 (1961) (holding unconstitutional an oath of office requiring affirmation of God); *School District of Abington Township v. Schempp*, 374 U.S. 203 (1963) (government may not invade the "citadel of the individual heart and mind," either to aid or oppose religion)]. Thus, the principle that persons must be free to make choices in matters of religion, and the propriety of measures to assure that principle, seem well grounded in tradition and case law.

It seems worth brief mention, as well, that both sides in the debate over cults invoke the rhetoric of self-determination. Defenders of these groups ask why young adults should not be free to join whatever religious organizations they wish, live as they wish, and adopt whatever life-styles seem right to them. Opponents answer that freedom of choice is exactly what the groups deny. Thus, self-determination values play a prominent role in public discussion about cults, as well as constituting basic normative limits on what religious organizations may and may not do.

Certain paradigms are associated with deprivation of choice. The most obvious is physical coercion or restraint: one person points a gun at another or keeps him or her imprisoned in a locked room. These forms are rarely, if ever, used by cults to recruit or maintain members. But there are other forms of volitional impairment. Informational deprivation or deception is one. If A offers B a ride in an automobile that A has painted yellow, B believing that it is a taxi, B has scarcely consented to the ride. Since the will translates information into action, manipulation of the will—such as through drugs, hypnotism, coercive persuasion, or extreme physical debilitation—can also impair autonomy. According to their critics, cults at times incorporate both forms of autonomy-negating influences into their recruitment/retention practices.

Legal rules pertaining to informed consent aim at protecting both elements of a person's choice-interests. In general, for consent to be valid, the individual must have had "knowledge" and been acting with "legal capacity." That is, the person making the choice must have possessed the relevant information concerning his or her choice, and he or she must have made the choice with an intact mind. If a person, at the time of a decision, lacked either knowledge or capacity, the requirements for an informed consent were not met.

Many cult recruits undoubtedly join the organization with full knowledge and capacity; they become cult members because they want to do so and are happy with their choice. For others, however, the decision to join and remain with a cult is not an autonomous expression of self, and does not meet the intent of legal-moral rules pertaining to consent. Two aspects, peculiar to the cult-joining situation, impel me to this conclusion. The first has to do with the manner in which knowledge and capacity are somtimes manipulated in cult recruitment. The second has to do with segmentation of the process into a series of stages, or steps.

The Relationship of Knowledge and Capacity in Cult Joining

Intuitively (as well as in law), for consent to be valid there must be knowledge and capacity. In the process by which a person becomes a member of a cult group, these two elements are sometimes manipulated so that they are in an inverse relationship. When capacity is high, the recruit's knowledge of the cult and its practices is low; when knowledge is high, capacity is reduced. When a newcomer attends his or her first meeting or training session, ordinarily the capacity to make a free, rational choice is unimpaired. The young person may be experiencing some rather ordinary life crisis (leaving home, attending college, breaking up with a boyfriend or girlfriend), but his or her faculties are generally intact. If, in this condition, the individual were confronted with the full truth about the organization—its name, leader, the demands it will later place on members—he or she would respond by leaving. Consequently, many groups conceal these items of information until the group perceives the recruit is "ready" for them.

Cult leaders disclose details of the cult's hierarchy, life-style, doctrine, and submission only after they perceive that the individual, through a process of peer pressure, stress, excitement, sleep deprivation, isolation from the rest of society, and in some cases abuse or threats, has lost the ability to absorb the information and act on it according to his usual frames of reference. By the time the recruit commits himself or herself to the group, his or her informational base has expanded, but only as his or her capacity has shrunk. Knowledge and capacity have thus been maintained, by design, in inverse relationship. When capacity is high (at the beginning stages), knowledge is low. Later, when capacity has been reduced, information is high. The two requirements of informed consent are not present at the same time.

A second characteristic, related to this manipulation of knowledge and capacity, is segmentation of the joining process into a series of steps or stages. The process by which a young person joins a cult is often deliberately segmented: first, the recruit attends an evening meeting and meal, then a weekend workshop, then a week-long retreat in the country, and so on. At each point, the individual's assent is given, at least nominally, to proceeding to the next stage. But the final stage or end result is concealed from view until the individual has reached the next-to-last step. As the individual progresses from one step to the next, the intensity of the peer pressure, indoctrination, guilt manipulation, and other influences used to generate commitment increases, as does the momentum of the process.

At each stage, the convert, if he or she asks, may be given a general idea of what is to take place at the next stage (retreat, workshop, training session), but at no early point in the process is he or she told where the entire journey leads. If he or she asks questions of this sort, they are typically put off with the excuse that they will be answered later. When the recruit reaches the penultimate step, he or she has been so softened up that committing his or her life and fortune to the group seems—and is— but a small step. Where they occur, both features—maintenance of an inverse relation between knowledge and capacity, and segmentation of the joining process—cast serious doubt on the voluntariness of the process by which young people join cult groups and suggest that remedies may be in order.

Since conventional religions do not incorporate these two elements into their proselytizing patterns, and since cult cases have begun reaching the courts only recently, there is relatively little case law concerning consent in religious settings. Currently the leading decision dealing with religious manifestations of questionable origin and authenticity is *Peterson v. Sorlien*, 299 N.W.2d 123 (Minn. 1980), cert. denied, 450 U.S. 1031 (1981), a

December 1980 decision by the Minnesota State Supreme Court. *Sorlien* is currently the highest-level "cult case" on record. In *Sorlien*, the parents of a young cult member tricked her into leaving the cult, ostensibly to visit a family friend. When they reached their destination, the parents confronted her, instead, with a team of deprogrammers, who attempted to engage her in "reality inducing therapy." For three days, the young woman strenuously avoided speaking with or listening to the deprogrammers, adopting the fetal position and blocking her ears with her fingers to avoid hearing what the deprogrammers were saying. Gradually, she opened up, spoke with the deprogrammers, reconsidered her decision to be a cultist, and opted to remain with her parents rather than return to the group. For a period of some weeks, she stayed with her parents and the deprogrammers, roller skating, taking trips, shopping, playing softball, and swimming. She was alone on several occasions but did not attempt to leave or rejoin the cult. Later, she expressed a desire to see her boyfriend, a cult member, with the object of persuading him, as well, to leave the cult. The parents and deprogrammers arranged a meeting, but the young woman subsequently rejoined the cult and sued the parents for unlawful imprisonment, a civil tort, and for damages.

The Minnesota Supreme Court found, as the trial court did, that except for the first three days, the young woman had been living voluntarily with her parents and the deprogrammers. Moreover, it found that during her period in the cult, the young woman had acquired a new temporary identity. It found that she had been subjected to "cult indoctrination . . . predicated on a strategy of coercive persuasion that undermines the capacity for informed consent" (299 N.W.2d 123, 129). It found, moreover, that in cult settings, "consent becomes a function of time," (id. at 128) and that other social institutions do not undermine consent so extensively as cults do. The court found the young woman's acquiescence in her life-style outside the cult "dispositive," and announced a new test of consent in cult settings; where the parents remove the child "and the child at some juncture assents to the actions in question," the entire course of conduct is deemed consensual and no unlawful imprisonment action will lie (id. at 129). The United States Supreme Court denied certiorari, 450 U.S. 1031 (1981), allowing the decision to remain undisturbed.

Sorlien thus constitutes legal recognition that there is something different, and troubling, about the voluntariness of the cult-joining process. It did not do so, of course, in connection with a search for remedies for cult-related harms; it merely gave the parents a defense to legal action directed against them for attempting a self-help (extralegal) remedy. Whether the same defects of consent noted in this paper and in *Peterson v. Sorlien* would justify an affirmative remedy of any of the kinds outlined in the first section of this chapter must remain, for now, an open question.

In evaluating any such affirmative remedy, whether of the preinduction or postinduction kind, courts will bring to bear a great deal of constitutional doctrine developed in First Amendment religious freedom decisions developed before cults became a reality. They will ask whether the remedy is supported by a compelling state interest, is narrowly tailored to avert the harm at which it is aimed, and does not intrude more centrally than necessary with religious functioning. The application of these technical doctrines and requirements will vary from case to case as different remedies are tested in different fact settings. Little generalization is possible at this point.

One piece of preliminary analysis can be undertaken, however. Some opponents of state intervention into cults argue that no form of intervention is permissible because it would be impossible to "draw the line," to distinguish between cult practices and those of other social institutions whose practices we tolerate.

Drawing the Line

The drawing-the-line difficulty does not seem insuperable. As this chapter, and the *Sorlien* decision, have noted, the cult-joining process contains elements rarely found elsewhere. Moreover, cults expose their indoctrinees to a greater variety of consent-negating techniques than do other groups, and apply them with greater intensity. Jesuit and other seminary schools may isolate the student from the rest of society at various stages of the training period, but the isolation is not continuous, nor does the training include physiologic depletion or deceit at initial stages—the young would-be seminarian is never in doubt about the identity of the institution he is entering nor the rigor of its demands. Most religious orders set out the demands and obligations of the calling clearly, even taking the position of "devil's advocate," urging the young candidate to consider whether he is really suited for the program. Nor do most major denominations concentrate, as some cults do, on the weak, the depressed, the vulnerable. Some orders use psychological screening to weed out those whose interest in the seminary or religious school is an expression of personal inadequacy, passivity, or emotional problems. A number require a waiting or "cooling off" period.

Outward Bound, military training, and high-pressure executive training programs all use peer pressure to induce new patterns of behavior or attitude, but rarely, if ever, seek to facilitate this acquisition by means of prolonged physiologic depletion, or induction of feelings of dread, doom, guilt, and sin. Private military schools enroll youths at an early age and isolate them from home and outside society for extended periods. But even here, the arsenal of thought- and behavior-modification techniques is not so extensive or so incessant as it is with cults. The students ordinarily return home for holidays and vacations and have at least limited access to the outside world through radio, television, and telephone. State requirements ensure that minimal standards of diet and sleep are maintained. Peer pressure is often manipulated to bring out conformity to the school's code, but it is generally applied on a simple reward-punishment basis rather than by means of sophisticated techniques aimed at tapping subconscious fears, anxieties, and guilt feelings, as is done in cults.

Consequently, few if any other social institutions approach either the intensity, sophistication, or unremitting quality of cults with respect to their induction and indoctrination processes. Society could institute measures to avert or abate the various physical, psychological, and autonomy-related harms associated with nonconsensual cult membership without fear of being accused of unfairness or intolerance—treating cults more harshly than other groups, not because of differences that set them apart, but merely because they strike us as peculiar or foreign-seeming.

Carefully tailored remedies, especially those of the relatively mild, preinduction sort, can help raise the level of public awareness of cult problems. They can also communicate to cults that deceptive, high-stress methods of recruitment that bypass the rational faculties of recruits will not be tolerated. The twin spurs of increasing public sophistication about cults and the adverse publicity that comes from legally sanctioned measures for intervention might well prompt cults to reconsider the necessity of some of their more extreme recruitment approaches. There is some evidence that cults are not beyond reach of such socializing forces and can, with firm encouragement, be made to moderate some of their practices. Some groups have reportedly already begun to do so. It may be that, over time, high-demand cult groups will mellow and begin to take on the look of mainstream groups. Legal measures like those discussed in this chapter may accelerate this trend on the part of groups that are reachable by social influence, and limit the harm caused by more extreme groups that are not.

Chapter 16

PUBLIC REACTION AGAINST NEW RELIGIOUS MOVEMENTS

David G. Bromley, Ph.D.
Anson Shupe, Ph.D.

The public reaction to new religious movements (NRMs) in the United States has now spanned more than a decade. Although the public response to NRMs has varied, the most striking qualities of the reaction have been intense hostility and the extent to which these disparate groups, popularly termed "cults," have been perceived as essentially equivalent. This chapter examines the sources, dynamics, and consequences of the public reaction. The reaction is found to have been triggered by conflicts of interest between major social institutions and NRMs. While conflicts of interest predictably lead to efforts by opponents to exert social control over one another, the "new religions" controversy evolved into a public scare. It was this social scare that determined the character of the reaction to NRMs. By "social scare" we refer to a climate of heightened fear and apprehension, growing out of social conflict, that basic values or institutional arrangements in the society are in imminent danger of subversion.

There is no set of criteria by which to identify the range of groups designated as "cults" or as manifesting "cultic tendencies." The only significant characteristic that these groups share in common is the designation "cult," and this label is differentially applied by oppositional groups (1, 2). While there seems to be broad agreement among anticultists that groups such as the Church of Scientology, Children of God, Unification Church, and Hare Krishna are "cults," Jewish organizations appear just as concerned with the Jews for Jesus and fundamentalist Christian groups would place Jehovah's Witnesses, Mormons, and Seventh Day Adventists in this category. This chapter therefore explores the causes and consequences of the labeling process through which such groups have come to be perceived and treated as essentially equivalent.

Public reaction is defined here not as "public opinion" but rather as the pattern of actions implemented by various major institutions that became involved in the controversy over new religions—family, religion, government, media. In fact, most individual Americans have had little if any direct contact with NRMs or their members, unless they were the object of a perfunctory streetcorner witnessing or fund-raising appeal. Public opinion, therefore, has been shaped largely by the actions of major institutions, which have been subsequently disseminated through the media.

In this chapter we examine the public response to NRMs in the United States. However, it is important to note that there has been a similar reaction in other Western industrial nations as well. Indeed, one of the prominent features of many of the NRMs is their international character. A number of these groups (such as the Unification Church, Divine Light Mission, International Society for Krishna Consciousness, Rajneesh) were first established in other countries and only later migrated to the United States and Western Europe. The public reactions within each nation have differed. The nature of the reaction to NRMs in the United States has been shaped in part by the constellation of institutions whose interests were threatened, traditional American conceptions of religion, the degree of religious diversity in the United States, and legal and constitutional protections granted to groups designated as religious. While the response of Western European nations also has been influenced by their unique sociocultural contexts, they have been parallel in a number of respects. Therefore, the information reported here on the United States is generally consistent with that reported for Western European nations (3–7).

A Historical and Comparative Perspective on Public Reactions to New Religious Groups

A brief review of the historical pattern of public reaction to new religious groups provides a useful perspective on the contemporary response. Religious groups new to the American scene, whether they have been indigenous cultural innovations or social transplants, typically have experienced opposition; some groups have even experienced lengthy periods of repression. Groups as conventional by contemporary standards as the Roman Catholics, Mormons, Jehovah's Witnesses, Quakers, Mennonites, and Christian Scientists at one time have been the objects of varying degrees of controversy and opposition. At some points the controversy surrounding Roman Catholics and Mormons generated a level of the public fear and apprehension comparable to or even exceeding that registered in the current cult scare, and thus the reaction to these groups offers a productive analogue for understanding contemporary events.

The rise of both Mormonism and Catholicism in the United States can be traced to macrocultural factors generated by nineteenth-century American society (8–10). The major source of growth in the Catholic population during the nineteenth century was the immigration encouraged by a need to consolidate settlement of the continent and to create an adequate labor pool to support the urban industrial revolution. Mormonism was born early in the nineteenth century as part of a period of widespread spiritual ferment, the Second Great Awakening. This period was characterized by a wave of religious revivals and the appearance of numerous millenial sects centered in a portion of upstate New York referred to as the "burned-over district."

As each group grew and achieved visibility, conflicts of interest emerged and opposition began to mount. In the case of Catholics the sources of tension included a carry-over of the long-standing Protestant-Catholic conflict in Europe, the traditional Catholic emphasis on integration of church and state, and the large and rapid influx of Catholic immigrants during the mid-nineteenth century who constituted an increasingly formidable voting bloc. The controversy surrounding Mormonism involved the Mormon plan to establish a theocracy, the rapidly growing number of Mormons which resulted from their recruitment abroad of convert-immigrants to establish Zion in America, the formation of a separate Mormon economy and independent military force, and theologically linked Mormon support for American Indians. In addition, Catholics and Mormons alike engendered charges of heresy as a result of their divergence from Protestant theological tenets, fears of the social exclusivism of the groups (even though this characteristic was at least in part a product of the hostile social response), and apprehensions about the potential political power of these growing churches.

Rather than being perceived as a series of specific political conflicts, however, Mormon-Gentile and Catholic-Protestant conflicts were cast as a threat to subvert the entire social order. The specific conflicts were caught up as well in the more general, pervasive cultural tensions that spawned reactionary Nativism (prowhite, pro-Anglo-Saxon Protestant, antiforeign prejudice). The result was a series of repressive formal and informal initiatives designed to control each group (8, 9). For example, various states introduced legislation to curtail immigration of both Catholics and Mormons. There were efforts to block the employment of Catholics and the charter of the Mormon Church was revoked by the federal government. A number of anti-Mormon and anti-Catholic organizations arose to lobby for formal state intervention and initiate their own informal control agendas. There were anti-Catholic riots in urban areas resulting in a loss of life and property while the Mormons were driven from New York to Ohio, Missouri, and Illinois before finally settling in Utah. Mormon leader Joseph Smith was murdered at the hands of an angry mob (10).

In addition, heightened public fear resulted in a wave of anti-Mormon and anti-Catholic sentiment in the media. Accounts of Catholic and Mormon life were filtered through stories, conveyed by apostates from those churches as well as in fictional literature, which portrayed these churches and their leaders as fundamentally exploitive, authoritarian, and immoral (11–13). One of the most inflammatory themes was sexual perversion. In the Catholic case the allegation was that convents were prisons in which young women were kept for the pleasure of sexually starved priests; in the Mormon case religious sanctioning of the polygamous family structure was depicted as simply a charade to conceal sexual exploitation of innocent women.

When new religious groups have appeared through American

history, they have often engendered precisely this type of response. The capsule descriptions of the Mormon and Catholic conflicts presented here are particularly instructive only in that they achieved national visibility, extended over a number of decades, and involved very high levels of public apprehension. Early in their histories NRMs frequently have come into conflict with an array of social institutions simultaneously. As a result, such conflicts have been characterized by substantial power imbalances; new religious groups have possessed little power and few allies compared with the institutional forces arrayed against them. Under these conditions, various specific conflicts have interacted with one another and have amplified the level of tension and antagonism. Given the relatively low power and legitimacy of NRMs, there has been little countervailing pressure against such conflict escalation. It has been in the interest of oppositional groups to accentuate these tensions since high levels of fear and apprehension coupled with a low level of restraint created the conditions for unilateral imposition of social control measures.

A key element in intense conflicts in which important cultural values or institutional arrangements have been perceived to be at risk has been the emergence of subversion myths (1, 13–16). These myths have created comprehensive, integrated explanations for the perceived danger posed by groups thought to be threatening the existing social order. Subversion mythologies are premised on the existence of a conspiracy. They posit a specific danger and a group associated with it, one or more conspirators who have planned and directed the plot, a set of base impulses that motivate the conspiracy leaders, a manipulative process through which the conspirators involve others in their conspiracy, an imminent danger for the entire society, and a remedial agenda that must be followed if catastrophe is to be avoided.

In the case of the Catholic scare, for example, Catholic immigrants comprised the dangerous group. According to nativists, the Catholic conspiracy was masterminded by the Pope and a group of unscrupulous, deployable agents—Jesuit priests. While most Catholics were viewed as simply innocent dupes with misplaced loyalties, there was also manipulation involved as priests wielded enormous power over individual Catholics through knowledge gained in confessions and through threats of eternal damnation. More coercive imagery was employed to describe Catholic nuns, who were depicted as virtual slaves. The primary danger to American society came from the political clout Catholics could wield if, as expected, they voted as a block upon papal instruction, although there also were widespread rumors during the nineteenth century that Catholics were forming an army in the West to launch a violent revolution. The analogous Mormon myth was built around a similar scenario of sexual exploitation of women and a military alliance with Indians which would threaten violence against all non-Mormon settlers.

Such myths have proven very resistant to refutation. For example, a number of convent captivity stories were demonstrated to be false soon after their publication, but they continued to be published and read decades later (9). Similarly, the inconsistency between Mormon men simultaneously enfranchising women (well before other American women received basic political rights) and simultaneously enslaving them was never explored in antipolygamy captivity narratives, and Mormon wives' testimonies on behalf of polygamous family structure were largely ignored. The tenacity with which such myths are defended in the face of strong counterevidence demonstrates that their function is an allegorical depiction of good and evil in culturally appropriate terms for the purpose of defending the social order based on that socially constructed reality.

The Contemporary Reaction to New Religious Movements

As in the case of the nineteenth century predecessors, a subversion myth has dominated the public reaction to contemporary NRMs. Currently it is widely believed that there exists a class of groups called "cults" which can be distinguished from any other type of group (17, 18). The distinguishing characteristics of cults include authoritarian leadership, suppression of rational thought, deceptive recruitment techniques, coercive mind control, a totalistic group structure, isolation from conventional society and former relationships, and exploitation of group members by leaders. Malevolent gurus are thought to be the driving force behind these pseudoreligious groups which have been cynically created to take advantage of religious liberty guarantees as a means of maximizing these leaders' power and wealth. The membership of these groups is comprised of young adults from the middle classes whose naiveté and idealism is being systematically exploited by these gurus. According to anticultists, cultic groups employ a combination of deception and sophisticated, coercive mind control techniques to subvert individual autonomy and free will. Thus the danger is rapidly growing and proliferating cults; gurus are the conspirators; the motives are power and money; the subversion mechanism is coercive mind control techniques; the imminent danger is legions of unquestioning followers in the service of unscrupulous leaders; and the remedy is formal or informal extrication of individuals from these groups along with revision of laws behind which they hide.

The subversion mythology interpretation of NRMs has largely obscured the sociocultural factors which led to the rapid growth of NRMs in the late 1960s and early 1970s (19, 20). There has in fact been a worldwide resurgence of religious movements, many of which have been associated with nationalistic fervor in developing nations. In the United States there has been rapid growth of fundamentalist, Pentecostal, and evangelical churches, and an outpouring of born-again Christian groups. Once facet of this religious resurgence has been the growth of youth-based movements that captured so much public attention during the 1970s. The sudden appearance of Eastern groups such as Hare Krishna, Divine Light Mission, Transcendental Meditation, and Rajneesh can be traced to a new missionary spirit among Asian religions, developments in western science (e.g., the emergence of parapsychology, the discovery of LSD, the spread of Jungian and humanistic psychology), and the repeal of the Oriental Exclusion Act in 1965 (which permitted the first substantial Asian immigration, including Oriental gurus, in several decades) (21). Other groups such as the Children of God, Shiloh Youth Revival Centers, and Alamo Foundation formed as offshoots of the youth-based Jesus Movement in the late 1960s and early 1970s. Still other well known NRMs, such as the Church of Scientology (22) and the Unification Church (23, 24), had existed in the United States for some years prior to the emergence of the cult controversy, awaiting a more favorable cultural climate.

Another factor was the growing prominence of the youth subculture during the 1950s and 1960s. The period between childhood and adulthood has been lengthening for some time, parental control has declined as an increasing proportion of youth pursued residential, postsecondary education, and there has been a widespread cynicism among youth about mainline institutions and their personal futures in them. One outgrowth of these conditions has been a large group of individuals without encumbering social commitments in search of alternatives for personal and social transformation. For some youth the focus of this search shifted to religiously based movements as the drug subculture and politically based movements began to lose their allure.

The public perception of a cult problem gradually emerged, therefore, out of what was actually a rather unconnected development of a diverse array of groups. A number of these groups such as Hare Krishna (25), the Unification Church (24), and Shiloh Youth Revival Centers (26) initially recruited members from the drug subculture or other marginal populations without great opposition. It was when recruitment began to move to college campuses and other centers of middle-class youth subculture that the visibility of these groups to families, the media, and political and religious leaders increased, and a concerted public reaction developed. The families of new converts initially organized to combat NRMs; only gradually did the broad-based institutional reaction to NRMs develop.

The nature of the reaction to NRMs can be traced to challenges to the interests of major institutions, including government, family, media, and churches. In addition, certain developmental qualities of NRMs also contributed substantially to the reaction as some movements sustained their symbolic identity and internal cohesiveness by rejecting conventional institutions and creating separate, encapsulating communities. It was out of the dynamics of the interactions between these NRMs and major institutions that the cult scare developed.

NRMs and the Societal Reaction

NRMs have always been in fact extremely diverse in terms of ideology, social organization, leadership style, and objectives (1, 14). Although anticult groups tended to lump disparate groups together, the anticult movement formed around and the most intense opposition was directed at groups such as the Children of God, Hare Krishna, and the Unification Church. These NRMs were organized communally, professed millennial, apocalyptic expectations, and recruited from the ranks of young, middle class individuals. There were some important organizational corollaries of such characteristics.

First, each of these groups functioned during the mid-1970s with an imminent expectation of world transformation (23). In order to prepare themselves for and contribute to this anticipated transformation, these groups withdrew from conventional society, which they deemed corrupt and moribund, and established spiritually based communities designed to be as independent of the larger society as possible. The outside world was primarily a source of converts, economic resources, and a model of immorality against which these movements' own utopian social orders could be contrasted. Second, recruitment was pursued aggressively as these groups perceived that world transformation was at hand. Total commitment was required to ensure salvation, and it was this type of total involvement which was so often interpreted as evidence of brainwashing. In this circumstance of heightened mobilization and absolute commitment there was little tolerance for questioning or dissent. Third, consistent with many other communal, utopian communities, these movements frequently employed familial metaphors (e.g., referring to fellow members as brothers and sisters and leaders as fathers and mothers) to organize and articulate normative interpersonal relations. Furthermore, in contrast to earlier NRMs, which had often recruited families as units, these groups recruited single individuals, which precipitated family conflict. Finally, the contempt for conventional society led to a lowered level of concern about conformity with the established normative order. The existing social order was perceived to be thoroughly corrupt and crumbling under the weight of its own decadence.

These characteristics contributed substantially to mistrust and hostility from the larger society. The contemptuous, shrill condemnations of society by these groups created both antagonism and apprehensiveness as they often were taken as indicators of probable behaviors rather than as of rhetorical, symbolic positioning. Parents of converts regarded the fictive kinship systems established by communally organized NRMs as an attempt to quite literally steal their children and usurp their rightful parental role. The accounts of disillusioned former members suggested a real disparity between the lofty idealism of the groups and the reality of infighting, ideological rigidity, and authoritarian leadership. Vindictiveness against dissidents and critics and violations of law and convention raised fears of violence and extremism.

A string of incidents confirmed this mistrust. Groups such as Scientology and Synanon harassed critics, dissenters, and former members. The more notable episodes involved Synanon members placing a rattlesnake in the mailbox of anti-Synanon crusader Paul Morantz, and Scientology's plot to falsely incriminate critic Paulette Cooper for planting a bomb in a public building. There were continuous incidents of Hare Krishna and Unification Church members engaging in deceptive fund-raising practices. The Children of God developed the practice of "flirty fishing" in which female members were encouraged to become "hookers for Christ," and the Rajneesh became notorious for sexual promiscuity and provocative confrontations with outsiders. And, of course, there were the chilling murder-suicides at Jonestown, Guyana. All of these incidents violated public mores, laws, or moral sensibilities. In the context of the cult subversion mythology, however, they appeared to constitute a threat of major proportions as they were perceived to be characteristic of "cults" rather than the product of specific groups and social contexts.

Families and the New Religions

Any analysis of the public reactions to NRMs must begin with the conflict between families and these groups. Although NRMs would certainly have engendered opposition from other quarters, it is unlikely that the intensity of controversy that has occurred would have transpired without the family conflict as its driving force. It was individual families and groups of families that banded together to form anticult organizations that coordinated the opposition to NRMs.

It has been widely observed that the functions performed by the traditional nuclear family have been gradually attenuating since the advent of the industrial revolution (27). Among the remaining functions of the contemporary American family, preparation of offspring for occupational and domestic careers are central. Mobility opportunities for offspring are the linchpin in family financial planning, residential location, and career management. Families seek to provide social and educational opportunities for sons and daughters so as to maximize the range of choices of career options and partners for family formation. Although families have retained both a real and perceived responsibility for socialization, managing this responsibility has become increasingly problematic as a result of the extended period of financial dependency, the increased importance of higher levels of education for achieving mobility opportunities, and the ambiguous boundary between adolescence and adulthood, which has reduced control parents retain during the latter stages of the socialization process. Of course, parental feelings of efficacy and family prestige also are involved in the successful negotiation of childrearing objectives.

Given the enormous investment families have in the outcome of socializing sons and daughters for career and family formation and the tensions inherent in that process, it is not surprising that decisions affecting future mobility opportunities are of the greatest consequence to parents. It is in this context that decisions by college-aged youth to join new religious groups must be understood. When some of the more prominent new religious groups began aggressive recruitment campaigns on college campuses and centers of youth subculture, many of the new recruits were at precisely the stage of career and family formation preparation for which their parents had so long prepared. When these individuals, often with little if any prior consultation with their families, decided to join a NRM and abandon their domestic and occupational plans, the reaction of parents was predictably negative (28, 29).

As Beckford has observed (30), the response of families was not uniform. He identified three types of response. The least frequent type of response was incomprehension and bewilderment. This reaction tended to occur where the recruit had grown away from the family and had been involved in other radical transformations of life-style, which left family members unable to predict the wayward individual's behavior. A second response was ambivalence, which occurred in families where parents regarded the new recruits as competent, self-directing, and responsible even if their choice of affiliation was unfortunate and ill-advised.

The third, and most common, type of response was anger and urgency. It was the most likely reaction in situations where parents felt unable to understand "how their best efforts to bring up children in what they regarded as a firm and fair fashion had resulted in an apparently sudden and unexpected rejection of the parental home and of all that it represented." It was this group of parents that, in the absence of any other explanation for unfolding events, was most likely to resort to the explanation that both recruitment and subsequent membership were the product of manipulation. This group is particularly significant in understanding the controversy over new religious groups because it was these families that possessed the motivation and determination to establish the organized opposition to new religions.

Parents of members of NRMs quickly formed as series of voluntary associations with names such as the American Family Foundation, the Citizens Freedom Foundation, and Love Our Children (2). These organizations served a number of functions. They operated as an information network and support groups for families with members in NRMs. Parents were able to share common concerns, use this network to attempt to locate offspring where relations had been strained or severed, and obtained information about specific NRMs' ideology and organization (although this information was refracted through anticult ideology). Further, anticult associations served as lobbying and "educational" organizations which sought to bring pressure on NRMs by enlisting the support of political, economic, religious, media, and educational institutions possessing greater resources and sanctioning power. Finally, anticult organizations served as the nucleus around which other services to families and former members clustered. Certainly the most unique of these services was the process of separating individuals from NRMs and returning them to conventional social networks, which came to be termed "deprogramming" (31).

It was out of this network of relationships that the subversion myth, based on the brainwashing metaphor, developed. Parents unable to account for the behavioral changes they observed in their offspring emanating from the role structure of communally organized NRMs concluded that those changes must have been coerced rather than voluntary. The first group of entrepreneurs who acted on behalf of parents to extricate offspring from NRMs, adopted the brainwashing explanation and conceived of "deprogramming" as the antidote for it. All that remained was to develop the techniques that would yield a reasonable rate of renunciations of membership, which became the standard for a successful deprogramming. Counseling services for individuals and lobbying services for the set of families soon followed. Embittered former members found roles providing public testimony on the dangers posed by cults, as deprogrammers and as counselors. Thus constructed, the anticult network became the most influential interpreter of NRMs, and its subversion mythology became the widely accepted explanation for the emergence and success of NRMs.

Churches and Religious Organizations

The response of established churches, ecumenical organizations, and religiously based oppositional groups was varigated given the diverse range of their interests (32). A substantial number of groups formed to oppose churches such as the Mormons, Jehovah's Witnesses, Christian Scientists, and Seventh Day Adventists had been in place and functioning when the NRM controversy arose. Many of these groups simply added the new groups to their lists of cults and used them as fresh evidence of the imminent dangers confronting the Christian community. A number of mainline churches defended NRMs in political and judicial forums where they perceived larger religious liberties issues were at stake (33); however, many churches or umbrella religious organizations also issued condemnations of the theologies and recruitment and socialization practices of certain NRMs (34).

In general, the fundamentalist, conservative Christian churches were more hostile in their responses than mainline denominations, and their ire was directed particularly at groups which drew on the Christian tradition such as the Children of God and the Unification Church. Many Jewish organizations also were stridently anticult. This extreme Jewish sensitivity stemmed from perceived antisemitism on the part of some NRMs, a belief that Jews were disproportionately represented in the membership of groups such as Hare Krishna and the Unification Church (35), and the conspicuous presence of individuals with Jewish backgrounds among the ranks of leadership in

NRMs such as the Children of God and the Unification Church. Much of the critique of NRMs from churches was theologically based, although it also incorporated manipulative recruitment and socialization practices. However, religious organizations and spokespersons generally did not support deprogramming, recognizing that if coercion (and particularly state-sanctioned deprogramming) were legitimated as a means of altering religious affiliation, the character of church-state and interfaith relations would be profoundly altered. Although the response from mainstream religious groups was not uniform, criticism and condemnation were widespread. As a result, NRMs were perceived not to be legitimate members of the pluralist religious community.

Local, State, and Federal Government Responses

The pattern of reaction by executive, legislative and judicial agencies reflected both a response to initiatives from family-based anticult organizations and to direct conflicts between governmental agencies and NRMs. Two of the most contentious issues at the local level have been public solicitation of funds and establishment of local NRM affiliates. Local governments have actively opposed public solicitation of funds by NRMs. There have been several thousand litigated cases in communities across the country over the last decade. Municipal officials have sought to inhibit NRM public solicitation as a result of the well-deserved reputations by such groups as the Hare Krishna and the Unification Church for deceptive fund-raising practices (36, 37), in order to make their communities generally less attractive to NRM proselytizers and fundraisers, as a means of reducing suspicion of representatives of accepted charitable organizations, and as an expression of support for local anticult groups. In general, federal courts have supported the right of NRMs to publicly solicit funds and limited restrictions to reasonable guidelines on time, place, and manner.

Localities also have attempted to block the acquisition of local real estate which it was feared would change the character of communities and create a permanent unwanted economic and political presence. Among the more publicized of these conflicts have been those between Scientology and the city of Clearwater, Florida; between Hare Krishna and the communities surrounding New Vrindaban, West Virginia; the Unification Church and the town of Gloucester, Massachusetts; and the Rajneesh and the community of Antelope, Oregon. In each case, the community has sought to defend interests such as property values, components of the local economy (in the case of Gloucester, defense of the economically fragile, local fishing industry), or governmental institutions themselves (in the case of Antelope, an unsuccessful attempt to prevent the Rajneesh from gaining sufficient electoral strength to take over the municipal government). For their part, NRMs have pursued the right to freely purchase property and establish businesses. While a number of these conflicts have proven rather intractable, tensions in some cases have eased through mutual accommodation. This seems to be the case in New Vrindaban, for example, where the surrounding area has benefited as that community has become the state's second largest tourist attraction and Hare Krishna leadership has sought accommodation with surrounding residents.

In addition, there have been numerous reported cases of local law enforcement officers and magistrates supporting families involved in forcible abductions and deprogrammings (2, 31). Police officers have permitted the abduction of members of various NRMs on the grounds that a family dispute was involved and magistrates have issued conservatorships under circumstances which have minimized the opportunity to contest those proceedings. Such cases have exacerbated community-NRM tensions. More recent judicial rulings against issuance of conservatorships and prosecution of deprogrammers have substantially decreased the number of such incidents.

At the state level the single most prevalent type of confrontation has come over the expansion of conservatorship provisions to encompass cases of alleged cultic brainwashing. Virtually all states have enacted conservatorship statutes which typically have been used to permit one individual (usually a family member) to petition a court for appointment as a legal guardian of another. Such provisions frequently have been employed to appoint a conservator for an elderly family member deemed incapable of making independent decisions. Anticult groups lobbied in a number of states to extend conservatorship provisions to include individuals putatively rendered incapable of autonomous decision-making by cultic mind control techniques. Although no bills have as yet become law, such legislation did pass both houses of the New York legislature on two occasions only to be defeated by gubernatorial veto. Legislative committees in several states also have conducted investigations of recruitment and socialization, financial, employment, and child care practices; however, these have usually eventuated in committee reports or legislative resolutions rather actual legislation. Such events have been important symbolically; however, as they allowed legislators to formally assert the public morality with which NRMs are perceived to be in conflict when the application of substantive sanctions proved politically untenable.

More recently, in part because of the failure to achieve legislative successes, anticult groups have been encouraging civil suits against NRMs. In these cases litigation usually is based on such generic charges as "infliction of emotional distress," but the actual allegations and testimony revolve around the brainwashing issue. For their part, unsuccessfully deprogrammed members of NRMs have brought infliction of emotional distress and false imprisonment charges against deprogrammers, often with the support of NRM leaders. To date verdicts have been mixed, and most cases involving large awards have been appealed. Nevertheless, these cases have all generated considerable media coverage and public debate of the various elements of the subversion mythology.

Much of the conflict between the federal government and NRMs is attributable to organizational differences between contemporary NRMs and traditional Christian church structure. In contrast to the historical pattern of Western Christian churches evangelizing in Asian nations, the appearance of Eastern NRMs (such as the Hare Krishna, Divine Light Mission, Unification Church, Transcendental Meditation, and Rajneesh) represented oriental evangelism of westerners. Missionaries from these NRMs possessed the same absolute assurance of the superiority of their own beliefs and often were no more knowledgeable of or committed to indigenous cultural arrangements than their historic Christian counterparts had been. Predictably enough the result has been antagonism and resentment. Conflicts over immigration were among those generated by the arrival of oriental groups as they imported members from abroad to consolidate and expand their newly established churches.

The latest crop of new religious groups also has adapted to current technological capabilities, international corporate organization, and a consumer-oriented economy. In the case of conservative Christian groups, popularly referred to as the "new religious right," for example, the use of media technology to establish "electronic churches," and the commercial-style messages to raise money to support these broadcasts, and political action committees to support ideologically compatible political candidates has aroused considerable controversy (38–40). Analogously, the Unification Church developed an international corporate network to fund its religious agenda (41); Hare Krishna has established a combined religious retreat and tourist center in New Vrindaban, West Virginia; Transcendental Meditation offers its meditative techniques as a leisure-time commodity and rehabilitative technique; and Scientology markets its religious auditing and related procedures as instructional classes. All of these organizational innovations produced suspicion and animosity, which were reflected in investigations and sanctions by various federal agencies.

Finally, some NRMs have developed political alliances or aspirations that have been a source of controversy. Much of this activity has been at the local or state level as exemplified by the Rajneesh's attempted takeover of Antelope, Oregon, and LaRouche candidates surreptitiously running for statewide office in Illinois on the Democratic ticket. On the federal level the most notable case has been the attempt by the Unification Church to develop political ties with political conservatives through its anticommunist activities. There also have been unsubstantiated allegations of political connections between leaders of the Unification Church and the Korean Central Intelligence Agency (42). In the late 1970s one of the federal government's concerns about Jim Jones's Peoples Temple was its overtures to socialist bloc nations.

These various conflicts have led to a succession of confrontations between federal agencies and various NRMs. For example, the Food and Drug Administration challenged the therapeutic efficacy of the "E-Meter" used in Scientology's auditing process. The Immigration and Naturalization Service has contested the status of both members and leaders of several NRMs. Ultimately it was over immigration issues that the Bhagwan Shree Rajneesh was deported from the United States. The Internal Revenue Service has challenged the tax exempt status and wage payment practices of various NRMs, and the relationship between taxable

322 CULTS AND NEW RELIGIOUS MOVEMENTS

and nontaxable purposes for numerous affiliate NRM organizations. The most publicized case of this kind resulted in the conviction and imprisonment of Sun Myung Moon on tax evasion charges. The Federal Bureau of Investigation has declined to become involved in deprogramming cases, even where forcible abduction and transportation across state boundaries have been involved, on the grounds that these are family disputes (2, 31). By contrast, federal courts have generally rendered decisions more favorable to NRMs, affirming their status as religious entities, limiting restrictions on fund-raising activities, and challenging the legitimacy of physically restraining members in the absence of substantial evidence of a clear and present danger to those individuals.

There have been, then, a steady stream of clashes between government at all levels and NRMs. Some have come at the initiation of anticult groups, others as a result of NRM-government conflict. In general, governmental units have sided with families, local businesses, and churches, even if only through symbolic actions. More substantive actions have been forthcoming where governmental interests were directly challenged. In a number of cases, however, the very real conflicts between governmental units and NRMs have been interpreted through the subversion mythology with the result that such clashes have been perceived as part of a generic "cult" problem rather than as discrete conflicts of interest.

Media Response to NRMs

Media coverage has been the single most important influence in the shaping of public opinion toward NRMs. Once NRMs had launched aggressive recruitment campaigns and anticult groups formed in the mid-1970s, the cult controversy became a major story. Newspapers and family-oriented publications published statements by parents or former members of NRMs warning readers of the imminent dangers posed by cults (43–45). Accounts of distraught parents unable to communicate with their children, a variety of culturally bizarre beliefs and practices, the specter of innocent youth being swept off the streets into virtual slavery through exotic mind control practices, and arrogant gurus who claimed or were attributed divine stature by followers all made sensationalistic copy. Journalists began competing with one another to publish the most sensational account, and cult stories soon were integrated into television shows, movies, and documentaries. The various other conflicts and events—anticult allegations, governmental investigations, radical acts by the groups themselves—provided the occasion for repetition of the subversion mythology.

The most influential types of account have been allegations by apostate NRM members; there have literally been hundreds of such stories reported in newspapers and popular magazines over the last decade (44). A high proportion of these individuals were involved in deprogramming or exit counseling, procedures that have been shown to be strongly associated with hostile attitudes toward the groups with which individuals were formerly affiliated (46). Many apostates exchanged loyalties as a result of these resocialization procedures, becoming as fervent in combating their former groups as they once had been in supporting them. For several years apostate reports were accepted and reported uncritically. The accumulation of a substantial body of participant observation research by social scientists provided an alternative source of data for media representatives. As a result, media coverage has become more balanced, sophisticated, and reflective of the various interest groups involved in the controversy.

Dynamics and Implications of the Public Reaction to NRMs

The reaction to NRMs is clearly grounded in sociocultural conflict. However, although numerous real conflicts of interest can be identified, the controversy over NRMs did not play out in those terms. Rather, the specific conflicts were joined together and treated as the product of a subversion plot. This escalation of the conflict into such global terms developed as a result of several factors.

One factor was the very real difficulty those confronted with emerging NRMs faced in interpreting their meaning. For example, families of converts to NRMs perceived that their function in socializing offspring for occupational and domestic careers was being usurped and, at the same time, they faced real difficulty in creating a meaningful interpretive framework for what they experienced as dramatic and unanticipated changes in long-standing plans and commitments. Similarly, religious and political leaders found NRMs challenging conventional understandings about the nature of religion and a church, the proper articulation of churches with other social institutions, and the type of commitments individuals normally make to religious groups. Not only did NRMs violate conventional conceptions of appropriate religious behavior, they also distanced themselves from conventional institutions, launched rhetorical attacks upon them, and paid limited attention to institutional norms underpinning the social order. NRMs exacerbated tensions as they often had no better understanding than outsiders of the developmental process in which they were caught up and they relied on tensions with conventional society to foster internal solidarity. As a result, for those faced with unexpected and escalating conflict, the cult subversion myth possessed much greater explanatory economy and appeal than a more complex structural analysis.

Another factor was the interaction effect among the various specific conflicts. The subversion myth fed off of the vagueness surrounding the use of the terms "cult" and "brainwashing." A motley assortment of groups and practices were subsumed under these umbrella terms. The result was a perception that there were hundreds or even thousands of dangerous groups, and the excesses of any single groups almost automatically were attributed to the others. Perhaps the single best example was the global fear that followed the murders-suicides at Jonestown when every NRM leader was viewed as possibly maniacal and every group was seen as a potential suicide cult (47). Institutions in conflict with NRMs found the cult designation useful because it provided additional leverage in their disputes. Allegations of economic exploitation, for example, gained force if enhanced by claims that those being exploited lacked free will. The result was that a variety of diverse conflicts became occasions for the repetition of elements of the subversion mythology.

Finally, the power imbalance between NRMs and their opponents allowed for the affixing of stigmatizing designations. A number of major institutions, each regarded as having legitimate rights and interests in their respective domains, were arrayed in opposition to NRMs. Where NRMs did gain allies it was almost always in support of civil liberties rather than the groups themselves. NRMs simply were not in a position to resist the more discrediting symbolic constructions of them which were in the interest of the coalition of anticult groups.

It was these elements in combination that elevated the controversy from a conflict of interest to a social scare. Yet despite the difficulties involved in gaining perspective on the cult controversy, there were from the outset strong grounds for skepticism about rhetorical brainwashing allegations, the central component of the subversion myth.

First, those making allegations about brainwashing generally ignored the conflicting theoretical perspectives and empirical assessments in the behavioral science literature on the exercise of extreme influence (48, 49) and vehemently resisted comparisons with comparable settings such as convents, monastaries, and military training academies (50, 51).

Second, as anticult ideology developed, brainwashing was stretched to fit an ever broader range of recruitment and socialization practices. Lectures, workshops, chanting, auditing, and meditating all were treated as simply variations on the mind control theme. It quickly became apparent that brainwashing served as a conclusionary value judgment rather than as an analytic concept.

Third, the rate of recruitment success registered by NRMs was so low as to be inconsistent with the notion of a process that individuals were unable to resist. Indeed, popular conceptions of runaway growth rates notwithstanding, most of the groups which triggered the cult scare never achieved an active membership of more than a few thousand individuals. Furthermore, membership size of a number of the more infamous groups declined significantly beginning in the late 1970s.

Fourth, the rate of defection was consistently high, even during the relatively brief time during which NRM membership was at its zenith. While it would be disingenuous to ignore the difficulty and pain associated with withdrawing from highly encapsulating social environments, it is misleading to portray such groups as psychological quagmires (52, 53).

Fifth, there was good evidence that the allegations of brainwashing levied against NRMs tended to come from individuals who had been involved in deprogramming. The clear implication of this research was that deprogramming in fact constituted a resocialization experience which invited individuals to reinterpret their former experiences through anticult ideology (46).

Sixth, the extremely narrow age band of NRM members left unanswered the question of why such techniques were effective only on young adults.

Seventh, the social scientists who undertook field research on NRMs such as the Unification Church (3, 23, 24, 54), Hare Krishna (25, 37, 55–57), Divine Light Mission, (58), and Scientology (22, 59), in part because of the controversy, did not report such findings. Nor did the substantial body of psychological and psychiatric literature on NRM members produce findings of any pattern of deleterious mental health effects associated with group membership (60–66). The very limited anticult-associated research has either provided very little empirical substantiation or has yielded unimpressive results (67–70).

Eighth, the social science research on NRMs is filled with accounts of deep and protracted schisms between various elements of NRM leadership and membership. These ongoing conflicts hardly were consistent with the conception of an all-powerful leader surrounded by a band of hapless, subservient followers.

Finally, the brainwashing notion implied that somehow these diverse and unconnected movements had simultaneously discovered and implemented highly intrusive behavioral modification techniques. Such serendipity and coordination was implausible given the diverse backgrounds of the groups at issue. Furthermore, the inability of highly trained professionals responsible for implementing a variety of modalities for effecting individual change, ranging from therapy to incarceration, belie claims that such rapid transformation can routinely be accomplished by neophytes against an individual's will.

The elevation of the new religions controversy into a scare has had several implications which derive from the nature and dynamics of scares as social phenomena. One has been a tendency toward continual expansion of the dimensions and boundaries of the "cult problem." A wide variety of groups have become equivalent by virtue of being labeled "cults" even though there is no systematic, research-based knowledge about any but a handful of the largest, most visible groups. A diverse array of recruitment and socialization practices have been designated "brainwashing" as a result of being utilized by groups that are labeled "cults." The number of groups labeled as "cults" or as manifesting "cultic tendencies" has continued to mount as suspicions about particular practices are voiced (71). The number of individuals associated with NRMs has been enormously exaggerated as a result of inflated estimates of the number of "cults" and acceptance of the brainwashing ideology. Another outgrowth of the scare has been the conceptual reduction of the "cult problem" to unidimensional causality based on the subversion motif. Accumulating information about NRMs is simply integrated into this preexisting conceptual framework. Finally, there is a ritualistic distancing of NRMs. This takes place as they are perceived to constitute a categorically distinct and pathologic type of group operating on the basis of distinct principles (i.e., brainwashing as opposed to conversion, manipulation as opposed to commitment). Complex patterns of motives and actions are reduced to stereotypical qualities. These groups thus require special handling. Deprogramming, for example, involves a highly ritualized processing of subjects until they agree to share the discourse of the deprogrammers. The result of these dynamics, of course, is that the mythologies underpinning scares are highly resistant to refutation.

The subversion-myth-based response to NRMs has had a number of social consequences, both for the NRMs and for their opponents. In the short run there have been a number of visible effects on NRMs such as the substantial economic costs to these groups resulting from boycotts of businesses affiliated with various groups and opposition to public fund-raising, extraordinary legal expenses growing out of suits and investigations, diversion of movement efforts from goal-oriented to defensive activities, and increased difficulty in recruiting. The longer-term results are less clear as the public response seems to have engendered both separationist and accommodationist responses. On the one hand, the scare reaction has simultaneously increased the defensiveness and radicalism of some NRMs already committed to withdrawal from and rejection of conventional society and diminished the ability of mainline institutions to exert any but coercive social control over these NRMs. For example, deprogrammers came to serve as real-life examples of the constant threat to NRMs and their members, and unsuccessfully deprogrammed members developed accounts that increased group solidarity and created heroic status for individuals who had resisted these attempts at "faithbreaking." Deprogramming offered reinforcement for the conviction that their true motives were not understood, that only a thoroughly corrupt social order would allow such an obvious contravention of basic human rights to go unpunished, and that no amount of communication with outsiders (even family members) could possibly bridge the chasm separating them (72).

On the other hand, the social control exerted against NRMs also has had the effect of fostering accommodation. For example, the Unification Church has moved toward finding alternatives to street solicitation for generating economic resources (41). The Church of Scientology dismantled its infamous Guardian's Office following revelations of harassment campaigns against dissidents and the conviction of some high-ranking leaders on charges stemming from burglarizing of federal government offices. Similarly, the International Society for Krishna Consciousness restructured its Governing Board and limited the authority of individual gurus following exposure of illegal activity in one West Coast temple. While all of these decisions involved numerous considerations, public controversy, the corresponding disputes that occurred within the movements, and pressure from groups upon which these NRMs depended for support were significant factors.

In the case of the anticult movement, the cult scare contributed significantly to the formation of an anticult "industry," developed and managed by moral entrepreneurs. The original informal network of parents' associations has gradually evolved into more formal organization (73, 74). The most sophisticated of these organizations is the American Family Foundation, which functions as the primary coordinating agency for the anticult movement by serving as an informational clearinghouse, providing a support network for families, publishing newspapers and reports on "cults," and conducting "educational" programs warning of the dangers of "cults."

More importantly, the anticult movement has begun to ally with a small group of mental health professionals as a means of creating legitimacy of its ideology. This alliance has taken the form of conducting research on deleterious consequences of NRM membership and offering counseling services to former members. Correspondingly, there has been a movement away from the early coercive deprogramming toward "exit counseling" services. The result has been a trend toward "medicalization" of the conflict (75). Attempts to combat NRMs through judicial and legislative initiatives continue, with the most recent development being the civil suits against NRMs. In part such suits simply reflect the trend toward litigiousness in American society, but they also constitute a conscious effort to generate a resource pool for future litigation, drain economic resources of target groups, and provide concrete victories in support of anticult ideology and solidarity.

It is particularly ironic that these developments in the anticult movement are taking place even as the groups that precipitated the scare have been receding. The Children of God left the United States for Europe in the mid-1970s. Since 1980 both Hare Krishna and the Unification Church have lost membership as a result of plummeting recruitment rates and high defection rates. Love Israel recently disintegrated amid internal conflict and schism. The guru Maharaj Ji disbanded the organizational apparatus of Divine Light Mission and now remains in touch with followers only through personal tours. A number of NRMs have made major efforts at accommodation. Although these initiatives have met with mixed success, involvement with representatives of mainstream organizations has produced a trend toward moderation and compromise. The public solicitation of funds, which ignited so much opposition, has declined as a source of NRM financing.

There is good reason to expect these trends to continue. The limited number of longer-term NRM members are now reaching middle age, and the priority accorded individual occupational, marriage, and family concerns has visibly increased. The appeal of NRMs to youth has declined as young adults in the 1980s have become more conservative and career oriented. The leaders of several major NRMs have died or are reaching advanced age, and it is not at all clear that these movements will be able to survive what historically has proven to be a major transition crisis. The response of the anticult movement to the receding visibility and size of the NRMs that sparked the initial controversy has been to expand the number of groups considered to be cults (or to manifest cultic tendencies) and to tie new themes to the cult controversy, such as child abuse, in order to rekindle public and media interest (76).

This continuation of the cult scare underlines what ultimately is probably its most significant legacy. Subversion mythology encourages the perception that social change is the product of personalized, conspiratorial forces, in this instance couched in medical pathology terms, rather than as the result of complex macrostructural factors in which individual actors have relatively little influence. Not only does this perspective disregard the total range of functions performed by social movements, some of which are positive for the social order (77), but it also undermines a society's capability to effectively calibrate the social response to the structural pressures for social change.

References

1. Bromley D, Shupe A: Strange Gods: The Great American Cult Scare. Boston, Beacon Press, 1981
2. Shupe A, Bromley D: The New Vigilantes: Deprogrammers, Anti-Cultists and the New Religions. Beverly Hills, CA, Sage, 1980
3. Barker E: The Making of a Moonie: Brainwashing or Choice? London, Basil Blackwell, 1984
4. Beckford J: The "cult problem" in five countries: the social construction of religious controversy, in Of Gods and Men: New Religious Movements in the West. Edited by Barker E. Macon, GA, Mercer University Press, 1983
5. Beckford J: "Brainwashing" and "deprogramming" in Britain: the social sources of anti-cult sentiment, in The Brainwashing/Deprogramming Controversy. Edited by Bromley D, Richardson J. Lewiston, NY, Edwin Mellen Press, 1983
6. Beckford J: Cults, controversy and control: a comparative analysis of the problems posed by new religious movements in the Federal Republic of Germany and France. Sociological Analysis 42:249–262, 1981
7. Shupe A, Hardin B, Bromley D: A comparison of anti-cult movements in the United States and West Germany, in Of Gods and Men: New Religious Movements in the West. Edited by Barker E. Macon, GA, Mercer University Press, 1983
8. Arrington L, Bitton D: The Mormon Experience: A History of the Latter-Day Saints. New York, Random House, 1979
9. Billington R. The Origins of Nativism in the United States, 1800–1844. New York, Arno Press, 1974
10. Heinerman J, Shupe A: The Mormon Corporate Empire. Boston, Beacon Press, 1985
11. Arrington L, Haupt J: Intolerable Zion: the image of Mormonism in nineteenth century American literature. Western Humanities Review 22:243–260, 1968

12. Cannon C: The awesome power of sex: the polemical campaign against Mormon polygamy. Pacific Historical Review 43:61–82, 1974
13. Davis DE: Some themes of counter-subversion: an analysis of anti-Masonic, anti-Catholic, and anti-Mormon literature. Mississippi Valley Historical Rev 47:205–222, 1960
14. Cox H: Deep structures in the study of new religions, in Understanding New Religions. Edited by Needleman J, Baker G. New York, Seabury, 1978
15. Robbins T, Anthony D: Cults, brainwashing and counter-subversion. The Annals of the American Academy of Political and Social Science 446:78–90, 1979
16. Sawatsky R: Moonies, Mormons and Mennonites: Christian heresy and religious toleration, in A Time for Consideration. Edited by Bryant DB, Richardson HW. Lewiston, NY, Edwin Mellen Press, 1978
17. Appel W: Cults in America: Programmed for Paradise. New York, Holt, Rinehart and Winston, 1981
18. Rudin AJ, Rudin M: Prison or Paradise? The New Religious Cults. Philadelphia, Fortress Press, 1980
19. Bainbridge WS, Stark R: Cult formation: three compatible models. Sociological Analysis 40:283–296, 1979
20. Stark R, Bainbridge WS, Doyle DP: Cults in America: a reconnaissance in space and time. Sociological Analysis 40:347–360, 1979
21. Melton JG: How new is new? the flowering of the "new" religious consciousness since 1965, in The Future of New Religious Movements. Edited by Bromley DG, Hammond PH. Macon, GA, Mercer University Press (in press)
22. Wallis R: The Road to Total Freedom: A Sociological Analysis of Scientology. New York, Columbia University Press, 1977
23. Bromley D, Shupe A: Moonies in America: Cult, Church and Crusade. Beverly Hills, CA, Sage, 1979
24. Lofland J: Doomsday Cult. New York, Irvington Press, 1977
25. Johnson, G: The Hare Krishna in San Francisco, in The New Religious Consciousness. Edited by Glock C, Bellah R. Berkeley, University of California Press, 1976, pp 31–51
26. Richardson JT: Stewart MW, Simmonds RB: Organized Miracles: A Study of a Contemporary Youth, Communal Fundamentalist Organization. New Brunswick, NJ, Transaction Press, 1979
27. Kilbourne B, Richardson J: Cults versus families: a case of misattribution of cause? Marriage and Family Review 4:81–100, 1981
28. Shupe A, Bromley D: The Moonies and anti-cultists: movement and countermovement in conflict. Sociological Analysis 40:325–366, 1979
29. Melton JG: The Cult Experience: Responding to the New Religious Pluralism. New York, Pilgrim Press, 1982
30. Beckford J: A typology of family responses to a new religious movement. Marriage and Family Review 4:41–56, 1981

31. Patrick T, Dulack T: Let Our Children Go! New York, Ballantine Books, 1977
32. Shupe A, Bromley D: The Anti-Cult Movement in America: A Bibliography and Historical Survey. New York, Garland Publishers, 1984
33. Richardson H: Constitutional Issues in the Case of Rev. Moon: Amicus Briefs Submitted to the United States Supreme Court. Lewiston, NY, Edwin Mellen Press, 1984
34. Horowitz IL, ed: Science, Sin and Scholarship. Cambridge, MA, MIT Press, 1978
35. Selengut C: Cults and Jewish identity. Midstream, January 1986, pp 12–15
36. Bromley DG, Shupe AD: Financing the new religions: a resource mobilization approach. Journal for the Scientific Study of Religion 19:227–239, 1980
37. Rochford EB, Jr: Hare Krishna in America. New Brunswick, NJ, Rutgers University Press, 1985
38. Hadden JK, Swann C: Prime Time Preachers. Reading, MA, Addison-Wesley, 1981
39. Frankl R: Television and popular religion: changes in church offerings, in New Christian Politics. Edited by Bromley D, Shupe A. Macon, GA, Mercer University Press, 1984
40. Latus MA: Mobilizing Christians for political actions: campaigning with God on your side, in New Christian Politics. Edited by Bromley DG, Shupe AD. Macon, GA, Mercer University Press, 1984
41. Bromley DG: The economic structure of the unificationist movement. Journal for the Scientific Study of Religion 24:253–274, 1985
42. Boettcher R, Freedman GL: Gifts of Deceit: Sun Myung Moon, Tonsong Park and the Korean Scandal. New York, Holt, Rinehart and Winston, 1980
43. Bromley DG, Shupe AD, Ventimiglia JC: Atrocity tales, the Unification Church and the social construction of evil. Journal of Communication 29:42–53, 1979
44. Bromley DG, Shupe AD, Ventimiglia JC: The role of anecdotal atrocities in the social construction of evil, in The Brainwashing/ Deprogramming Controversy. Edited by Bromley D, Richardson J. Lewiston, NY, Edwin Mellen Press, 1983, pp 139–160
45. Shupe AD, Bromley DG: Apostates and atrocity stories: some parameters in the dynamics of deprogramming, in The Social Impact of New Religious Movements. Edited by Wilson B. New York, Rose of Sharon Press, 1981
46. Solomon T: Integrating the Moonie experience: a survey of ex-members of the Unification Church, in In Gods We Trust. Edited by Robbins T, Anthony D. New Brunswick, NJ, Transaction Press, 1981
47. Shupe AD, Bromley DG: Shaping the public response to Jonestown: the People's Temple and the anti-cult movement, in Violence

and Religious Commitment. Edited by Levi K. University Park, PA, University of Pennsylvania Press, 1982

48. Richardson JG, Kilbourne B: Classical and contemporary applications of brainwashing models: a comparison and critique, in The Brainwashing/Deprogramming Controversy. Edited by Bromley DG, Richardson JG. Lewiston, NY, Edwin Mellen Press, 1983, pp 29–46

49. Scheflin A, Opton E: The Mind Manipulators. New York, Paddington, 1978

50. Ebaugh H: Out of the Cloister: A Study of Organizational Dilemmas. Austin, University of Texas Press, 1977

51. Dornbusch S: The military academy as an assimilating institution. Social Forces 33:316–321, 1955

52. Rothbaum S: Between two worlds: issues of separation and identity after leaving an alternative religion, in Falling From the Faith. Edited by Bromley DG. Beverly Hills, CA, Sage (in press)

53. Wright S: Leaving new religious movements: issues, theory and research, in Falling From the Faith. Edited by Bromley DG. Beverly Hills, CA, Sage, 1987 (in press)

54. Fichter JH: The Holy Family of Father Moon. Kansas City, Leaven Press, 1985

55. Cox H: Interview with Harvey Cox, in Hare Krishna, Hare Krishna. Edited by Gelberg SJ. New York, Grove Press, 1983

56. Judah JS: Hare Krishna and the Counterculture. New York, John Wiley & Sons, 1974

57. Shinn LD: Interview with Larry D. Shinn, in Hare Krishna, Hare Krishna. Edited by Gelberg SJ. New York, Grove Press, 1983

58. Dowton JV: Sacred Journeys: The Conversion of Young Americans to Divine Light Mission. New York, Columbia University Press, 1979

59. Strauss R: Religious conversion as a personal and collective accomplishment. Sociological Analysis 40:158–165, 1979

60. Galanter M: Group induction techniques in a charismatic sect, in The Brainwashing/Deprogramming Controversy. Edited by Bromley DG, Richardson JT. Lewiston, NY, Edwin Mellen Press, 1983, pp 182–193

61. Galanter M, Buckley P: Psychological consequences of charismatic religious experience and meditation, in The Brainwashing/Deprogramming Controversy. Edited by Bromley DG, Richardson JT. Lewiston, NY, Edwin Mellen Press, 1983, pp 194–199

62. Levine SV: Radical Departures: Dangerous Detours to Growing Up. New York, Harcourt Brace Jovanovich, 1984

63. Richardson J: Psychological and psychiatric studies of new religions, in Advances in the Psychology of Religion. Edited by Brown LB. New York, Pergamon Press, 1985

64. Ross MW: Clinical reports of Hare Krishna devotees. Am J Psychiatry 4:416–420, 1983

65. Saliba J: Psychiatry and the new cults: part I. Academic Psychology Bulletin 7:39–55, 1985

66. Ungerleider JT, Wellisch DK: The programming (brainwashing)/deprogramming religious controversy, in the Brainwashing/Deprogramming Controversy. Edited by Bromley DG, Richardson JT. Lewiston, NY, Edwin Mellen Press, 1983, pp 200–212

67. Conway F, Siegelman J: Information disease: have cults created a new mental illness? Science Digest 90:86–92, 1982

68. Singer M: Coming out of the cults. Psychology Today, January 1979, 72–82

69. Singer M: Therapy with ex-cult members. National Association of Private Psychiatric Hospitals Journal 9:15–19

70. Kilbourne B, Richardson JT: The Conway and Siegelman claims against religious cults: an assessment of their data. Journal for the Scientific Study of Religion 22:380–385, 1983

71. Conway F, Siegelman J: Holy Terror. New York, Doubleday, 1982

72. Barker E: With enemies like that: some functions of deprogramming as an aid to sectarian membership, in The Brainwashing/Deprogramming Controversy. Edited by Bromley DG, Richardson JT. Lewiston, NY, Edwin Mellen Press, 1983, 329–344

73. Shupe AD: The routinization of conflict in the modern cult/anticult controversy. Nebraska Humanist 8:26–39, 1985

74. Shupe AD, Bromley DG: Social responses to cults, in The Sacred in a Secular Age. Edited by Hammond PE. Berkeley, University of California Press, 1985

75. Robbins T, Anthony D: Deprogramming, brainwashing and the medicalization of deviant religious groups. Social Problems 29:283–297, 1982

76. Rudin M: Women, elderly and children in religious cults. Cultic Studies Journal 84:8–26, 1984

77. Robbins T, Anthony D, Curtis T: Youth culture and religious movements: evaluating the integrative hypothesis. Sociological Quarterly 16:48–64, 1975

INDEX